WHAT YOUR DOCTOR MAY *NOT* TELL YOU ABOUT™ FIBROMYALGIA

REVISED AND UPDATED

The Revolutionary Treatment That Can Reverse the Disease

R. PAUL ST. AMAND, M.D.
and CLAUDIA CRAIG MAREK

WARNER WELLNESS

NEW YORK BOSTON

PUBLISHER'S NOTE: The information herein is not intended to replace the services of trained health professionals or be a substitute for medical advice. You are advised to consult with your health care professional with regard to matters relating to your health, and in particular regarding matters that may require diagnosis or medical attention.

Warner Wellness
Hachette Book Group USA
1271 Avenue of the Americas
New York, NY 10020

Visit our Web site at www.HachetteBookGroupUSA.com.

Warner Wellness is an imprint of Warner Books, Inc.

Printed in the United States of America

First Edition: January 2006
10 9 8 7 6 5 4 3 2

Library of Congress Cataloging-in-Publication Data

St. Amand, R. Paul.
What your doctor may not tell you about fibromyalgia : the revolutionary treatment that can reverse the disease / R. Paul St. Amand and Claudia Craig Marek.— Rev. and updated.
p. cm.
Includes bibliographical references and index.
ISBN 0-446-69444-4
1. Fibromyalgia—Popular works. 2. Fibromyalgia—Treatment—Popular works. I. Marek, Claudia. II. Title.
RC927.3S73 2006
616.7'42—dc22 2005017749

I dedicate this book to my wife, Janell, who endowed me with her support and love while sparing me time from the companionship I should have provided. I have burdened her frequently with my tales of fibromyalgia. I have required much understanding and acceptance. She gave me both.

—R. Paul St. Amand, MD

To my husband, Lou (who cooked me many dinners), and to my sons, Malcolm and Sean, for giving me the gift of time to write this book. To my sisters and parents for their love and support this busy year and all years. To all our patients and the members of Guai-Support for their eloquent stories and insightful wisdom—I could not have done this without any of you.

—Claudia Craig Marek

Contents

Foreword ix

Preface xiii

Acknowledgments xix

PART I. The Plan for Conquering Fibromyalgia 1

Chapter 1. An Invitation to Join Us and Find Your Way Back to Health 3

Chapter 2. The Fibromyalgia Syndrome: An Overview of Symptoms and Causes 19

Chapter 3. Guaifenesin: How and Why It Works 40

Chapter 4. Meet the Enemy: Aspirin and Other Salicylates, Natural and Otherwise 72

Chapter 5. Hypoglycemia, Fibroglycemia, and Carbohydrate Intolerance 98

Chapter 6. The Protocol 145

PART II. Distinguishing the Many Faces of Fibromyalgia 171

Chapter 7. The Brain Symptoms: Chronic Fatigue and Fibrofog 173

Chapter 8. Musculoskeletal Syndrome 187

Chapter 9. The Irritable Bowel Syndrome: Fibrogut 198

Chapter 10. Genitourinary Syndrome 217

Chapter 11. Dermatologic Symptoms 240

Chapter 12. Head, Eye, Ear, Nose, and Throat Syndrome 256

Chapter 13. Pediatric Fibromyalgia 270

PART III. Strategies for the Road Back 289

Chapter 14. Medical Band-Aids: Currently Promoted Treatments for Fibromyalgia—What You Don't Know Can Hurt You 291

Chapter 15. Coping with Fibromyalgia: What Will Help While Guaifenesin Heals Your Body? 329

Conclusion: One Author's Last Word 357

Appendix 361

Notes 372

Resources 377

Index 403

Foreword

IN 1988, WHEN I was an intern in the Bellevue Hospital Medical Clinic, I would see many patients who complained of generalized joint and muscle pain. Although these patients expressed tenderness at my touch, I could find no other abnormalities. I ordered many X-rays and prescribed a lot of Tylenol and Motrin, and eventually became frustrated with my inability to help these patients—or even understand their illness. My colleagues had no better results—even the supervising faculty could not understand why the patients were experiencing chronic pain, and using terms like *total body pain.* Three years later, while studying for my medical boards, I came across the term *fibromyalgia.*

I immediately realized that many of the patients I had seen were suffering from the disease. I also realized that my lack of understanding of this illness had caused me to order many unnecessary tests, and prescribe medications that were of no help. There were a large number of doctors doing the same, and I knew that if I learned how to effectively treat fibromyalgia, I could make a difference in a lot of people's lives. After finishing a fellowship in rheumatology, I began my practice at the New York University Medical Center. I took an interest in treating fibromyalgia and soon began to see many patients with the illness. Although I had some success in treating my patients with a variety of muscle relaxants, sleep medications, antidepressants, and painkillers, there were still many who remained ill. Frustrated by the limitations of these mainstream treatments, I began to look for other ways to help my patients. Textbooks and journals offered no help. Then I decided to search the Internet. Initially, this increased my frustration—most sites either offered toxic medications that appeared unlikely to help, or were poorly disguised ads trying to sell something. But then I came across Dr. St. Amand's Web site. At first, I was skeptical that a medication as simple as guaifenesin could produce such impressive results. However, I was impressed with how well thought out Dr. St. Amand's protocol was and intrigued that I might be able to help my patients with this safe, inexpensive drug.

I immediately began treating a few of my patients with guaifenesin. At first, due to the fact that I did not realize such a large number of products contained salicylates—substances that hinder guaifenesin from working—I had a low success rate. But then some of my patients began to get better, and the few who were able to completely avoid salicylates improved dramatically. A turning point in my treating fibromyalgia occurred when I finally spoke to Dr. St. Amand. I called him one day, and despite not knowing me, he immediately took my call. He explained how he began using guaifenesin, how to adjust the dosages, and what one needs to do so as not to prevent the medication from working—avoiding salicylates.

Armed with this new information, I began to treat many more patients with guaifenesin. Remarkably, after an initial period of worsening, many of these patients began to improve. They experienced not only decreased pain but also less fatigue and an increased level of concentration. The difficult part was teaching patients to properly avoid salicylates.

As you can imagine, I was being bombarded with questions

about salicylates and which products contained them. But Aileen Goldberg and Kristen Walters, two of my patients, came to my aid and formed a support group for fibromyalgia patients in New York City. There was now a resource for my patients' questions (in addition to Dr. St. Amand's site on the Internet). Besides information on salicylates and other treatments for fibromyalgia, the group also offered great support to other sufferers when they were in the midst of painful cycles.

My patients continue to improve with guaifenesin and every day I am grateful I have the opportunity to use this powerful medication. I am also grateful to have learned from such a dedicated man.

Finally, I had the opportunity to meet Dr. St. Amand. It was an honor to speak with such a compassionate and caring man, one who has devoted his life to helping patients with fibromyalgia. I had a chance to learn his mapping techniques and to "fine-tune" my use of guaifenesin.

While many of the other medications I use may improve the pain and fatigue of fibromyalgia, guaifenesin offers patients the possibility to actually reverse the illness. This book should be the beginning of the road to health for many with fibromyalgia.

Bruce M. Solitar, MD
Clinical Assistant Professor of Medicine
Division of Rheumatology
New York University Medical Center

Preface

THE FIRST EDITION of this book was written with some hesitation. The focus of my practice had always been on helping the patients who came to me directly. In the past, I avoided publicity for my work because of the controversy I knew would arise from treating a no-name illness that other doctors didn't believe existed. Because of this, I even hesitated to discuss this strange illness with my colleagues and the large medical group I headed. But I soon realized that I had no choice but to ignore their skepticism, because results are what really count in medicine—and I was getting them. I can now write this revision with enthusiasm, since success has bred even greater success.

In those early days, however, I was on my own. I drew sketches to help my patients better understand their disease and the course of treatment I recommended. When the "fibrofogged" needed something written to review and bring home to their families, it became necessary to write descriptive papers. These were frequently copied and circulated among many others with or without fibromyalgia. I could not have anticipated the number of people these papers would stimulate to come to my office, first from all over the United States and eventually from around the world.

When the name *fibromyalgia* was coined twenty-some years ago, I gratefully adopted this classification—misnomer though it was! A terribly common illness had previously existed only in obscurity, but was now endowed with a name. Though it was not immediately embraced, it inspired acceptance for the condition from some open-minded members of the medical community. This emboldened me to more militantly champion the illness. Although my approach seemed unconventional, I had already been using it for more than twenty years.

While a consensus party line for patient management was slowly developing in rheumatology, I already had a healing protocol developed with the patience and help of a group of dedicated patients. I was increasingly asked to speak and write about my experiences with fibromyalgia and its associated conditions, the most prevalent being hypoglycemia (or low blood sugar). I was breaking through!

As I studied and learned more about this newly named fibromyalgia, I realized that I also had it. Later, I was able to identify the condition as one of my father's legacies. It was he who carried the gene and passed it on to my two sisters and me. Over the span of a few years, I also realized that, one by one, each of my three daughters was developing the same symptoms as she grew older. Illnesses have a way of taking on special significance when they strike near to home. Thus, my family's health concerns drove me to hone my skills a bit more sharply.

Over the ensuing years, I had found four effective medications, but side effects kept me ever watchful for something safer. I now have that in the compound guaifenesin. You can easily imagine how success with the very first medication I tried would stir me to ask why it worked. This *why?* led to possibilities and then to theories, which I occasionally modified, and I continue to do so. Of course, a theory is merely a supposition based on as much fact as can be garnered. This search keeps me poring over esoteric papers looking for insights on cellular physiology to maintain or alter my hypotheses as new data might require. It should be evident that whatever errors might exist in my theories do not diminish the efficacy of the treatment. Perhaps a simpler statement is: What works, works. In fact, the heart of my approach is so basic that it can be stated in a simple quartet of phrases:

1. There is an inherited disease known as the fibromyalgia syndrome (FMS)—a misnomer because of what it doesn't include.
2. There exists an effective, safe treatment using a very common medication, guaifenesin.
3. The inability to generate adequate energy in affected tissues explains the spectrum of the illness.
4. Hypoglycemia, or low blood sugar, is a frequent co-condition.

This book was first written and is now revised from the stimuli of both despair and dedication. Despair has come from describing what I have observed in nearly fifty years of medical practice: how desperate was the need for help, for understanding, and for answers. Dedication translates into the need to disseminate information to the millions of patients who have never had the chance to validate their symptoms. Most of my life has been spent in treating fibromyalgia, and now it's time for patients to take responsibility for their own treatment. With any chronic illness, it's unrealistic for patients to lean totally on doctors without helping themselves. We are sharing our protocol with those who want to listen, and who are willing to strive hard to make it work.

There will be those who will claim that we wrote this book only for its commercial value. Others, more academic in their criticism, will point to the fact that our treatment protocol using guaifenesin has not been subjected to a successful, double-blind study. More technically skilled critics will wonder how we can assume so much by delving into the realm of deep-seated biochemistry, yet using so little evidence. Additional skeptics will feel that we are utterly simplistic in recommending a very unsophisticated medication to reverse a terribly complex disease.

Let me respond to each criticism in turn. First, we do trust this venture will be somewhat profitable—though not particularly cost effective. Second, we did attempt to show the success of our treatment with a double-blind study. It was carried out at the University of Oregon. The effort failed due to distinct errors—errors we now know how to fix. I was a consultant to the project, and I must share the blame for this misadventure. At that time, I had no idea how easily certain commonly used compounds could block the benefits of guaifenesin. Also, a strongly confounding mistake was made in not identifying patients with hypoglycemia and immediately omitting them from the project. So, to date, we still lack the gold-standard data that medical journals require for publication. We are doing what we can to remedy that matter, but in good conscience we want to share what we know works to help those who need it now.

Lastly, I would also like to address the concerns of the chemically sophisticated minority. The science we invoke is up to date only as of this revision. We know chemical energy is lacking in fibromyalgia, and we believe that future developments in biochemistry will prove us reasonably correct. Thus, with this foundation, we are hoping that some of the mysteries surrounding fibromyalgia will soon be unveiled.

We were inspired to write this book by the millions of untreated patients, many of whom suffer terribly and are desperate for knowledge. Though we must leave time to see our own patients, we try to answer the hundreds of letters, e-mails, and phone calls that flood our office. Thankfully, our success rate has improved as we have learned from our patient-teachers. Their perceptions of seemingly insignificant nuances and their eagerness to share their experiences have proved invaluable. So it is that I dedicate this, my life's work, to the ever-growing group who continue to stand by us during these formative years. They were and are the flesh and blood of my concepts of fibromyalgia and "fibroglycemia." They've been invaluable in providing you with the lifesaving program outlined in this book. You will surely join me in saluting them with deserved affection as your health is restored.

—R. Paul St. Amand, MD

Acknowledgments

I BOW TO my nurse and coauthor, Claudia Marek, who has filled this book with her intelligent perceptions. She has provided years of inspiration, not only for me, but also through her dedication to our patients. She has done this with her caring and deep-seated knowledge of these illnesses. In the book world, I must thank Mari Florence for her wisdom and expertise in helping me simplify often complicated medical jargon. Diana Baroni, our editor at Warner Books, labored with skill and enthusiasm to help us, and we appreciate all her efforts. There's not enough room to express gratitude to all of our friends and families, especially Janell, Lou, Malcolm, and Sean, who patiently added their art and observations while allowing us to steal monumental time from our relationships. Lastly, another stands out as a mighty contributor: my secretary, Gloria Martinez, who has efficiently and uncomplainingly assumed many mundane and technical duties that freed nurse and doctor to pursue this endeavor.

Part I

The Plan for Conquering Fibromyalgia

The first part of this book is an invitation. We address fibromyalgia as a compilation of what several thousand patients have described over the years. We will explain what we do and why and how we do it.

Many of you already know you have the illness. A like number will make your own diagnosis after reading this book and will seek confirmation from your doctor. In the end, only you can decide for yourself if you are a candidate for our protocol. Even if you opt out, you will have learned a lot about your illness and what it is doing to your body. We will also devote pages to describing the medication we use, and what you need to know before you start treatment. So many fibromyalgics have carbohydrate intolerance that we have written a full chapter describing low blood sugar, or hypoglycemia. Though there is no corrective diet for fibromyalgia, you can learn for yourself if you might feel better by avoiding some carbohydrates. The last chap-

ter in this section will provide a concise step-by-step explanation of our protocol. We understand that many patients have what's called fibrofog—difficulty understanding and remembering what you've just read. For that reason, we've tried to keep our explanations and advice simple and to the point.

Chapter 1

An Invitation to Join Us and Find Your Way Back to Health

> "Having fibromyalgia means many things change and a lot of them are invisible. Unlike having cancer or being hurt in an accident, most people do not understand even a little about this illness and its effects, and of those that think they know, many are actually misinformed."
>
> —*J. M., Texas*

IT CAN START off subtly: a bit of muscle pain, along with some generalized aches and stiffness. Then there are periods when concentration is impossible, a day or two of overwhelming fatigue, and maybe a little dizziness, some cramps, and diarrhea. Symptoms come and go at first, and it's easy to chalk them up to a mild case of flu that never quite hits. You may blame stress or overexertion for these strange little complaints.

Then, one day, you realize one part or another of your body always hurts. You're often confused, short of memory, unable to concentrate, and you're always stressed and feeling as if you're at the end of your rope. You wake up tired every morning no matter how much sleep you've had the night before. Your symptoms begin to worsen, and you notice new ones: depression, numbness and tingling of the hands, leg cramps, headaches, abdominal pains, cramps, constipation taking turns with diarrhea, or bladder infections. Now you notice that you can no longer sleep through the night. Sometimes pain keeps you awake; most of the time, though, you don't know what causes the insomnia or what keeps waking you up. And what causes your craving for sugar and starch? Why is it that you don't eat very much but you still gain weight? Then, before you know it, bad days outweigh the good ones, and eventually you just cycle from bad to worse. By this time, nobody has to tell you that you haven't felt right in a long time.

> "It feels like coming down with the flu, yet it never manifests fully. It's like being fluish, achy and tired, and embarrassed and discouraged about it because you don't know why or what you can do to make it better or what you did to make it worse. Everyone gives advice but they don't have a clue as to what it's really like. Having people tell you to eat differently and exercise more and not focus on your health makes you just want to isolate yourself because you've already experimented with every possible food plan, supplement, and idea."
>
> —*Miki K., Hawaii*

You become increasingly immobile. Gradually and almost without realizing it, you stop making plans with your family and friends because you have no idea how you'll feel tomorrow. The simple task of going to the supermarket can be an impossible chore that you dread. By now you've visited more than a few doctors, many of them specialists. Your hopes have been dashed each time despite many tubes of blood offered up and too many tests that each came back normal. None of your doctors was able to set things right, and maybe one or two of them have even admitted that they had nothing else to offer you. Or maybe you've spent more money than you have on miracle supplements or medications your insurance won't cover that promised relief—relief that never materialized.

Your life has entered a vortex, a downward spiral into more pain, depression, and fatigue. For some of you this feels like rock bottom, and you reproach yourself: It must all be due to your inadequacies or poor coping abilities. You feel guilty for all the things you can't do and all the people you are letting down when you don't feel well yet again.

Relationships are suffering now: You are not the person your spouse married. You fret about almost everything, but nothing is as upsetting as your inability to care for your children the way you want to. On your worst days, you may even contemplate suicide.

At this point, you've had many diagnostic tests and spent hundreds, perhaps thousands of dollars, even though you may be lucky enough to have medical insurance. Your friends and relatives have suggested using vitamins and nutritional aids that cured so-and-so whom they know well. But you've tried that, tasted that, and spent that and yet never improved beyond the initial, placebo days. Maybe you've heard the word *fibromyalgia.* Perhaps you've been fortunate enough to have an official diagnosis. That may have validated your symptoms and eased your guilt—but now where's the treatment?

> "It feels like everyone around me is normal and happy and having a good time and I'm so different. I want to have a few normal days. I don't fit in anywhere because no one understands. People laugh and say 'You look fine' but I'm dying inside and I can't explain it to them. I'm so tired of pretending I'm okay when I want to scream. I have kept a positive attitude for so long but it's exhausting and I just can't do it anymore. I wish I could just go away somewhere and hide."
>
> —*Susie, California*

Fibromyalgia is prevalent in all ethnic groups in all parts of the world. In North America, it is estimated that about 5 percent of the adult population suffer from this disease, although we believe the actual rate is higher. Conservatively, then, some twenty million Americans suffer from fibromyalgia and its related disorders—most are women, with the ratio to men at about five to one. There is some evidence, mostly anecdotal, that this statistic may be skewed due to the fact that men are often either misdiagnosed or less likely to visit a doctor. Rheumatologists say fibromyalgia is the most common disorder they see.[1] Another twenty-five million people suffer from chronic fatigue syndrome, which I (and most other physicians) believe is the same disease. In addition, we have good reasons to conclude through our work that today's fibromyalgia is the prelude to tomorrow's osteoarthritis. (That attack on joints seems to strike about 40 percent of older people to various degrees.) Adding up these rather indeterminate numbers suggests that one third of our population will, however mildly, suffer some of the symptoms of fibromyalgia in their lifetimes.

> "My rheumatologist told me I was too old to have FMS. At that time I was fifty-four, never mind the fact I had had symptoms most of my life. The disease had become 'full blown' when I was about fifty-one. . . . After another year of suffering, I diagnosed myself via the Net. My DO (Doctor of Osteopathy) sent me back to the same rheumatologist because he is the only board-certified one in our area. At that time he told me I was too old to have FMS but even if I did there was nothing that could be done. . . . I have since been diagnosed with FMS by three other doctors, all of whom have told me the only thing they could do was treat my symptoms. I was as good as I would ever be and would get much worse."
>
> —*Betty, Texas*

In 1843, a physician named Robert Froriep first described the condition now known by the name *fibromyalgia* as "rheumatism with painful hard places" that could be felt in many locations on the body. Unfortunately, the word *hard* (swollen) is mostly ignored nowadays during the examination of patients. In the early 1900s, Sir William Gowers in London began studying his own lumbago and a cluster of symptoms in his patients, and dubbed this disease fibrositis. (This name stuck for the next eighty years or so despite the fact that it was subsequently revealed that the inflammation the name implies was not present.) Dr. Gowers observed that his patients were also exhausted and that the disease was "so painful it would make a strong man cry out." He tried everything he could think of in an attempt to relieve this pain, including injecting cocaine into the tender points (it didn't work very well). He also gave his patients a newly discovered drug, aspirin, and noted that it didn't work very well, either.[2]

Fibromyalgia, a Greek word meaning "pain in the muscles and fibers," has now replaced the previously popular names *fibrositis* and *rheumatism*. On New Year's Day 1993, the World Health Organization (WHO) as part of the Copenhagen Declaration officially declared fibromyalgia a syndrome. It was described as the most common cause of widespread chronic muscle pain. Because of this action, the illness was given an ICD code (International Statistical Classification of Diseases and Related Health Problems), further validating the entity. Henceforth, doctors could credibly bill insurance companies or even declare patients disabled if worse came to worse. The WHO also incorporated the American College of Rheumatology's 1990 distinguishing features of fibromyalgia as penned by Drs. Muhammed Yunus, Hugh Smythe, Frederick Wolfe, and others.[3] Their efforts had determined the common location of eighteen so-called tender points symmetrically dispersed, nine on each side of the body. The criteria they established also called for unexplainable pain in all four quadrants of the body, which had lasted for a period of more than three months.

But the World Health Organization went a little farther. The Copenhagen Declaration added: "Fibromyalgia is part of a wider syndrome encompassing headaches, irritable bladder, dysmenorrhea, cold sensitivity, Raynaud's phenomenon, restless legs, atypical patterns of numbness and tingling, exercise intolerance, and complaints of weakness." It also recognized that patients are often depressed.[4]

Today, thousands of medical articles later, fibromyalgia is almost universally recognized as a distinct illness. Sadly, there remain a few, increasingly rare doctors who still tell patients it is simply a catchall name for a collection of symptoms shared by a group of neurotic women. Despite much research and more speculation on the subject, much of fibromyalgia remains poorly understood. It is a complex and chronic disease that causes widespread pain and profound fatigue. Its range of symptoms makes simple, everyday tasks daunting, difficult, and often impossible.

> "Once upon a time, a lifetime ago, I was a gymnast, played in tennis leagues, golfed, played on a softball team, and panned for gold in the Colorado mountains. . . . Now I am lucky if I can walk to my mailbox—usually I have to drive. If I can make the stairs, I go down to check on the laundry situation, or go upstairs to see if the dust has carried away the entire floor."
>
> —*Gloria, Florida*

Fibromyalgia doesn't dependably cause the same complaints in everybody. Symptoms affect widely disparate parts of the body. This can make it difficult for doctors to grasp the connections among a foggy brain, pain in the neck or knee, frequent bladder infections, brittle nails, and poor hair quality, and understand them as relevant symptoms of the same illness.

People who enjoy semantics will argue whether we are dealing with a condition, illness, syndrome, or disease. If you are unwell, you have a condition that causes your illness. *Disease* suggests lack of ease. Fibromyalgics are certainly qualified to wear that name. Symptoms and findings that regularly appear together often enough are regularly grouped in medical parlance as *syndromes.* Lucky you: Fibromyalgia is that, too.

Many publications have listed the symptoms of fibromyalgia, most of them incompletely. Yet despite this litany, it remains a phantom illness that has few confirmatory physical findings obvious to the untrained examiner. There are no validating laboratory, X-ray, or scanning techniques to provide sound footing for physicians. The breadth of symptoms and unreliable physical targets greatly deter diagnosis and relegate the illness to a ghost-like domain. For these reasons, fibromyalgia is often described as an "invisible disability."

A well-conducted history will illuminate the chronology of cyclic and progressive symptoms that strongly point to the diagnosis. The currently used physical examination has shortcomings and is not always supportive because of frequently unreliable findings. (We authors are dedicated to altering or supplementing the current approach by using an old-fashioned, hands-on technique called mapping. We search the body for any swollen joint, muscle, tendon, or ligament.)

> "There is no doubt in my mind that there is a genetic predisposition to FMS. My eighty-six-year-old father has had it since my teen years. My mother recently told me when I asked about his leg pain that the doctor said years ago that there were lumps in his legs."
>
> —*M. Bush, Alabama*

Although fibromyalgia is not a terminal illness, it is a demoralizing and debilitating one. The symptoms can be unbearable—so much so that the so-called Suicide Doctor, Jack Kevorkian, helped a few patients end their suffering. In 1997, one of these fibromyalgics was forty-year-old Janis Murphy. After her death, her father spoke out about his daughter's struggles with her illness. "Over the years, I've seen my daughter experience intractable and unrelenting pain," he said. He hated losing his only child, but "there are things in this world worse than death." Such a solution is not acceptable—not when something can be done. Our purpose in writing this book is to make a solution clear and widely available.

The most popular advice given to patients by their doctors is to exercise. It's astounding how few can tolerate doing even a token amount. This advice is usually administered with a series of chemical Band-Aids to temporarily soothe a few of the ever-growing list of symptoms. Medical professionals unwittingly promote eventual disability when they prescribe ever-stronger medications that, sooner or later, further deplete energy and deepen the mental haze. Yet for the most part, they have nothing else to offer and defend the practice by simply stating that they cannot sit by and watch people suffer pain.

To make something very bad even worse, long-term disability insurance companies have now entered the fray. They are not disinterested parties. On the contrary, they are very, very interested. It is to their advantage to insist that fibromyalgia and all of its variations stem from psychiatric disorders such as depression. They have no difficulty in finding a well-compensated psychiatrist who will agree. Since the vast majority of insurance policies do not cover mental disability beyond a specified time, there is a great deal of money at stake. Insurance companies defend themselves by pointing out that fibromyalgia cases have reached epidemic proportions in the form of U.S. Social Security disability claims, workers' compensation, and accident litigation. As many as 25 percent of American fibromyalgia patients have received some form of disability or injury compensation.[5]

We are the first to agree that the country can ill afford to swell these ranks. Indeed, when compensation has been granted, we want to get that patient motivated to heal and reenter the workforce. Yet we can't turn our backs on very real suffering, either. We see only one solution to this dilemma: Get to the sick ones much sooner, and get them well.

The basic problem for patients and physicians is that there is no consensus regarding the cause of fibromyalgia. Considerable sums have been spent, and no one agrees on anything. However, we think there is an answer. The purpose of this book is to present our findings and the observations of our patients in simple terms. As we already suggested, fibromyalgia stems mainly from an inherited problem. We strongly suspect the trait leads to faulty renal excretion and hence, retention of a compound known as phosphate.

The vast majority of physicians are skillfully trained, well intentioned, and dedicated to their oath-driven principle of trying to help patients. Fibromyalgia is such a systemwide illness with so many seemingly unconnected, rapidly shifting complaints that doctors are understandably confused. Add to that the professional frustration they experience when they're stymied at every turn no matter what newfangled medication they prescribe. They eventually respond by referring patients to another doctor who should know more than they do about some "new" symptom. In the process, patients receive a fast-track medical education as they go from specialist to specialist.

It's no wonder that most of our colleagues consider fibromyalgia incurable. All they can do is relieve symptoms as best they can by fully deploying drugs from the latest issue of the *Physicians' Desk Reference*. With no known cause to treat, it makes total sense to attack each symptom with whatever it takes. Polypharmacy soon emerges, making use of NSAIDs (nonsteroidal anti-inflammatory drugs), various analgesics, antidepressants, sedatives, tranquilizers, and the ultimate enlistees: narcotics, whatever their potency. The process is unstoppable. Patients get sicker and forced by their medications into a far worse limbo state than before treatment. For many, the picture is truly bleak.

> "What do you do when Fibro is causing your whole life to come apart? Your money situation is gone from bad to worse because you can't work and you can't think well enough to budget. You forget to make a deposit or your lights get turned off because you forgot to pay. Your husband wants to know when you'll get better because he feels lonely when all you can do is drag yourself through the day let alone make passionate love all night. Your kids are having trouble in school and you can't help them because you can't think. Neither can you skate with your daughter or play basketball with your sons. You look at your laundry piled up and you can't imagine sorting it let alone carrying it over to the laundry room. I can't think, can't talk, can't feel. I feel dead."
>
> —*Debbie, California*

In my forty-nine years as an internist and endocrinologist, I've devoted forty-plus to the diagnosis and treatment of fibromyalgia—even before it supposedly existed. I have found that there is an effective, safe treatment for the condition, one that I had to use for myself. The illness entered my life when I was in the armed services in 1945. I was hospitalized with the diagnosis of "possible rheumatic fever" because of my red, swollen leg joints and painful muscles. All my tests came back normal. After six weeks, everything cleared spontaneously. Cycles of various symptoms appeared sporadically over the ensuing years but with much lighter intensity. I was hit in earnest in my early thirties with many new symptoms but never again with the earlier joint swellings. I had no idea why this developed; I had never been taught about such a ridiculous condition. I assumed I was not emotionally geared for the stresses, long hours, and general tribulations of private medical practice. I tried to pace myself and relax as best I could. That didn't help, of course, so I was convinced I needed to work harder at it! Only after I stumbled onto and began treating patients with what was later named fibromyalgia did I realize that theirs was a misery I shared. I simply began treating myself. Who else was going to do it?

Over the years, I have explored the many facets of this illness mainly through observation and compilation of data from my patient-teachers. They willingly joined me in our trial-and-error approach that lacked any other scientific credentials. It has taken me many years to reasonably grasp the full extent of this illness and to comprehend just how insidious, infuriating, and debilitating it can be.

We have used several different drugs to treat fibromyalgia. In the past, we prescribed exclusively gout medications that were thoroughly effective. Unfortunately, each had certain side effects that left a small group of patients in a treatment limbo. In 1992, our search led us to try guaifenesin, a widely available medication. It is well tolerated and has no known side effects. It is available over the counter without a prescription. Some short-acting varieties are well made and effective. Prices vary among these preparations, and despite the fact that the cost has gone up in recent years, the drug is inexpensive when compared with most other medications.

We've used guaifenesin as the mainstay of a treatment protocol that actually addresses basic disturbances caused by defective genes, and does not work by merely covering over resulting symptoms. This book is the culmination of more than four decades of research and hands-on examinations. We have treated thousands of patients who have traveled from all over the world seeking relief from this enervating disease. With this treatment, symptoms and pain reverse and disappear completely in most patients. Other individuals resume normal lives with minimal residual problems. This is not to say that recovery occurs immediately. Not only is it necessary to find the effective dosage of guaifenesin, but there are also other crucial factors that influence the success rate of our protocol.

In order for guaifenesin to work, it must have unrestricted access to receptors in the kidneys. These are like little garages where the medication must park and unload its contents before it will be permitted to work. Many ingredients in the products we use every day—pain medications, lipsticks, muscle balms, nutritional and herbal supplements, skin care products, toothpastes, deodorants, sunscreens, and even the sap of plants—contain a chemical known as salicylate. This little devil is capable of hogging all of the parking spaces in the kidney receptors where guaifenesin needs to work. This is nothing new for us. All of our previous medications had the same problem. We stress for patients: The main thing our protocol demands is the avoidance of salicylates.

It also must be understood that approximately 30 percent of female fibromyalgics have hypoglycemia, or low blood sugar, with symptoms that greatly overlap those of fibromyalgia. To be successful, then, treatment must address both conditions simultaneously. If this connection is overlooked and patients fail to make required dietary adjustments, fatigue, cognitive, and intestinal symptoms of hypoglycemia will remain even though fibromyalgia itself will reverse on guaifenesin.

As we will expound in this book, our protocol must be followed very carefully if patients are to achieve the positive results we describe. You can imagine our frustration when we hear, "Oh, I tried this treatment and it doesn't work." We've heard too often from patients and physicians alike who missed the mandatory step of cleaning out all sources of salicylates.

We would like to take up twenty pages of bold print with caps repeating the mantra *Don't use salicylates!* Enough said?

We will share our knowledge of fibromyalgia throughout this book. We know firsthand the nature of the disease: the cognitive distress, the unrelenting exhaustion, and the pains that cumulatively induce deep depression and finally even suicidal thoughts. We know about how hard it is to be understood in a healthy world, where perfect specimens are all around you, when (dare we say it?) "you don't look sick!" We've poured our hopes into yours in the succeeding chapters. We'll try to explain simply and discuss clearly all of the important lessons you must learn if you plan success. We'll stress what you must change, because for most of you more is needed than just a pill to get you fully energized and relatively pain-free. Patients of any age can follow our protocol, which is designed to reverse fibromyalgia in far less time than it took to develop the illness. Despite damage in later years from osteoarthritis that guaifenesin cannot reverse, clear thinking, restored energy, and eased bowel and bladder symptoms can be achieved.

The use of guaifenesin in treating fibromyalgia is not yet accepted in mainstream medicine. We have been unable to publish in medical journals for lack of a successful double-blind study, as we will later explain. However, word of our protocol has spread from grassroots support and the militancy of the patients it has helped. Thus, many physicians and other practitioners do use and support our protocol. Exactly how many are included in this growing infantry is beyond our knowledge. We get frequent letters from patients who have either recruited their physicians or been urged by them to adopt our protocol. We have spoken to many gatherings of physicians, individuals who've called our office, and face-to-face with those who've come to us for hands-on training. Many more have written for information. Claudia and I speak at medical meetings, patient–doctor mixed groups, guaifenesin support groups worldwide, occasional television programs, and more frequent radio interrogations to deliver our simple message. During these events, we regularly extend invitations to join us in fighting the battle. In short, we preach to anyone who'll listen. Whether through this book or in person, we repeat over and over, "Guaifenesin works. We plead with you; just follow our instructions!"

> "I have never contacted an organization or a website for any reason so I'm not sure what I'm doing. I just hope you receive this. I do not know what else to do. I'm divorced, single mother of two daughters, 16 and 10. I've been through some extremely stressful years while trying to work, raise my girls and go to numerous doctors some of which claim they specialize in Fibromyalgia. I don't know what to say next except I'm hoping you can help me. I'm forty-two-years old and for the past few years I feel like I'm seventy-two. I'm always exhausted, experiencing pain, irritable, dizzy, issues with my bowels, skin problems . . . I've always lived my life feeling that no matter what was handed to me my glass was always half full but now it feels like my glass is empty. I want my life back. I want to be the person I was in the past."
>
> —*Lisa, Maryland*

We suspect each of you already knows that you must take charge of your own illness. Physicians will forever have trouble coping with salicylates in products other than prescription drugs. None of us can expect doctors to hop around cosmetics counters using magnifying glasses to scan labels. No one will hover nearby to slap your hand when you reach for a piece of pie when you should be on the hypoglycemia diet. But we ask you to see it this way: Not reading labels or cheating on the diet will not only harm you but also discourage your doctor, who might be watching, hoping to assess positive results and acquire a method for treating other patients. Even if your physician feigned disinterest and only allowed that guaifenesin can't hurt you, he or she will start taking notice as you begin to feel better. The fact that you are reading this book says a lot. You're still motivated to try despite all of the previous setbacks. That fact alone speaks volumes. For each one who picks up this book, we know that there are many who put it down because it "looks too hard" and they "feel too sick."

> "I have coped with this disease for over 20 years and have lost as much as anyone else. This disease cost me my marriage, my children and my livelihood. All the things we are supposed to have. You reach a point where you must stop mourning and build a new life. It is so painful—I know, I know. I remember pacing the floor in a cold house (those terrible heat bills) in that terrible pain not knowing if my last hundred dollars was a lot or a little. When you are at the end of your rope that poster of the kitten hanging on to the rope knot isn't funny. But you still have choices. Forgive me for recalling the sixties but 'tomorrow is the first day of your life, and you can do what you want with it.' "
>
> —*Bev, Hawaii*

We invite all fibromyalgia sufferers (and their loved ones) to embark upon a journey back through time to improved health. Let us be your tour directors. We're passionate about providing you with the information you need. We've both done it, paid our dues, and are eager to share what we know. Realize up front that this journey is not for the faint of heart. For most of you, the road back to good health will seem long, with days of pain and discomfort. In the beginning, this may be more severe than what you have suffered to date. But the destination is golden.

This treatment is designed to flush the body of the metabolic debris that's junking up your energy-producing factories, tiny mitochondria buried deep inside all your cells. While that's happening, your emotional and physical pain will most likely increase. But with time, you'll notice symptoms easing to evoke some good hours, eventually better ones, and ultimately great days. You'll actually bounce back after an illness, injury, or hard work, just as you once did. Most welcome is the ability to participate in activities with the energy and enthusiasm that have eluded you for years. By following our treatment regimen to the letter, along with your doctor's advice, this is all within your reach. We want you to resume living your life to the fullest. The best definition of happiness we've ever heard is: "Happiness is freedom from pain." Wipe out mental anguish and constant pain, and life is a joy.

Chapter 2

The Fibromyalgia Syndrome: An Overview of Symptoms and Causes

> "Fibromyalgia is real, Fibromyalgia hurts, and Fibromyalgia intrudes into lives and relationships in a real way. The two basic challenges that face a newly diagnosed patient are the following: learning about your illness so that you understand it and then explaining it to everyone else in your life so that they do as well."
>
> —Claudia Marek, *Fibromyalgia Is Real*

WHAT IS FIBROMYALGIA?

What is fibromyalgia? The medical community and patients are still looking for the answer even twenty-something years after the condition was named. My coauthor, Claudia, asked her son, Malcolm Potter, that question when he was about ten years old. His response was: "It feels like all my muscles want to throw up!" That intuitive response still seems as descriptive as anything else that's been offered. Another one is: "The irritable everything syndrome," coined by Dr. Hugh Smythe of Toronto, Canada. From ten-year-old to prominent researcher—two phrases that pretty well cover it, wouldn't you say? You'll have to judge if we do any better.

Fibromyalgia is different from other illnesses. If we were to describe thyroid diseases, diabetes, or rheumatoid arthritis, for example, we could easily recite their distinguishing characteristics. Most conditions have a single set or series of lab tests to help confirm the diagnosis. Often, one major organ or gland is the culprit. That's not so with fibromyalgia, however, because it doesn't pick on just a single type of cell or limited body part. Instead, it shows up with myriad seemingly unrelated symptoms in endless combinations. At first glance, the only thing these complaints seem to have in common is that they coexist in a single human being. Symptoms don't neatly fit into diagnostic categories. Perversely, they spill profusely over the borders that define any particular medical specialty. That's made the illness elusive and treacherous, troublesome to pin down and worse to treat.

Despite this lack of an obvious pattern, fibromyalgia worms its way through individuals with enough nuances to eventually lend cohesiveness to a certain number of complaints. These characteristics make patients seek help from whatever specialist seems best suited to handle the most pressing problem. Specialists, by definition, work in somewhat limited spheres, and thus get easily trapped into a focus, which forces them to view only symptoms germane to their field. Because it's not their job to expand their perspective to include the whole patient, they end up treating just a few symptoms as if they were the entire disease. Therefore, irritable bowel syndrome, interstitial cystitis, vulvar pain syndrome, chronic fatigue syndrome, chronic candidiasis, and myofascial pain syndrome are often treated with narrowly focused methods. To us, though, they're simply facets of fibromyalgia. Hearing patients speak about any one of them alerts us to look for the others. So it is that physicians in family practice, internal medicine, and rheumatology who more routinely perform complete patient evaluations are often more adept at catching all the nuances of this illness.

I've already described the environment in which I practiced for much of my career. I was visited by patients with numerous complaints, who had seen many doctors, and had taken many medications. They still weren't well and were progressively more frustrated. Their family doctors had examined and tested them, often in memorable detail—"everything normal." Now the diagnosis seemed assured: "nothing wrong but a bad case of nerves." Family and friends soon echoed that conclusion and accepted the fact that their loved one was neurotic, a hypochondriac. I, too, believed this in my earliest years of medicine, because I was taught that way and had no evidence to contradict it.

What was being missed was the connecting thread among patients. Glaringly obvious was the sheer volume of complaints. Sure, many patients found it difficult to pinpoint exactly when their symptoms had begun. Most had great trouble discerning the order in which they appeared. They wilted under questioning as if they were being cross-examined and a wrong answer would result in jail time. Migraines, fatigue, depression, muscle aches, dizziness, nasal congestion, gas, diarrhea, breaking nails, numbness, bladder infections, and on and on. Shouldn't someone along the line have caught on sooner? All of them were repeating the same things!

> "Some mornings I would wake up and feel so lethargic it was all I could do to make it to work. For several years, I'd attributed my muscle pain to the few fender benders that I'd been in. I'd thought the migraine headaches were hereditary. And I would tell myself I'd caught a 'bug' when the dizziness and fatigue became a problem. The strange thing was the symptoms seemed to get worse as time went on, not better, despite the treatment I'd received from traditional MDs, chiropractors, holistic practitioners, acupuncturists, masseuses, and herbalists.
>
> "About a year ago, I was so frustrated I rattled off all my re-

curring symptoms to my [previous] doctor and demanded, 'I've been here before with these problems. What's wrong with me?' To which she replied with annoying frankness, 'I don't know.' "

—Michelle, California

Not unlike other illnesses, the severity and impact of fibromyalgia differ from patient to patient. Some are able to lead relatively normal lives. Often they live with a number or irritating symptoms for years when suddenly the hesitation is over and the full-blown, unrelenting disease hits. Others become considerably debilitated early on or even homebound. There are those who feel well until traumatized by an accident, surgery, extensive dental work, or emotional stress. They single out those events as triggers that were the cause of their illness. In most cases, with a careful history we can elucidate earlier complaints. But for the vast number of people, symptoms sneak up insidiously, wax and wane, gradually intensify, and eventually never go away.

In addition to the physical complaints, the vast majority of patients also have difficulties with memory and concentration—cognitive difficulties that have been nicknamed fibrofog. This embarrassing condition possibly takes a heavier toll on patients than do the aches and pains. They raise fears of premature and serious brain deterioration, and we are asked daily if we think these symptoms might be Alzheimer's. Only rare patients have never feared they're losing their minds. You can appreciate the severity of the neurological component by reading the following description.

"I sit at a computer at work with a headset on, answering calls from people about computers of all types. . . . I have to solve their problems, at the same time 'teach' them. Many times I have found myself not knowing who I am talking to (man or woman?) and what we were talking about. It is like just waking up from a dream. So I have to keep notes of what I'm doing on my calls, or just plain ask the person to repeat what they just said. This will eventually cost me my job . . . I don't know what my future holds. I've gotten in my car and forgotten how to turn the lights on, or where the windshield wipers are. Sometimes I can laugh about it, later. But it's getting more frequent and I'm not laughing anymore."

—*Cyndi S., Arkansas*

In my early days in practice, I knew of no disease that would include all of the weird symptoms being expressed by this group. From the sheer number who presented with the same complaints, however, I became progressively more certain that some new disease had to exist. The frequent cycling from good to bad days in the early phases of the illness made it very unlikely that I was dealing with a neurosis. I noticed that with most of these patients, the tensions and stress levels at home or work made little difference as to when the sick days would strike. Neurotics are always neurotic; they don't suddenly experience great days out of nowhere. The fact that my patients were inexplicably better at times despite living under identical conditions made me more attentive to the repetitious nature of their symptoms.

There was no doubt that these patients were emotionally upset, frequently at the end of their ropes. They complained of varying degrees of pain, at least some stiffness, affecting many parts of their bodies. That seemed pretty tangible and at least represented specific locales for me to start searching. I began trying to feel for abnormalities in the painful areas people designated. Not only did I find them, but they were regularly riddling the body with easily detectable swellings. I soon made the connection that worse-pain days meant worse-everywhere complaints. It wasn't long before I realized that the entire symptom cascade was interrelated. It became obvious that pain hurts whether it stems from an emotionally floundering brain or from a gut in spasm, a burning and irritated bladder, or a headache. It was indeed all one great big mess! I was literally feeling my way and reinforcing my ever-growing conviction that everything was linked and had to have a single cause. What on earth could it be?

THE SYMPTOMS OF FIBROMYALGIA

By and large, fibromyalgia symptoms can be grouped into the following categories: central nervous system, eye-ear-nose-and-throat, musculoskeletal, dermal, gastrointestinal, and genitourinary. There are a few other, isolated problems that don't fit easily into any classification other than miscellaneous. We'll look at all of those affected areas and present you with a tableau of fibromyalgia. Each of these biological systems earns its own chapter later in this book. We'll separate them just to make the full ramifications of the disease more comprehensible. But please remember, they are all very much connected, all stem from the same cause, and are all equally restored by one medication, guaifenesin.

Cerebral—Fatigue, irritability, nervousness, depression, apathy, listlessness, impaired memory and concentration (fibrofog), anxieties and suicidal thoughts, insomnia, frequent awakening and nonrestorative sleep.

Musculoskeletal—Pain and generalized morning stiffness in the involved muscles, tendons, ligaments, and fascia that may arise from such structures surrounding the neck, shoulders, upper and lower back, hips, knees, inner and outer elbows, wrists, fingers, toes, and chest as well as from injured or old operative sites. Pain can assume any form and intensity, such as throbbing, burning, stabbing, stinging, grabbing, or any combination of these. Joints may be swollen, red and hot, or just painful as in the temporomandibular joint (TMJ). Numbness of the extremities or face and tingling anywhere arise from contracted structures pressing on nearby nerves. Facial and head pains spring from the neck or skull bone connections (sutures). Tiny parts of muscles often twitch, and the restless leg syndrome makes it impossible to find a comfortable position. Patients also complain of feelings resembling electrical impulses in their muscles, and a feeling of general weakness. Leg and foot cramps are common.

Dermal—Undue sweating; various rashes may appear with or without itching: hives, red blotches, acne, tiny red or clear bumps, blisters, eczema, seborrheic or neurodermatitis, and rosacea. Nails are often brittle, or they peel or chip. Hair is of poor quality and either breaks or falls out prematurely, sometimes in bunches. Strange sensations are common, including cold, heat (especially of the palms, soles, and thighs), crawling, electric vibrations, prickling, supersensitivity to touch, and flushing that is sometimes accompanied by a somewhat pungent and irritating sweat.

Gastrointestinal—Irritable bowel syndrome, leaky gut, spastic or mucous colitis, fibrogut. Transient nausea, gas, pain, bloating, constipation alternating with diarrhea, mucus in stools, and sometimes hyperacidity with reflux.

Genitourinary—Pungent urine, frequent urination, bladder spasms with very low (suprapubic) abdominal aching, burning urination (dysuria) with or without repeated bladder infections or so-called interstitial cystitis. Vaginal yeast infections without the usual cottage-cheese discharge are mimicked by vulvodynia (vulvar pain syndrome), which includes vulvitis (painful, irritated, burning, and sometimes raw vaginal lips), vestibulitis (same symptoms deeper into the opening), vaginal spasms or cramps, burning mucous discharge, increased menstrual-uterine cramps, and painful intercourse (dyspareunia).

Head-eye-ear-nose-and-throat—Headaches that are labeled "migraines" when they're severe enough; dizziness, vertigo (spinning), or imbalance; dry eyes as well as itching and burning with or without sticky or a gritty discharge (sand) first thing in the morning; blurred vision; excessive nasal mucous congestion and postnasal drip; painful, burning, or cut tongue; abnormal tastes (bad or metallic), scalded mouth; brief ringing (tinnitus) or lower-pitched sounds in the ears; ear and eyeball pains; sensitivity to light, sounds, and odors. Late-in-life-onset asthma and hay fever are sometimes related.

Miscellaneous—Weight gain; low-grade fever with night sweats; lowered immunity to infections; morning eyelid and hand swelling from water retention that slowly gravitates to the lower extremities and by evening stretches tissues, impinges surface nerves, and causes the restless leg syndrome.

Tender Points

> "You are tired of being consumed by pain. The unending pain and frustration is just too much to take any longer. Fear of the unknown: 'Is it going to get worse than this?' hovers over you."
>
> —*Carol, Texas*

Ever since the 1840s, when "painful hard places" were described in certain patients with rheumatism, doctors and patients have been fascinated by them. These painful spots are now referred to as tender points or trigger points, the latter term usually reserved for areas that cause myofascial pain. The official American College of Rheumatology (ACR) criteria for the diagnosis of fibromyalgia are based to a degree on finding tenderness in eleven out of eighteen predetermined sites when appropriate pressure is exerted by an examiner. These spots have been mapped, poked, prodded, biopsied, injected, and scanned. They're frequently assessed using a contraption called a dolorimeter. This is a spring-loaded device that measures how much pressure must be applied before a patient cries out or flinches.

When questioned, most patients confirm tender areas throughout their bodies. Most are located on or near muscles, tendons, or ligaments. Painful spots seem to move around a lot, but they don't actually vary all that much. The reality is that the most painful site of the day takes precedence and drowns out the screaming by the others. Swelling changes with fluid content, and pain is determined by what pressure is put on neighboring nerves. That's why small swellings can sometimes hurt much more than the bigger ones. Pain sensitivity is largely inherited and varies in a spectrum of tolerance.

The tender-point concept has always seemed a bit arbitrary for us. What do we do with someone who has all the symptoms of fibromyalgia but only nine tender points in the locations we're supposed to check? What if the patient has twenty palpable sore areas in other places, but few among the predetermined sites? People with high pain thresholds may feel no tenderness or only negligible sensitivity anywhere, including the designated sites. That's not uncommon, especially in athletes. This raises the obvious question of what to do with a mostly nontender individual who's loaded with swollen tissues, but nevertheless has all of the fatigue, cognitive, bowel, and urinary tract symptoms of fibromyalgia. The lack of tender points shifts such persons away from the true diagnosis and into the realm of chronic fatigue syndrome.

Obviously the tender-*point* concept is unduly limiting. After taking a patient's history, we begin our search for any involved tissue in the process we call mapping. This manual examination turns up many large and small spastic zones, sometimes involving an entire muscle bundle. These spots are distinctly swollen; most are also painful but not always. We simply call them the lumps and bumps of fibromyalgia. We record each of these by noting its location on a map or drawing of the body. (See chapter 6 for a more thorough description of mapping, and a blank body map.) There are patients we can hardly touch, whereas others can be prodded with seeming impunity. Our method of examination doesn't rely on what they will feel. They've already recited their observations and their pain distribution. To keep our findings purely objective, we record only the involvement that we palpate without including any further inputs from the patient.

WHAT CAUSES FIBROMYALGIA?

Given the broad spectrum of bodily functions and tissues affected by fibromyalgia, it's only natural to wonder: What kind of illness could affect so many systems of the body? How can it be so pervasive? Can brittle nails and migraines really be connected? Why can't we find any abnormality on diagnostic tests? These are some of the perplexing issues that physicians and patients alike address and contemplate. Even those of us who have studied fibromyalgia for years don't agree on the answers.

In light of controversies in the medical community about the nature of fibromyalgia, I might as well join in and expound my own theory. Luckily, I can rely on and make use of my own experience. I've seriously studied the concepts others have proposed. Just like the treatments that have been offered, none of them holds up too well in the examining room. Before delving into detailed nuances, here is my authentication: I've gathered firsthand evidence from more than ten thousand patients and continue adding to those numbers daily. I've examined every single one of them personally, and fibromyalgia is the only disease I currently treat. Therefore, I feel very secure in using the words, *in my experience.* What we're about to tell you makes the most sense from a physiological and biochemical perspective. We repeat what we said earlier: The concept fits, and the treatment works.

Here we ask the reader to bear in mind that a theory is nothing more than a set of assumptions based on as many facts as can be gathered. When you encounter a theory, you should immediately recognize that there are undoubtedly errors and oversights. Ours will surely be improved upon as we learn more about the biochemical mechanisms that we believe are at the root of this illness. So we ask that you please proceed with us patiently. We fully recognize that what follows is just a theory, and should be rigorously challenged and tested. We have proven to our satisfaction that fibromyalgia can be treated successfully with our approach. Yet we still aim to find out how and why our medications work—particularly guaifenesin, the most successful to date.

Many dispute our assertion that *chronic fatigue, chronic candidiasis, vulvar pain,* and *myofascial pain syndromes* are all names for the same disease. Symptoms we've described in this chapter are distinctly those of fibromyalgia. It isn't a physician's prerogative to extract only preselected complaints and leave a host of others in limbo.

We wish we could choose a more descriptive name that would fit all of the symptoms. *Fibromyalgia* works quite well to describe pain in muscles and fibers, but is clearly inadequate for the rest of the illness. *Chronic fatigue syndrome,* the second most commonly used moniker, focuses mainly on brain exhaustion and malfunction. For most patients, both labels apply at various times during their illness but can't be easily combined into one classification. At times, the symptoms of one entity are prevalent and tilt the scale to one or the other diagnoses. However, it just takes a careful history and appropriate examination to make it indisputably clear that we're dealing with one and the same condition. It's merely a matter of tissue sensitivity, disease intensity, and individual pain threshold.

For these reasons, fibromyalgia badly needs a new name—not that this is likely to happen. We proposed *dysenergism syndrome* (faulty energy) in our first edition. Since then, a learned Greek colleague used his prowess with his native language to suggest *energopenia,* meaning "dearth of energy." This term fully encompasses patient fatigue and cellular failure as due to the same basic metabolic problem. Our treatment is designed to restore vitality by releasing the body from a biochemical blockade we're about to describe. When this is accomplished, the symptoms of the illness disappear. I can say that in my own case, at seventy-eight I'm able to do things I couldn't have done in my thirties. Sadly, however, much as we'd love to change the name, we have to go along with common usage and stick with *fibromyalgia.*

THE MALFUNCTION JUNCTION OF FIBROMYALGIA: A BIOCHEMICAL THEORY

What in the world could be the metabolic difficulty that springs up to cause such a bodywide failure? The block of symptoms we've listed above surely signals that many bodily functions have gone on strike all at the same time. You and your doctors may have been just looking at the surface effects of fibromyalgia. There certainly has to be some type of fundamental breakdown. Aches and pains arise from spasms; the brain is obviously too tired to remain functionally alert. But why do the bladder, skin, intestinal tract, eyes, nose, throat, and more all join in? All of those parts are nothing but a bunch of cells that should work smoothly. There must be some altered chemistry behind all this—a truly basic connection.

We believe that fibromyalgia is caused by an excess of a specific biochemical substance that enters individual and interconnected cells. This process begins at birth and accrues until the body's safety nets are overstretched and become porous.

The inherited malfunction is predominately in the kidneys, which allow excess accumulations of some normal body constituent. There is a dictum in medicine that either too much or too little of a given element will interfere with function. Not surprisingly, cells work within a very narrow range for each of their chemical contents. Wisely, and to preserve itself, the body distributes surpluses among a variety of cells, and this occurs in a logical order. Reaching a critical concentration, our theoretical bad guy ultimately induces a marked energy deficit—the hallmark of fibromyalgia. The time from birth until sickness varies with the genetics of each individual.

Every bodily function needs energy—not only moving, running, exercising, and speaking, but also simply growing hair, breathing, digesting food, fighting illness, and, especially, using the brain. Eighty to 90 percent of our food must be converted to life-giving fuel. Each cell must produce a currency of energy, known as adenosine triphosphate (ATP). Every chore we've just listed and whatever else a body does all dearly depend on this vital compound. That's even true for anything else that's alive: plants, bacteria, and all animals large and small. This process involves extremely complicated biochemical mechanisms. Many of the compounds and enzymes that play significant roles in energy production are already known.

In order to understand how fibromyalgic cells malfunction, we need to study how energy is produced in everybody. In properly functioning cells, the concentration of all the substances integral to energy formation is meticulously maintained. Tiny power stations called mitochondria where raw materials are processed are where our story is now focused. These are present in all cells of the body, but they are stacked especially high in brain and muscle cells. They're complex little factories that convert 80 percent or more of our foods into ATP, adenosine triphosphate—three phosphates (*tri*) hooked onto a single molecule of adenosine. When a cell must perform some function, it rips one high-energy phosphate off adenosine, and expends it for the activity. Such chemical reactions provide almost all of the energy required by living tissue. Electrons are released almost magically in these bursts and are somehow directed to the right place to do the right job at precisely the right time. That's somewhat like the gasoline in your car's tank: ready for burning. It's also like plugging in an electric cord: The energy's been there all the while, just waiting for a signal to connect. Electrons flow through cells, charge up various enzymes, and run electrical currents in tissue "appliances." In normal bodies, cells seem to have an almost unlimited supply of ATP. In fact, within thousandths of a second, cells can produce new energy from a series of reservoirs.

So how does an energy deficit occur in fibromyalgia? We know that this is the problem. It had been suggested much earlier, but a study reported in 1989 actually measured ATP levels in tissues of fibromyalgics.[1] Two Swedish researchers, Drs. Bengtsson and Henriksson, found a 20 percent reduction in muscle biopsies taken from such sites. They sampled bits from the swollen and tender trapezius, a muscle located at the top of the shoulder. Adjacent, normal tissue was also biopsied and studied but showed no similar ATP deficits. A few years later, low ATP levels were found in red blood cells of affected individuals. These studies, along with the more technical magnetic resonance spectroscopy that can probe inside living cells (see appendix), support our theory of inadequate energy as the cause of fibromyalgia.

We like having our theory validated, but the question still arises: Why this depletion? What has interfered so stressfully to suck out ATP? The body is superbly geared to *prevent* such an occurrence, since major losses would mean cellular death. Obviously, that doesn't happen in fibromyalgia. Something must be lacking or have entered and accumulated to gunk up or idle the generators.

It's well known in physiology and biochemistry that phosphate excesses in the inner core of mitochondria, the matrix, gear down these power stations. Eventually, this not only eats up surplus ATP, but strains basic production as well. Blocking ATP generation means there won't be enough high-energy phosphates available for the cell to do any real work beyond simple surviving. Cells with the highest activity are the first hit and worst affected by this shortage. The more cells are pressed into service, the more seriously are they affected. Small wonder that brain and muscle are the heaviest hit! Optimal function is permitted only when energy is sufficiently replenished. Is any of this news to a fibromyalgic? It's why the condition should be renamed energopenia, to truly reflect the obvious: Tired cells yield exhausted patients.

But phosphate is not the only problem. It can't pile up indiscriminately inside cells without causing permanent damage. Because each phosphate ion carries two negative charges, electrical equilibrium can only be maintained with counterbalancing (buffering) by a cohort that sports two positive charges. Enter calcium, the preferred companion for phosphate. Whenever and wherever phosphate goes, so does calcium.

Calcium normally sits quietly inside storage bins, known as the endoplasmic reticulum, or lurks just outside the cell's wall. When a stimulus arrives, a command is given to the endoplasmic reticulum to release calcium into the main fluid chamber of the cell, the cytosol. The amount released is just enough to perform the desired task, no more and no less. If more is needed to amplify the signal, liberal amounts can be imported from the readily available external pool. Focus on the fact that calcium is the final battery terminal—the ultimate messenger that commands any cell, *Get going and do what you're told!* (See figures 2.1 and 2.2.)

Calcium won't quit its demands for performance as long as it sits in the cell's liquid interior, the cytosol (known as the

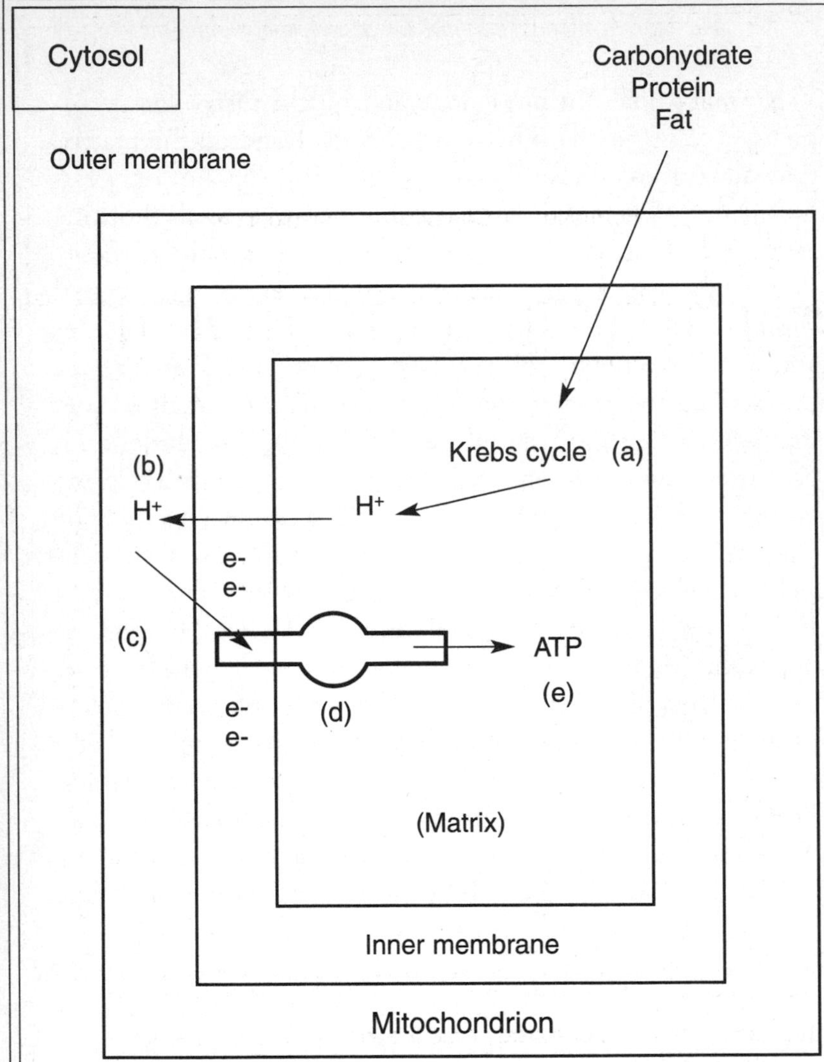

(a) Foods enter Krebs cycle; process releases hyrogen ions (H^+).
(b) H^+ is driven out to the outer chamber.
(c) H^+ enters space within inner wall of mitochondrion and releases electrons (e-).
(d) H^+ is driven through proton pump back into the matrix.
(e) Process produces ATP.

Figure 2.1

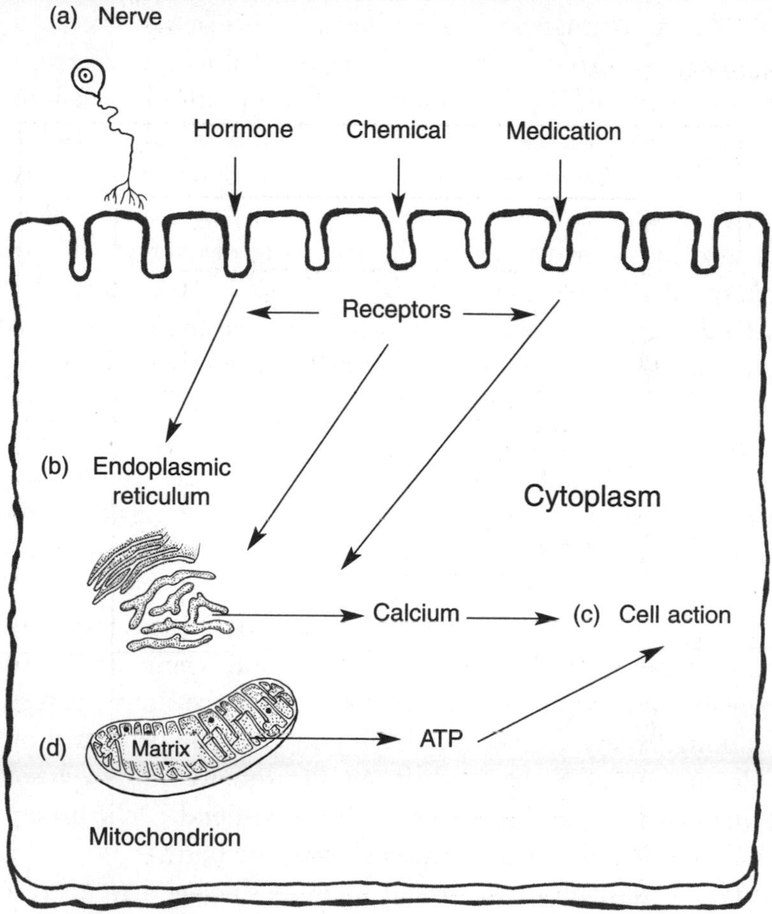

(a) Nerve, hormone, chemical or medication signal endoplasmic reticulum (ER).
(b) ER releases calcium into cytosol.
(c) Calcium initiates cell action.
(d) Mitochondrion produces ATP that provides cell with energy to perform whatever it is told to do.

Figure 2.2

sarcoplasm in muscles). So the poor cell must strive to keep up working as instructed until it's relieved of duty. To interrupt go-ahead signals, calcium must be either pumped back into storage within the endoplasmic reticulum, or totally extruded from the cell. There are actual enzyme pumps that are used just for this purpose. And as we already know, any function performed by the body uses ATP as its source of energy, so these pumps also must be empowered by it. Some 40 percent of a cell's energy is expended simply moving calcium in and out of internal storage or shoving it externally. Lack of ATP in fibromyalgia permits calcium to sit too long where it's no longer needed. Simply put, there's not enough energy to fully man the pumps, and insufficient calcium is being baled out. As a result, tissues affected by the errant metabolism are totally overworked and continue to work day and night to the point of exhaustion.

The numerous lumps and bumps we feel when we examine patients are found in muscles, tendons, and ligaments. These palpable areas are in a contracted state—they're simply tissues working twenty-four hours a day. This can only be caused by calcium, out of storage and sitting dictatorially in the cytosol (sarcoplasm) of a cell. This friend-turned-fiend is chemically shouting for unremitting action all over the body.

It's not difficult to accept this premise, since patient distress points directly to the core of the basic abnormality. There isn't much else to consider as a logical explanation for the overwhelming tension state caused by this disease. Readers with fibromyalgia know without being told how many seemingly unrelated structures are affected. "My whole body is tired; it aches; my bladder is irritated, my gut doesn't work, my brain is addled, and even my fingernails keep breaking." The extent of these common complaints should alert my profession to the fact that the malady is fundamental and strikes at the very heart of life. The widespread metabolic mayhem can all be explained by inadequate sources of ATP. The nature of the illness is most easily grasped if it is viewed as an accumulation of overworked systems that, true to their design, continue to heed unchecked calcium signals well unto collapse.

We tend to focus on the brain deficits and musculoskeletal pains of fibromyalgia and ignore the facts confirming that they, too, are victims. They just suffer louder than the rest of the body in their demand for relief. Multiple studies have attested to isolated problems within other tissue producers of various molecules, hormones, and neurotransmitters. They've been found at higher or lower levels when compared with normal controls. Here's more than you want to know: With frequent disagreement, researchers have reported low test results for growth hormone; insulin-like growth factor 1; serotonin; free ionic calcium; calcitonin; free urinary cortisol; certain amino acids; neuropeptide Y; T cell counts with faulty activation; and thyroid stimulating hormone response to TRH.

Hoping you're not too easily bored, higher levels of certain factors are also suggested: prolactin; substance P; angiotensin converting enzyme; and, in one study, hyaluronic acid. Skin biopsies have shown disrupted mast cells, which release histamine, among other things (cytokines), into the skin. At these same sites, an excess of immunoglobulin G was accumulating in the dermis, the deepest layer of the skin. We're not listing these scattered and seemingly unrelated findings in preparation to discuss each abnormality individually. People sometimes quiz us about these reported "facts"—"Did you see . . . ?" We aren't going to expound on their technical significance, and we don't even want to sound superbright. We simply want to illustrate how many different tissues and systems must be affected to alter so many scattered laboratory results. None of these preceding tests helps to make the diagnosis of fibromyalgia. Findings are also inconsistent and often refuted by subsequent research papers. It's probable that many new confounding values will be found emanating from the multiple systems we know are affected. It's also certain that more subtle testing will find disorders in tissues we currently think have been spared.

Energy deprivation is certainly at the root of this illness. No matter what pops up in the future, the shortage of ATP will continue to explain the disturbance. So many capable MD and PhD investigators are looking for a culprit that something quite unexpected may well emerge. Any new theory would need to propose a similarly enervating disturbance, serious enough to decimate what was once a smoothly functioning body. Only restoration of normal ATP production can give patients back their mental and physical energy.

In genetics, polymorphisms speak of multiple variations in a single gene. We're quite certain that there is more than just one such perpetrator in fibromyalgia. In defense of our position, we've treated several patients under the age of five, but also many individuals who displayed neither the symptoms nor characteristic findings until later in life—even one who began at the age of seventy-four. This last observation suggests the presence of one or more less vicious genes. Adding these kinder (recessive) genes to the less gentle (dominant) ones would permit all types of combinations (permutations), which in turn determine when the illness is first expressed. If both parents have the defect, their mutual children could not escape.

I erroneously predicted in our first edition that the X chromosome would be the likely site for the major genetic defect. However, in our book about children, *What Your Doctor May* Not *Tell You About Pediatric Fibromyalgia*, Claudia realized that prior to puberty we had equal numbers of boys and girls (ninety-three and ninety-four, respectively). So why is it that, postpubertally, women make up 85 percent of the fibromyalgia population? It dawned on us that bones and muscles require huge amounts of phosphate to sustain rapid growth.

That timing put to rest the myth of "growing pains." These pains occur mostly in the preteen years when growth is slow, and usually disappear during the spurt that signals puberty. Testosterone-fed male tissues beef up and sustain lifelong phosphate requirements. That's likely what offers men more protection from the onslaught of fibromyalgia.

The human genome has now been mapped, and though there are yet slots to fill in, it shouldn't be very long before the defective genes are identified. The fear is that so many people have fibromyalgia, geneticists might at first consider the variations as normal subtypes. The search is under way: We and our patients are currently involved in one such study with a premiere research institute in Southern California. We strongly suspect that this trait will be encoded by defective enzymes that are normally dedicated to precision phosphate or, possibly, other ion control. Those protein molecules would be acutely responsive to bodily needs and easily able to retain or eliminate phosphate with great precision. Initially, the defects would still allow the body to tuck retained excesses into receptive sinkholes, particularly in bones. The daily retention would be minute, but we believe that "tuckability" is eventually exceeded. Other cells must take up the slack even though they get sick doing it.

Enough preliminaries? It's time to discuss our treatment for reversing fibromyalgia.

Chapter 3

Guaifenesin: How and Why It Works

> "I will consider changing my medications, my physical therapies, and even my exercise routine, but I will not consider going without guaifenesin, nor will I take anything that might block its effect. It's too important to my well-being."
>
> —Devin Starlanyl, author of *The Fibromyalgia Advocate*

AS OFTEN HAPPENS in medicine, I stumbled upon the treatment for fibromyalgia quite by accident. I was young and equally naive, but I was lucky. It all began with a patient's chance observation. In 1959, long before our illness had been officially defined or given a name, one of my patients, Mr. G, came in to see me on a revisit. He suffered from gout and was taking the only drug available at that time, probenecid (Benemid). He was now feeling fine but unexpectedly said, "Hey, Doc, does this medication take tartar off your teeth?" Without much display of social grace, he scraped off bits and pieces of tartar (clinically referred to as dental calculus) and flicked them to my office floor. Though I was not particularly pleased with his uncouth newly discovered skill, I responded the way a poised physician should. I harrumphed appropriately and said, "I don't think so."

Yet my curiosity was piqued, and I began to reflect on this

slightly disgusting finding. I awakened two nights later asking myself what his flaking prowess might indicate.

Since my knowledge of dentistry was limited, I consulted a textbook that had a page or two devoted to dental calculus. I found out that the mineral backbone of tartar was mainly calcium phosphate in a chemical structure called apatite. Tartar develops from saliva, which in turn derives from the serum of blood. Water, all varieties of minerals, proteins, abundant calcium, and phosphate are leaking out of blood plasma into the salivary glands. These glands modify and manufacture their own proteins, such as mucus and digestive enzymes. They then mulch and concentrate such things with the above elements to make saliva. My search taught me that salivary phosphate concentrations were four times that normally found in blood. The level of salivary calcium, on the other hand, is just about equal to what's inside the body. Chemically speaking, this makes for a very unstable solution. We multiply the calcium level by that of phosphate and produce a number called the solubility constant. At this point, crystals form and deposit on teeth and under the gum line as tartar. Though dental calculus can wreak havoc on the gums, teeth, and oral hygiene, that was all the information I could find in that impressive tome. I knew not everyone created dental calculus, and that some people produced the stuff at variable rates. My quest was to learn what was metabolically different about tartar formers. I began by looking more closely at those with gout, since it was a gout medication that made my tartar-flicking patient such an able performer.

Gout—A metabolic disease unrelated to fibromyalgia. It is diagnosed with a blood test, which will show high uric acid level. Aspirations of the joint show uric acid crystals.

Gout is treated with two types of drugs: uricosuric drugs such as sulfinpyrazone and probenecid, which cause the kidneys to excrete more uric acid; and more commonly now allopurinol, which inhibits the formation of uric acid. Gout has many symptoms, the most common of which is a red, hot, or swollen joint. It is inherited, and ten times more common in men than in women, where it is usually seen only after menopause.

I had been interested in gout and suspected that there was more to the illness than merely joint pains and swelling. I reread the original description Thomas Sydenham had written more than three hundred years before, in 1683. He described gout as a disease with joint pain and one manifested by "great mental torpor," "suffusion of the sinuses," generalized flu-like aching, and malaise or fatigue, along with many other complaints, all in the dramatic language of his day. In other words, there were systemwide effects that were often overshadowed by the severe pain and throbbing of the red-hot joints.

Uric acid—A waste product from the breakdown of nucleic acids in body cells; it is also produced in the digestion of some foods. Most uric acid passes by way of the kidneys into the urine and is excreted, although some is passed through the digestive tract. When the kidneys do not excrete uric acid properly, high levels can build up in the body. This can lead to gout or, to a lesser extent, kidney stones

Gout is usually inherited, and we know the cause. In susceptible individuals, accumulations of uric acid crystallize and form deposits in certain joints. Sydenham's description of systemic symptoms preceding the joint attack made me wonder if there might be a gout syndrome. Only elevated blood levels of uric acid would alert physicians to the possibility of this new syndrome. In this scenario, people would have all of the preliminary symptoms of gout without arthritis. The condition would appear in cycles due to mini deposits in certain tissues such as the brain and the gastrointestinal tract. Muscles would be dusted only lightly and joints spared altogether until very much later in the disease.

I soon found a few patients whom I thought might have these pre-gout symptoms: cyclic bouts of fatigue, irritability, nervousness, depression, insomnia, anxieties, and loss of memory and concentration. They also described generalized, flu-like aching and stiffness (mainly in muscles), headaches, dizziness, numbness and tingling of the extremities, and leg cramps as their most prominent complaints. Indigestion with a sour stomach, gas, and flatulence completed the picture. Blood tests revealed the anticipated culprit: higher-than-normal levels of uric acid (urate). When I treated these patients with gout medication, their uric acid precipitously dropped to normal. I was exhilarated by the fact that their symptoms also disappeared. Oddly enough, although patients quickly felt better, they relapsed off and on. I noticed, however, that they suffered less intensely and with fewer symptoms during each subsequent attack. I'd always known that treating gout by lowering the blood uric acid often precipitated acute gouty attacks. As uric acid crystals come out of the joints, they seem to cause the same pains as they did going in. My gouty-syndrome patients also suffered reversal symptoms similar to those they had experienced before treatment. It was exactly the same as Sydenham had described—except, I must stress, that there was no joint involvement. This was gout at its best, before there was gout!

Flushed as I was with success, my confidence in my new "gout syndrome without gout" was soon shaken. Here came another group of patients who certainly had all of the symptoms that suggested my new creation. Yet no matter how many times I tested their blood, they didn't have an elevated serum uric acid. Another difference was that their aches and pains seemed to emanate from the entire musculoskeletal system. They had tenderness and swelling in tendons, ligaments, and especially muscles. I decided to put them on gout medication anyhow. They also began recycling their symptoms, just as those with elevated uric acid had. I grew suspicious that somehow they were clearing something out of affected tissues, something totally different, because uric acid testing had never shown abnormalities. Gradually, cyclically and progressively, they began experiencing more good days than bad ones; ultimately, they went on to complete clearing and remained well as long as they stayed on the medication. In short, results were identical in all three groups: those with the classic symptoms of gout who displayed red, hot, and swollen joints; those without joint symptoms—the gouty syndrome; and now this other condition that had neither finding. One drug was effective for all three, but what in the world was the cause of this third thing?

I tried to concentrate on what was different about the last group. They suffered from many aches and pains, but overwhelming fatigue was almost always there. I soon realized that women greatly outnumbered men in this new group. I knew gout was predominantly a male disease and fairly uncommon in women—almost nonexistent before menopause. These facts made it ever more likely that there was no connection with gout or the uric acid group except in the similarity of symptoms and the fact that probenecid worked to reverse them. My sleeping brain must have been mulling this over, since I woke up one night with the thought: *Could there be an entirely new disease that acts like the gouty syndrome and is somehow connected to Mr. G's tartar show? Are there people who retain some ion*—a particle with an electrical charge—*other than uric acid that causes the same bunch of symptoms?*

I found it difficult to stop thinking about this idea. Without a named disease (*fibromyalgia* has only been around since the 1980s, and at the time the name *fibrositis* had fallen into disuse), I had previously been relegating all of these patients, except those with classic gout, to the trash heap of medicine. I was taught to consider these people as psychological misfits; they were my languishing hypochondriacs and anxiety neurotics. Standard medical thought held that these women were suffering from unbalanced hormones, unhappy marriages, empty-nest syndrome, inadequate upbringing, or just plain social maladjustment. When I began to elicit symptoms somewhat more methodically, however, I became fascinated by how similar their stories were. If these women really had a psychosomatic illness, how could they all invent nearly identical complaints? The most common symptoms were pain, fatigue, emotional and cognitive defects, spastic colon, cramps, numbness and tingling of various parts of the body, and insomnia. That's the short list. Just go back to my description of syndromes; these patients had them all. Yet not one of them had gone to a school that gave accreditation to neurotics!

They didn't know each other; they represented every ethnic group; they came from all over the country and from widely disparate socioeconomic demographics. Yet their monotonous symptoms were nearly identical! They told me about pains, fatigue, and cognitive complaints that came and went without rhyme or reason. In the earlier phases of their disease, they had good and bad days. Whether they were well or sick, they had the same marriages, the same children, ugly dogs, stress, and fun times, yet they cycled through good and bad days. I knew it was ludicrous to continue in my belief that all of this was due to their nerves, no matter what the books suggested. I knew I might as well accept it: There existed a heretofore unexplored and real disease, even if it had never been described.

When I first used the gout medication, probenecid, I met with variable success. The first two patients began the cyclic reversal I had learned to expect in the gouty syndrome. My enthusiasm was soon dashed when I failed with the next three patients. After some initial teeth gnashing (mine), something told me to try these three misfits on a higher dosage. I did so, and the rewards were swift: All three patients began the hoped-for reverse cycling. It now seemed even more likely that there actually was a tartar, or apatite crystal, syndrome—as I first named it. Equally obvious was the fact that uric acid had no part in the condition, since I could never detect abnormal levels in any of these people. Later, I realized that even tartar had no direct relationship to the disease, though that was how Mr. G had first drawn my attention to a strange phenomenon.

As I found progressively more patients who fit the mold, I felt certain I was peering into a major illness, far more common than gout and affecting women far more than men. This was a debilitating disease, cyclically but inexorably consuming energy, and ultimately utterly destructive to the quality of life. Large numbers of these patients quickly swelled my practice and helped me to expand the parameters of the illness. Soon I realized how often these symptoms seemed to run in families. Older family members related their own horror stories and an even greater litany of complaints. The difference was that now, nearly all of them also had to contend with osteoarthritis.

As I got to know and began to listen more to these patients, I was touched by their years of suffering, and this further motivated me to refine my treatment. Although the nuances in their stories made each patient a bit different, there was no question that each was ill with the same sickness. One woman spoke of a large area in her back that had been stiff and painful for twenty-four years. Another told me that she hadn't been able to have sex for seven years because of pain and spasm in the vulvar area. Sometimes it seemed I would need a calculator to tabulate the visits to doctors, the tests they had run, and the almost equal number of diagnoses that these patients had accumulated. I can repeat most of those, but let's shorten the list. I've heard: "It's a bad menopause," "depression," "inner ear disorder," "defect in your neurotransmitters," "rheumatic arthritis," and "migraine syndrome." Many women were eventually told: "It's all in your head; you need a psychiatrist." Some seriously considered suicide, so compromised was the quality of their lives. They were regularly frustrated and guilt-ridden about not being able to care for their families. Most of them were acutely aware that they were different from other people without ever knowing why. When I told them I thought they were suffering from a real illness, most of them started to cry.

> "I have had fibro since I was a little kid but I did not know that I was ill—at least not beyond the allergies, migraines, etc. that I had accepted as part of my family heritage. Our first child came when I was twenty-one. It did not take me long to realize that I was different from other young mothers. They got more done than I did. They were not sick all the time like I was with almost weekly migraines and multiple bouts of bronchitis. Even when I was not sick I did not get to the end of my work before I crashed, just out of steam. Even with all of that I often thought I could cope if I could just think straight, but I couldn't. I would forget things that I knew. I lost important things. I couldn't remember people's names. My husband became so disgusted with my behavior that he avoided me more and more rather than trying to help. He worked odd shifts and I was pretty much left alone to tend to myself and the kids. . . . My husband was slow to believe the diagnosis. It was just an-

other 'excuse' for substandard behavior as far as he was concerned."

—*Mary Lee, California*

Some years later, a new uricosuric medication, sulfinpyrazone (Anturane), became available. Later, there were others with trade names such as Flexin and Robinul. All successfully lowered uric acid and were strong enough to treat gout. I've used each of them for that disease, for gouty syndrome, and for fibromyalgia. These drugs have only one thing in common: each forces uric acid excretion by an action on a particular area of the kidney where probenecid is known to act. But remember, fibromyalgia is not connected to uric acid. I feel I must repeat this because of confusion in some circles. Several articles and books have printed that I believe uric acid is involved. I emphatically do not think that, I never have, and I have been constant in this statement for more than forty years. It's definite that uricosuric medications work extremely well for fibromyalgia. Therefore, whatever they do at the known site of their action (proximal renal tubule) is greatly beneficial. Something obviously different from uric acid is being excreted at the same kidney level. Whatever it may be, it is what our defective genes have made us retain and what we must expel in the urine for successful treatment.

Many patients also began flaking tartar, confirming the clue provided us by Mr. G. It didn't seem to matter which drug I used; the calculus effect was the same. Monitoring the teeth was not very helpful. Changes were too inconsistent, and dental technicians kept attacking it. Nevertheless, the patient observations proved extremely helpful. They caused me to strongly suspect that the body was improperly handling either calcium or phosphate. Patients also commonly described chipping and peeling of their fingernails in cycles. Nails are predominantly calcium and phosphate—the same as tartar. I quickly realized that nails attracted similar excesses at their root. It is similar to the layering of concentric rings in trees; crystal excess in nails cause chipping when the defect reaches the tip. That's why several nails seem to break at the same time.

Within a few weeks, I was able to absolve calcium as the villain. It actually proved helpful when I gave it with meals as a supplement. Furthermore, calcium allowed me to use somewhat lower dosages of reversing drugs. Calcium, unlike urate, is an ion with a positive charge. If the problem wasn't calcium, then, it seemed logical to look at the other element in tartar, phosphate. Collectively, there are certainly solid biochemical reasons for suspecting phosphate. Phosphate, like urate, has a negatively charged ion. I knew taking calcium helped patients feel better. Calcium binds chemically to phosphate in the intestine, and both are then eliminated in the bowel movement. As a result, less phosphate is presented for absorption, and it doesn't flood the system so intensely.

Although the drugs I was using to treat fibromyalgia were successful, they did have side effects. Sulfinpyrazone could raise stomach acidity enough to cause ulcers. Probenecid is a sulfa drug, and if allergy develops, the resulting hives could last for weeks. Robinul caused dry mouth or eyes, made some patients more tired or slightly spacey, was contraindicated in glaucoma, and caused major urinary retention in men with prostate enlargement. I was always on the lookout for a more effective, better-tolerated medication. In 1992, more than thirty years after I began my initial research, I got lucky. My nurse's ten-year-old son, Malcolm Potter, had been on our treatment for fibromyalgia since the age of seven. As he grew, he needed somewhat larger amounts of his medication, sulfinpyrazone (Anturane), to continue his reversal. As mentioned above, this drug causes hyperacidity and gastric upsets in 8 percent of patients. As my young patient grew taller, he finally raised his dosage to a level too toxic for him, and, sure enough, his stomach began to hurt. I didn't want to try the other medications since I worried about their particular side effects. Remember, this was a kid who would need some drug possibly for the rest of his life. So I intensified my search for a safer substitute.

Luckily, it wasn't long before I recalled a little clipping about another drug that could ever so slightly lower uric acid. I was able to confirm this in a newer edition of the *Physicians' Desk Reference*. The effect of this medication on uric acid is far too weak to successfully treat gout.[1] But you'll recall that anything I'd used so far with that effect had also worked for fibromyalgia. A bit later, I came upon a corroborating article in an old copy of the *Journal of Rheumatology*.[2]

The FDA-approved use of guaifenesin is for producing and loosening mucus in various respiratory infections. Thus, it's found in many cold preparations. It originated somewhere around 1530 as a tree bark extract called guaiacum and, believe it or not, was widely used for rheumatism.[3] It was even used to treat gout. In 1928, a medical paper extolled its virtues for treating growing pains in children. It also relieved several symptoms we would now recognize as fibromyalgia related. Guaiacum was later purified to guaiacolate, and made its first appearance in cough mixtures about seventy years ago. It was eventually synthesized and about twenty-five years ago was pressed into tablets and named guaifenesin. Its original use isn't completely ignored, however. In the *PDR for Herbal Medicines, Guaiacum officinale* remains a medication indicated for rheumatism.[4]

The standard guaifenesin dosage for loosening phlegm in bronchitis, asthma, and sinusitis is two tablets in the morning and two in the evening (2,400 mg per day). In liquid form, it is still one of the active ingredients in many cough medications and expectorants. The drug is no longer under patent and is sold without prescription, making it widely accessible and affordable. For many years, guaifenesin was a prescription drug in the form of 600 or 1200 mg tablets. For thirteen years, we used the 600 mg tablet almost exclusively. Now it's all nonprescription and available in 200, 300, 400, and 600 mg short-acting forms, as well as combined short- and long-acting, 600 and 1,200 mg tablets—known as Mucinex. There are liquid forms with 100 and 200 mg per teaspoon that we've used for children who could not swallow tablets. Guaifenesin is quite well absorbed from the intestinal tract at rates that differ among preparations.

> "*Guaifenesin* (gwy-FEN-e-sin) is an expectorant that thins mucus and helps to loosen phlegm. Guaifenesin is quickly absorbed from the gastrointestinal tract, and is rapidly metabolized and excreted into the urine. Guaifenesin is also known to lower uric acid levels. No serious side-effects have been reported."[5]
>
> —*Physicians' Desk Reference*
>
> To read more about guaifenesin, you can ask your pharmacist or doctor for the package insert or consult the *Physicians' Desk Reference (PDR)*. This is the doctor's guide to medications and has a complete description of guaifenesin. This book can be found in the reference section of libraries, bookstores, or on your pharmacist's and doctor's shelves.

Let's go back to my willing test subject, Malcolm, who had been off his original medicine for some time due to his irritated stomach. I surmised that I'd see some kind of reversal symptoms within a few days if guaifenesin was effective. Lucky for all of us, on the second morning after beginning guaifenesin, Malcolm stumbled out of his bedroom moaning, "Mom, I can't walk—even the bottoms of my feet hurt!" So pervasive were his stiffness and aching that we knew we had found a safer and more potent weapon. Since guaifenesin has no significant side effects, his surge in symptoms could only mean that we were purging his fibromyalgia. Happily, despite the full-blown torture, he was back on the road to recovery!

HOW DOES GUAIFENESIN WORK ON FIBROMYALGIA?

Do you remember our discussion in chapter 1 about the lumps and bumps of fibromyalgia? We find them on every patient with the disease, and we draw them on a body caricature, or map, to keep track of them. These swollen places are for the most part tender. They're also located in tendons and ligaments, but mostly in muscles. Ninety to 95 percent of the swelling is simply water that has collected under considerable pressure. We suspect this fluid has been sent into cells because of the unwelcome presence of a slight excess of phosphates, calcium, and probably other constituents such as sodium and chloride. Our bodies dispatch water to these areas in an attempt to dilute these ions and keep them from crystallizing inside the cells. This tactic succeeds and keeps the tissue accretions in solution. This permits cell survival, but at the expense of losing some normal functions. The worst part of this process is that swelling presses on nerves and they transmit messages of discomfort to the brain, which is the only organ that can feel pain. Only when each ion is neatly tucked into the safest storage areas possible is some of the water allowed to leave and actually make the bump smaller, easing pain somewhat.

Why did getting worse tell us that Malcolm was improving? The reason is simply reversal: the opposite of how the disease develops. This time, however, the body can't pull concentrates out into more diluted areas because this would defy the body's dictum of equilibrium, or balance. When reversal begins, water has to reenter the ailing cells, wherever the cleaning out is about to start. That extra fluid causes swelling all over again, exerting more pressure on nerves to renew the message of pain. Thanks to guaifenesin, when an area is being purged, newly accumulated fluid quickly reverses its direction and is pulled out from cells. This time, it lugs out some of the excess phosphate, calcium, and whatever else was added to expand the miseries of fibromyalgia. Depending on the amounts of water-borne material being extracted from a given site, the bloodstream suffers varying degrees of flooding by the same debris.

So when cells do spring cleaning, they simply sweep their rejected phosphate and fellow travelers out into the blood. This results in an added burden for that system; it's now loaded with the very substances it has been trying to dump for years. Large batches of these excesses are delivered to the kidneys, but those organs can't just process the inflow instantly. You'll recall our theory postulates that fibromyalgia occurs because the kidneys are sluggish when it comes to expelling phosphate. Therefore the flood pouring out of cells is also more than they can immediately handle. Since the urine is the main elimination route, debris piles up a bit and must wait its turn to get out of the body. The blood is impatient and, meeting renal resistance, responds by sneaking mini deposits all over the body. Muscles knuckle under the pressure and suck up a fair share, which causes generalized, flu-like aching. The brain also cooperates and scoops up enough debris to intensify fatigue, cognitive impairment, irritability, depression, anxiety, and insomnia. It's as if the disease were heading entirely in the wrong direction. In fact, it seems worse than ever, since purging is moving debris out of cells at least six times faster than it had been allowed to enter. It's déjà vu all over again! The difference this time, however, is that the kidneys are now working in the right direction, thanks to guaifenesin. They're in overdrive trying to eliminate the excess phosphate, calcium, and whatever at full capacity. The symptoms of fibromyalgia thus disturbingly worsen until the kidneys finally catch up.

What begins streaming out in the urine are the accumulated energy blockers that caused fibromyalgia. Guaifenesin will pull one batch of phosphate after another out of the tissues now that the kidneys are able to cooperate. Added to all of the above symptoms, patients also describe unpleasant tastes, bad breath, burning perspiration, and urine as the body dumps the acidy phosphate into all bodily fluids. Even tears and vaginal secretions may sting. During this leaching-out period, people often notice small amounts of particulate matter or bubbles in the urine. Each cycle ends when that's all that can be done metabolically for the time being.

Between reversal cycles, relative rest periods often follow. They could last for just a few hours, sometimes days, or even weeks depending on the amount of offending substances left to be purged. Even during more peaceful periods, it's likely that some reversing is going on at a subliminal level. What patients experience varies greatly since so much depends on individual pain thresholds and ability to cope. Only one thing is sure: Dependably and suddenly, the crescendo mounts as more cellular debris is offered up for cleansing and becomes available for recycling. It soon becomes clear that the next attack is under way. Over time, these repetitive onslaughts gradually diminish in intensity and frequency. It's much like a roller-coaster ride. The first few hills can be medical thrillers! It's also like shooting a rapid: Peril lessens, and patients fairly swiftly get ever closer to restoring their health. Reversal symptoms, however intense, should reassure that guaifenesin is working because the drug has no known side effects. Given to a normal individual, even in large amounts, no symptoms would appear.

It's these attacks, along with improving body maps, that confirm to us that restoration is under way.

> "I have already started guaifenesin 300 mg twice a day. I have not seen my family doctor yet (I am waiting for the new insurance year to start) but I have visited with my old chiropractor friend and trusted advisor who knows so much about muscles and tendons—more than my family doctor or any specialist I have seen yet, and who, when I discussed the guai treatment and Dr. St. Amand's explanation of the cause of FMS nodded his head and said 'Yes, I think you are on the right track.' I am having him map my 'lumps and bumps' with help from your website. Even though I called a local endocrinologist to enquire about your treatment and was immediately told by the receptionist that 'we don't treat Fibromyalgia' I have hope for the future."
>
> —*Jean, Illinois*

As we've commented earlier, including guaifenesin, we've now described benefits from five totally different chemical compounds. All they have in common is that they act in a certain area of the kidney, the renal tubule. One of the things they do there, in very different degrees, is urge the kidney to excrete uric acid. But we've already explained how we quickly figured out that fibromyalgia has nothing to do with urates. This effect was a clue, not an answer. I had measured the urinary output of phosphate, calcium, and urate before and during treatment using probenecid in the early years of our protocol. Now we appropriately retested patients using guaifenesin and got virtually the same results. We found a 60 percent increase in phosphate excretion and a lesser (30 percent) unloading of oxalate and calcium with both drugs. But whereas the gout medications significantly increased uric acid excretion, only minimal increases in urate output occurred with guaifenesin.

How does guaifenesin purge phosphate from the body? Well, it's somewhat like opening a spigot that lets the kidneys drain out the problem. Think of your home water system. You open the tap; water flows from your pipes and collects it from the main line. This in turn pulls a relatively small amount from the entire system. Ultimately, the reservoir is lowered by the amount you used at home, no matter the distance between the two locations.

We can use this analogy to explain our version of fibromyalgia. Those of us with one or more defective genes have otherwise perfectly normal kidney function. We think the problem arises because our inherited trait makes us produce some slightly crippled proteins called enzymes. Good-quality specimens normally allow smooth opening of the spigot whenever the bloodstream offers up waste for renal filtering. You recall our theory postulates that the kidneys badly direct the fate of inorganic phosphate (symbol: P_i). Our genetic malfunction causes fibromyalgia because it doesn't let the tap open fully; phosphate still leaks out, but only sluggishly. There may be considerable daily variability, but that back-damming effect will eventually send uneliminated P_i for redistribution throughout the body. It's only a matter of susceptibility of certain tissues that determines which ones best scoop up excess phosphate.

The blood brings all sorts of metabolic debris to the kidneys to be filtered out through their small tubules. Water and no-longer-needed substances are extracted and join in the formation of urine. The first tiny flushes have concentrations of mineral, chemical, and water almost identical to those of the blood—with some notable exceptions. Inorganic phosphate is one. Almost all of the huge amounts in our foodstuff are absorbed. Most of it is used to make energy, but there are some leftovers, too. Every single body activity sucks out some energy that's locked inside cells as P_i and frees it up inside cells. This phosphate is mostly recycled, but here, too, there are tiny sur-

Kidney Phosphate Control

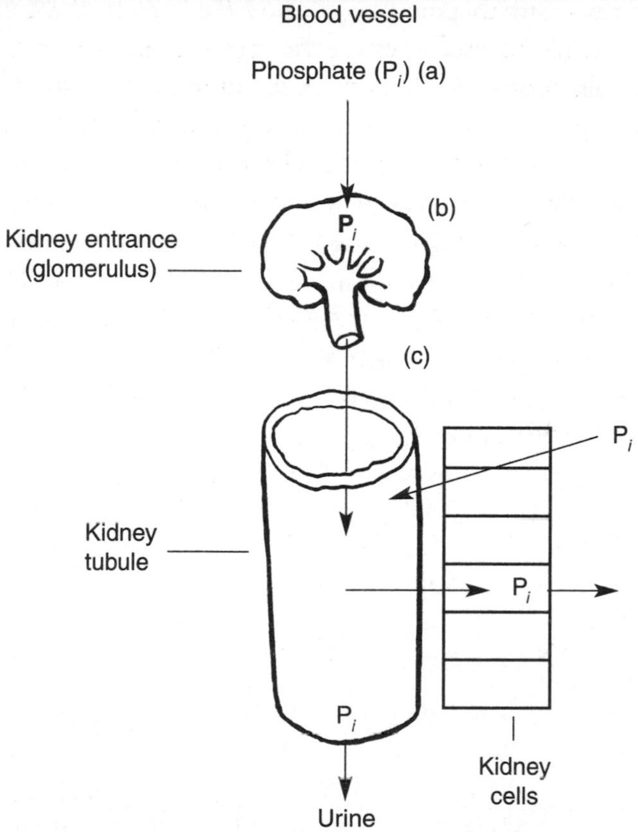

(a) Blood brings inorganic phosphate P_i to the kidney.
(b) P_i is filtered through the glomerulus and is delivered to the tubule.
(c) P_i can also be delivered directly through the blood and through the kidney cells into the tubule.
(d) P_i can go two ways from the tubule:
1. Out into the urine.
2. Reabsorbed from the tubule into the kidney cell and back into the bloodstream.

This is how kidney cells "decide" to keep or eliminate phosphates according to what the body needs.

Figure 3.1

pluses. What our metabolism considers excess baggage slips out into the blood and floats downstream for elimination.

Metabolic debris travels to the kidneys, which are the command center when it comes to designing urine. At some point, cells lining the walls of the renal tubules must make a decision. They normally solicit nerve or hormonal advice before letting all of the filtered phosphate escape into the bladder. If impulses arrive indicating a newfound need for P_i back in the body, tubules are perfectly capable of reabsorbing to send it back. The outside of the cells face the urine stream and work from there. Those same cells also have undersides that look the opposite way, interfacing with a bunch of tiny blood capillaries. They can choose to stop or continue pulling phosphate out of the blood. They can also open their particular side gates and allow P_i retrieved from the urine side safe passage right through the substance of the cell straight back into the bloodstream. You can see by figure 3.1 how this works.

So basically, phosphate has two ways to go. Both are through the bloodstream's capillary walls. The first system shoves it directly into the fluid that's about to become urine. The second extracts it from the blood straight into the tubule-lining cells from one side and ejects through the other side into the urine. This does sound like an unnecessarily duplicated effort. However, these two venues are under different yet synchronized control. Phosphate concentrations are sensed; nerve and hormonal suggestions are respected to please the body's requirements. *If you're soaked in* P_i*, let's get rid of it. You need a bit extra? We know how to get it, and we'll absorb some for you.* It sounds simple, but these activities count on enzymes responding correctly to the body's needs. In fibromyalgia, it is probable that one or more of the involved enzymes could be genetically defective or malformed. This would fit with our theory: Fibromyalgics just can't get rid of enough phosphate to keep out of trouble. We've ended up with some bad plumbing and can't get spigots open enough to rid ourselves of accumulated metabolic trash.

Now we can choreograph the whole scene. Cells work so we can live, and require a huge amount of energy in the process. Most of our food is expended to create ATP in the many mitochondria that sit inside each cell. Once formed, this adenosine triphosphate can flip off attached phosphates one at a time and make metabolic things happen. The fact is, it's energy-expensive to make all those parts function. The normal wear and tear of cells adds more waste phosphate to join any dietary surpluses that weren't earmarked for immediate use. As we've just seen, excesses and waste materials are transported by the bloodstream to the kidneys. There they come face-to-face with the downstream blockage that is fibromyalgia. Things come screeching to a halt.

The body won't tolerate P_i accumulation in the blood, because it's a reciprocal to calcium. This means that when phosphate rises, calcium must fall. There are four parathyroid glands in the neck that won't permit such an imbalance. Their purpose is to pour out hormones to protect calcium levels. So phosphate can't escape in the urine, and it isn't even allowed to stay in the bloodstream. There's now no choice: In some predetermined pecking order, certain tissues must help clear the blood by accepting some phosphate excess. Bones are the most adept at tucking it in, but eventually they become saturated and refuse to soak up any more. Muscles and sinews must help, and they do. That's how inorganic phosphate gets driven back into cells all over the body. At some point, excesses finally slow down mitochondrial generators, and soon energy production fades badly. It's chemically necessary that water enter cells to dilute concentrations of incoming phosphate and its fellow traveler, calcium. Other unwanted substances surf along and, everything combined, cause considerable swelling. These are the lumps and bumps of fibromyalgia that squeeze nerves to signal the brain into expressing the many sensations of pain:

burning, crawling, tingling, and numbness. We've sketched this sequence in figure 3.2.

Earlier we explained how excess phosphate interrupts energy (ATP) production in mitochondria and causes the symptoms of fibromyalgia. All we have to do to solve the problem is help our kidneys purge the excess phosphate, and our cells will again produce all of the ATP we need. ATP-controlled pumps efficiently siphon calcium from where it doesn't belong and stuff it neatly into storage. Rid of misplaced calcium, cells have periods of unfettered relaxation. This rest subsequently energizes our dysfunctional systems to what they once were. We believe that guaifenesin is the best and safest agent to help our enzyme spigots open wide and let us get on with the business of robust living. (See figure 3.3.)

The most difficult aspect of treatment is what patients must go through during reversal. They've already been disappointed too many times by promises of cures that never materialized. They enter the initial recycling phases desperate for their bodies to show them a glimmer of hope with a flash of a few better hours. We've told each of them that such inspirational moments will be their assurance of the success to come. If the body is capable of providing them with a few significantly better hours or days, it will eventually do so on a permanent basis. But until they feel this first breeze of well-being, they can only hope that we've not lied and that guaifenesin will work for them as it has for so many others. It takes guts and perseverance when they're being confronted by all of the sometimes intense early reversal symptoms. Though later cleansing cycles can also be tough, by then patients have had a taste of recovery, a series of good days with much less pain and fatigue. That makes it easier to keep the faith and stay the course. But at the start of the next reversing cycle, concerns rise fast, and it's easy to fret that those better moments were only a mirage—a rainbow that has permanently faded from the horizon.

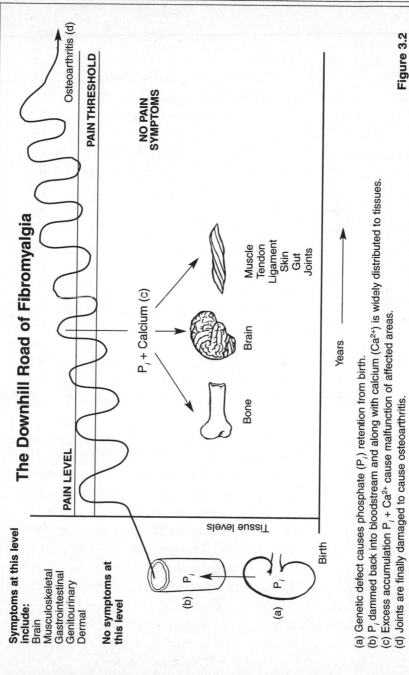

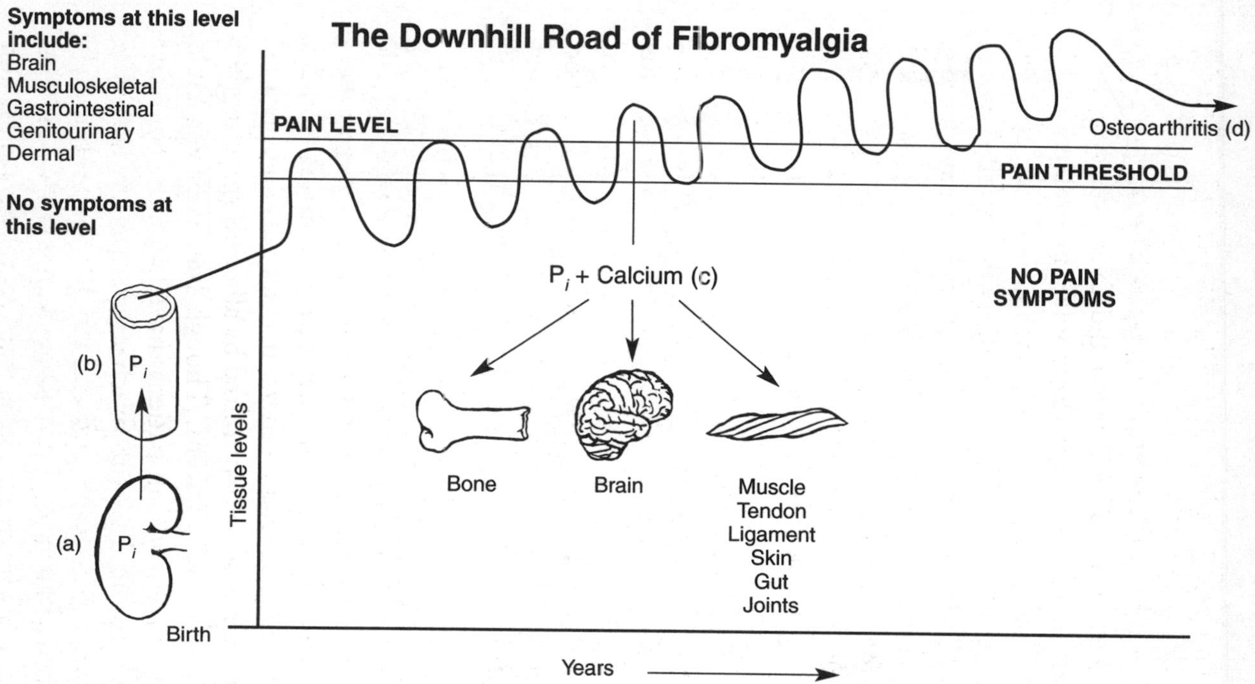

(a) Genetic defect causes phosphate (P_i) retention from birth.
(b) P_i dammed back into bloodstream and along with calcium (Ca^{2+}) is widely distributed to tissues.
(c) Excess accumulation $P_i + Ca^{2+}$ cause malfunction of affected areas.
(d) Joints are finally damaged to cause osteoarthritis.

Figure 3.2

The Road Back from Fibromyalgia

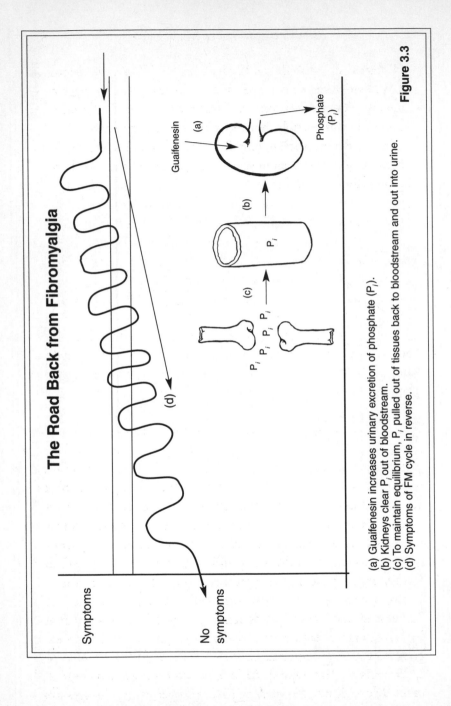

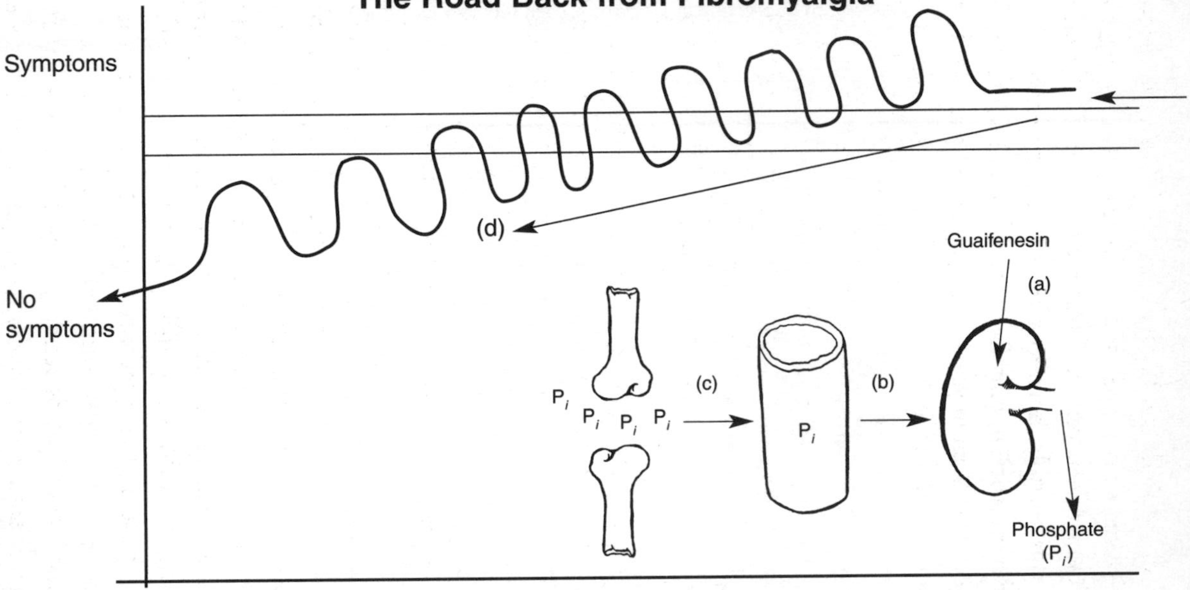

(a) Guaifenesin increases urinary excretion of phosphate (P_i).
(b) Kidneys clear P_i out of bloodstream.
(c) To maintain equilibrium, P_i pulled out of tissues back to bloodstream and out into urine.
(d) Symptoms of FM cycle in reverse.

Figure 3.3

> "I started on guai in mid-January 1998. I had experienced FMS symptoms since childhood. I am thirty-four years old and as of January was very ill. I had the gamut of FMS symptoms and was horribly, horribly fatigued and depressed. Now, I am a different woman, only five months later. I am so much better than I have been in years. . . . Fatigue and pain are drastically diminished, and in certain areas I have no pain anymore. Mood has improved. I sleep much better as a rule. My sex life is wonderful. I'm thinking more clearly. Not to say that the road has been easy, no, no, no. Sometimes I couldn't see the light at the end of the tunnel. But now, it's only five months later and so much is behind me."
>
> —*Julie O., Canada*

Another common reaction is for patients to feel that their body is somehow different from those of other fibromyalgics. They have trouble overriding the fear that their case is too far gone ever to get sustained benefits. But as treatment progresses, confidence mounts, and relatively soon they become old pros at the ins and outs of their disease. They know the good days will return in progressively greater numbers. They also learn that attacks will be milder and far more bearable, and fewer and fewer areas are left to purge. Though the initial reversal cycles might have attacked ten to twenty places at one time, later reversals may work on only one or two sites simultaneously. This alone greatly diminishes the severity of subsequent attacks. In addition, purging phases get progressively farther apart, making these setbacks minor by comparison.

Every patient asks: "How long will it take to clear me up?" There's no easy answer. It depends on several things—primarily how long patients have had the illness and to which dose of guaifenesin they respond. Low-dose patients (300 or 400 mg twice a day) clear rapidly in intense and almost constant attacks. More slowly responding patients need larger dosages and spread their reversal rates over a spectrum of possibilities. We rely on a well-tested rule that the *slowest* of our patients will clean out one year of fibromyalgic debris every few months. The clock doesn't start ticking, however, until they've found the proper dosage and become totally salicylate-free. Yes, it's gradual for some and unbelievably fast for those lucky quick responders. What's most heartening to us is the visible improvement in just about all of our patients' lives

> "I have been on guaifenesin for seven and a half months. I have had painful FMS symptoms since July 1991, following whiplash and a concussion during an auto accident. Since being on guai my quality of life has greatly improved. I have less pain overall, even when cycling. I used to have trouble riding in the car, even for a few miles, because the vibrations felt greatly magnified to me. This has lessened slightly. The severity and frequency of my headaches have diminished significantly. My MPS (Myofascial Pain Syndrome) is gone. I have periods that my skin doesn't hurt when someone touches it lightly, I used to hurt all the time from a soft touch or rub. I am capable of doing much more day-to-day things like loading the dishwasher and watching our children during the day. I need to rest quite a bit less. . . . I have had a full three weeks with virtually no pain. This is the first time in seven years that this has happened. This treatment is our one great hope."
>
> —*J. M., Texas*

Another patient who went through years of hardship with fibromyalgia, and had difficult cycling during treatment, recounts her experience:

> "I want to brag about my second thirty-mile bike ride. I am very proud of myself. I want you to know how far I've come. I am forty-eight years old and suffered all my life with progres-

sively more and more pain and depression. I have been on most of the powerful painkillers and antidepressants over the years. I closed my business and quit working in 1994. My mind was worthless, the fatigue and pain made getting out of bed impossible on most days, and I had horrid insomnia for years. The symptoms would come and go, and most of the time I 'looked normal,' although I put on a lot of weight. Life has always been a fight against body and mind pain. In February of 1997 I was hit hard. My entire body swelled, my skin burned all over, my mouth burned badly and I salivated constantly. My stomach contorted. My mind went crazy. Most of my muscles were in spasm. I couldn't move without sweating profusely."

—G. M., California

FREQUENTLY ASKED QUESTIONS

Before we leave the subject of guaifenesin and end this chapter, let's deal with some of the questions we're most commonly asked.

Does guaifenesin have side effects?

Other than infrequent and transient nausea in the early treatment stages, guaifenesin has no known side effects. Even that sensation is such a frequent part of the irritable bowel that most times, we can't blame the drug. Also, upset stomachs may be just part of cycling. Some people have difficulty with any medication. We urge them to buy or cut tablets into sizes that will fit into gelatin capsules, which can be purchased in any pharmacy or health food store. Since the stomach can't digest gelatin, the capsule slips the drug into the small intestine, where it's released. Very rarely, we've seen individual sensitivities to some filler in the tablets or to an added dye. Pharmacists can suggest different brands that are dye-free and contain different fillers. The pain, numbness, and host of other symptoms you might feel while taking guaifenesin are due to the anticipated reversal process. Even occasional hives or other rashes are almost always part of the disease and are due to purging of the skin, not to allergy. All of these cleansing symptoms are great clues that guaifenesin is at work.

Which guaifenesin should I use?

Guaifenesin is an ingredient in many cough mixtures and decongestants. These items contain too many other substances that either block the kidney benefits of the drug or will make you even sicker. Any pure guaifenesin free of added medications such as pseudoephedrine and dextromethorphan will do just fine. We've restricted our use of liquid guaifenesin to children, since the concentrations are too low for adults unless they're willing to drink nearly a bottle a day. That's a bit pricey.

Can I get guaifenesin over the counter?

Guaifenesin is available in 200, 300, 400, 600, and even 1,200 mg tablets. Currently, all are being sold over the counter. Some are twelve-hour acting (600 and 1,200 mg), and others are short acting (400 or less). Powders are also available, but may have lost potency before being pressed into tablets or while being stuffed into capsules due to excess handling. We mistrust some imports, which take too long to get to patients. We continue to use Mucinex, Pro Health, Grace Fibro-Smile Solo Guai, and freshly compounded guaifenesin—but others likely exist. The situation is truly buyer beware; we can only vouch for the ones we've used successfully. Our Web site, fibromyalgiatreatment.com, tries to stay abreast of changes.

We don't particularly recommend self-treatment unless there's no alternative. There are many symptoms in fibromyalgia that could easily mask some other condition. It's certainly best to exclude these before starting our protocol. Once that's done, you're correct in expecting physicians to consider the diagnosis of fibromyalgia and knowing how to confirm their suspicions by physical examination. However, not enough doctors know about our protocol. You the patient could help educate them. If you luck into a doctor who knows how to find the lumps and bumps of the disease, work on the reversal together. We'll soon tell you about selected parts of the body that regress within one month, and quickly help identify the correct dosage. If your doctor knows how to palpate these areas, it will provide you great reassurance in the early stages of treatment. Furthermore, you might need professional help down the line if strange symptoms pop up. Assistance is also essential should you stop improving or actually regress and need help in finding some hidden source of salicylate.

Are there any special instructions for storing guaifenesin?

The medication should be stored in an area that has a temperature between fifty-nine and eighty-six degrees Fahrenheit, not in the refrigerator or in a very warm room. Avoid getting your supplies wet. Tightly pressed tablets have a longer shelf life than capsules, and powder has the shortest shelf life of all. If you are filling capsules in your own home, make sure you purchase the powder in small amounts so that it remains potent.

Do I need to drink lots of water with my guaifenesin?

That's not necessary. Pushing fluids was urged mainly for people taking guaifenesin for lung or sinus problems. The extra fluid intake further helps them loosen mucus. You're more interested in its kidney effects.

Should I continue my other medications when I start guaifenesin?

Since guaifenesin mixes safely with anything, your doctor will undoubtedly let you continue your other medications. Only salicylates block the renal effect of guaifenesin, though not its ability to liquefy mucus. Just to name a few, you must avoid

Soma Compound (replace with plain Soma), Darvon Compound (replace with Darvocet-N), Fiorinal (replace with Fioricet), Empirin, and Percodan (replace with Percocet). You'll have to make do with Tylenol (acetaminophen) and the nonsteroidal anti-inflammatories (NSAIDs such as ibuprofen and naproxen), since even tiny bits of aspirin (salicylates) will stall your progress. We'll tell you more about such things as Pepto-Bismol, toothpastes, Ben-Gay, and others in chapter 4. You should not discontinue or change the dosage of any prescription medication without consulting with your physician.

Some people refer to the guaifenesin protocol as detoxification. Is that correct?

There are no toxins in fibromyalgia. Accumulating research and extensive testing have found no abnormal factors. Whatever is causing FMS doesn't appear to be a substance foreign to the body. The body mounts no inflammatory response or antibody attack. We think fibromyalgia is caused by customarily friendly phosphate—there's just too much of it in the wrong places. Therefore, since there are no toxins, guaifenesin does not "detox."

Is it beneficial to cleanse the body of yeast and/or parasites before starting guaifenesin treatment?

We do not ascribe to the diagnosis of chronic candidiasis as it's currently being made using plasma antibodies or stool cultures. Antibodies are our friends and are present because we've encountered a particular infection in the past. They're poised to pounce on the offender at any time if it tries to reenter the body. Also note that the so-called anti-yeast diet is the one we prescribe for hypoglycemia. That's why patients improve on low carbohydrate intake—not because of any theoretical effect on *Candida*. Similarly, parasites are too often blamed for fibromyalgia. It's not something we've observed. "Herbal cleansing" ingredients block guaifenesin, so if you feel you must, go ahead do it and only later begin our protocol. Remember that the immune system is slightly depressed in fibromyalgia, and therefore infections may be more common.

Is guaifenesin safe to take if I get pregnant?

Guaifenesin has actually been used to help women get pregnant. It was thought to be helpful solely for its ability to liquefy the mucous plug that normally sits at the opening of the uterus. Later findings have identified spermatocidal qualities of this mucus in certain fibromyalgic women, a defect also corrected by using guaifenesin. We suggest each woman discuss this issue with her own doctor. We advise our pregnant patients to stop and, with the permission of their obstetrician, resume treatment after the sixth month of pregnancy. (The baby is fully formed by that time.) This way, fibromyalgic women avoid the sudden burst of symptoms that quickly follow delivery.

Am I at greater risk of osteoporosis when taking guaifenesin?

The calcium excreted by guaifenesin is limited to the inappropriate surplus temporarily locked within your cells. So you don't have to worry about causing osteoporosis. Remember, the medication is more than four hundred years old in some form or other. Problems should have shown up by now.

Can guaifenesin cause kidney stones?

No, there are no connections among kidney stones, guaifenesin, or fibromyalgia. Most stones are calcium oxalate, some are sodium urate, and a smaller number are calcium phosphate. As I just stated, guaifenesin has been in use for many years and has never been linked to kidney stones except for one tiny study. If you read this study carefully, you will be able to see what was confirmed to us by the authors: The patients in this study were not taking pure guaifenesin but rather were abusing combinations of guaifenesin and pseudoephedrine (methamphetamine manufacture). As a result, they were taking huge amounts of both drugs.

Is it okay to drink colas while taking guaifenesin?

We have not had to restrict colas when we treat fibromyalgia. They do contain phosphoric acid, and phosphate is the ion we're trying to purge from the body, but we've seen no problem with such drinks. Guaifenesin appears to overcome that small added load rather easily. It also overcomes the amounts contained in nearly all plant foods as long as patients are compliant with the protocol.

If I have asthma, can I take guaifenesin?

Guaifenesin is frequently used for asthma. It's actually marketed as a "mucolytic" agent—something that helps cells produce a bit more though softer and less tenacious mucus. This cuts down on wheezing by making it easier to raise phlegm. Whenever you have other medical conditions, you should always ask your personal physician if he or she objects to the addition of any medication.

We're sure you're more than ready to move on to learn more about the protocol. The next few chapters will describe lots of things that will help you understand and successfully treat fibromyalgia.

> "After the initial onslaught of the illness, there was disbelief. I sat in my chair for hours not believing I could possibly be living in such a broken body. The pain came in waves, rendering life an unpredictable nightmare of perceived uselessness and anger. I gave up my role as a wife, a mother, a daughter and a therapist. I had loved each of those roles. [The depression began] so long ago I don't even remember. I prayed to God.

Then I quit praying. No strength for it. I gave in and gave up and spent most of the time doing nothing. It is so easy to get stuck right there doing nothing, not caring, not wanting to live, hoping not to die. It is hard work to be sick. It's harder work to get well . . . but getting well is the best thing there is, and guaifenesin is the way to do it."

—Gretchen, South Carolina

Chapter 4

Meet the Enemy: Aspirin and Other Salicylates, Natural and Otherwise

> "You can manage to get by without salicylates. In the beginning, if you are unsure and too confused to understand, just use fewer products. It's funny that we do without so many things when we are sick, but then want to argue about giving up mint toothpaste. There's no point in reading the book and getting guaifenesin and hoping that you'll get better if you don't do your homework about salicylates. There are many resources to help you and now there are many companies that make special products. Don't throw up roadblocks of your own when you've spent years complaining about an illness and people with no understanding who have gotten in your way."
>
> —*Gloria, California*

A BRIEF HISTORY OF SALICYLATES

Guaifenesin and the other medications we've used for fibromyalgia have only one enemy, a chemical compound known as salicylate. This substance blocks the action at the kidney level, precisely where we need guaifenesin to do its work. It's important to know that there are no known drug interactions between guaifenesin and any other medication. Taking guaifenesin with salicylates will not make you ill. It will still help liquefy your mucus, and make a cough more productive, but it will be rendered impotent against fibromyalgia. The fact that there is no outward manifestation is both good and bad news. While it means that you will not feel sick if you make a mistake, it also means that you will have no immediate sign that you've goofed. Only in time, when your map shows a lack of progress or your symptoms haven't reversed as you expected, will you suspect the problem. By then, valuable time will have been lost. That's why it's so absolutely necessary to read and review this chapter until you understand what's written here. As we've said repeatedly, our protocol's chances of reversing your illness are at the mercy of how completely you observe what follows. Unless you avoid salicylates as we instruct, no amount of guaifenesin can do anything to heal you.

Salicylates have been used medicinally since about 1500 BC. A recipe for dried myrtle leaves was recorded by ancient Egyptians to relieve back pain. In the fifth century BC Hippocrates, known affectionately as the father of medicine, used a juice extracted from the bark of willow trees to treat aches and pains. Around the world, diverse cultures such as the American Indians made the same discovery and used barks and meadow grasses to prepare topical and internal preparations for the same purposes. During the late Middle Ages, a willow bark concoction for pain and fevers was so popular in Europe that it had to be outlawed because it was wiping out the trees used by the wicker industry faster than they could be replanted. It was not until 1806 that this law was repealed, because the only alternative, quinine from Peru, was stopped by Napoleon's blockade.

Whenever plants are found useful in treating disease, a search begins to find the active chemical that's responsible. Then it can be extracted, purified, and made into doses that are uniform in potency. In 1823, in Germany, the chemical salicin was successfully extracted from the bark of the willow tree and named for the Latin moniker of that plant: *Salix*. Later it was also extracted from meadowsweet and many other plants.

Once the chemical was identified, a race was on to synthesize the molecule—that is, to make it from scratch in a laboratory. It was hoped that this process would be easier, be less expensive, and, of course, result in a successful capitalistic venture that wouldn't require the continued deaths of trees to treat human pain. In 1853, this was accomplished but then abandoned because the substance was too acidic.

A few years later, a German chemist, Felix Hoffman, began searching for a form of salicylate to help his father, who suffered from arthritis and could not take the natural compound because it upset his stomach. When Hoffman's work yielded a product that helped, he convinced his employer, Bayer, to market it. In 1899, aspirin arrived as a prescription drug in the form of a powder. A tablet soon followed; in 1915, it was made available without prescription. It has been widely used since then for fever, arthritis, rheumatism, lumbago, and neuralgia.

Aspirin has extensive effects on the body, some of which have never been explored fully and others that have only recently become known. We all know it as a good pain reliever, especially for arthritis, backache, and headache. It works by reducing the body's ability to form prostaglandins, compounds that induce inflammation. Aspirin also lowers the risk of repeat heart attacks and certain kinds of strokes in men and older women. It accomplishes this by making platelets, the elements of the blood that initiate clots, less likely to stick together. Aspirin may help prevent certain types of cataracts as well as affording some protection against colon and rectal cancers. Because it is so easily and inexpensively produced, it is very commonly used in many types of products. In its concentrated form, salicylic acid is used to remove warts and corns. The acid is also commonly applied in creams and lotions for treating acne and dandruff. It's used as a cosmetic chemical peel by dermatologists. Women often unknowingly use the agent as an ingredient in their facial cleansing creams, where it provides an exfoliating action and removes dead skin. In sunscreens, it offers a small amount of UVA protection. (It does not protect against skin cancer.)

Salicylates are fairly praised for their usefulness and therapeutic benefits. Unfortunately for fibromyalgics being treated with guaifenesin, this means that they appear in many products, so some diligence is required to avoid them. Another subset of chemically sensitive people can't use them because they're common allergens implicated in attention deficit disorder (ADD) and illnesses such as asthma. A nationwide organization, the Feingold Association, was named for the doctor who first postulated this connection. It is an invaluable resource for children and their families who must avoid salicylates at all costs. Its research has also greatly expanded our knowledge of the chemical's effects.

WHY SALICYLATES BLOCK GUAIFENESIN

Why do salicylates cause such problems for our protocol? The answer isn't very complicated. There is a particular area in the kidneys where our older medications and now guaifenesin must be allowed to work unimpeded. Unfortunately, it's precisely the same location where salicylates also attach to targeted cells: in the renal tubules. These cells have surface areas that house thousands of receptors. It's easy to visualize the process if you think of each receptor as a custom-made garage designed for use only by a certain specially shaped car. Each garage will allow parking only for cars that fit that perfectly. In the human body, every receptor on every cell is precision-made to accommodate only specific hormones or chemicals. For any medication to succeed, it must somehow find and neatly fit into a garage, even though that space was designed for a natural molecule. This is what the science of pharmacology is all about. Drugs are manufactured to occupy natural receptors that will either trigger an action or have a blocking effect. Once medications are correctly parked, cells under their influence will perform or not perform specific actions. Unfortunately, guaifenesin and salicylates are competitors for the same receptors, or garages, and the latter are a better fit and so get preferential parking. It takes very little salicylate to occupy the few available sites, and that leaves no place for guaifenesin to make contact with the cells. None of the drugs we've used, regardless of the amount, has been able to overcome this discriminatory behavior by the kidney receptors. Once the parking garage is full, it shuts down, hangs up a CLOSED sign, and does not accept any new vehicles. In the presence of salicylates, guaifenesin still successfully liquefies mucus because it can fit slightly different receptors in other areas even when the kidney sites are closed. *But its benefit for fibromyalgia is nonexistent.*

We've struggled with this problem—we call it blocking—for many years. We knew enough to avoid aspirin from the very beginning, because it's contraindicated with the uricosuric gout medications, including the very first one we ever used, probenecid. That fact is well documented in medical resources. We never had to discover that aspirin was a problem—and knowing this fact afforded us important clues early in the game and helped us to figure out and learn what follows.

A number of studies have demonstrated how effectively salicylate is absorbed through the skin. It's obvious, of course, that it is, because otherwise topical pain creams wouldn't provide any relief when applied to the skin over a muscle that hurts. What was less appreciated when we first started treating fibromyalgia is how widely distributed throughout the body things rubbed into the skin end up. When our suspicions were aroused because of the lack of progress by a patient using Ben-

Gay (methyl salicylate), we were able to find a study of what happened when it was applied to the trapezius, a muscle at the top of the shoulder area. One and a half hours later, biopsies were taken from that muscle and from the opposite shoulder.[1] Blood levels of salicylate were nearly identical in both, even though the cream was rubbed into the skin on only one side.

Now in the days of nicotine patches, sprays, and gum, birth control and pain patches, nasal sprays for headaches, and gels or creams that deliver therapeutic levels of hormones, this realization seems dated. It's hard to believe that until only recently, our idea that relatively small but concentrated amounts could be absorbed through the skin in medicinal amounts was ridiculed. In the ensuing years, pharmaceutical companies have learned that there are actual benefits from delivering medications through such a direct route. Now it is well understood that this method allows for lower doses, since drugs don't have to wander down the intestinal tract and face degradation by digestive juices.

> "I have a dear friend who is a chiropractor and very involved in a new procedure to check antioxidant levels and to supplement them to enhance overall health and destroy free radicals. She dispenses a product that is supposed to raise antioxidants but I told her that if there is any hint of salicylates in that product that I would rather have lower than optimum levels than start redepositing. My greatest issue with FMS was exhaustion from lack of restful and restorative sleep. It was only a short time on guai before I was able to actually suggest going out to a movie on Friday night after a long week at work, and I have continued to have high levels of energy from good quality sleep."
>
> —*Marsha, California*

There are physicians who scoff at our insistence that what they consider to be inconsequential amounts of salicylates can block guaifenesin. To this we say, nonsense! We've created thousands of maps on our patients that graphically illustrate the complete reversal of previous improvement when errors have been made. Ignore any and all voices to the contrary; salicylates block with devastating efficiency.

Sensitivity to blockade is genetically determined, but since none of us knows our personal susceptibility, we should meticulously abide by the protocol. There is no need to further belabor this point. To our fibromyalgic readers, we plead—do your job and give guaifenesin a fair chance. Go to our Web site for help if your medical professional doesn't fully warn you or you don't feel secure in your ability to check your own products. If you have taken the time to read this book and invested in guaifenesin both financially and with your hopes, do the protocol correctly. It doesn't make sense to do otherwise.

AVOIDING SALICYLATES

Since my first day in medical school, I've had a love affair with medicine. It's a love that has endured without waning. That is, not until it was severely strained by several years of almost daily torment trying to guess the new source of salicylates blocking a particular patient. It's certainly been a learning curve! Claudia and I spend time every day cautioning patients on how to avoid various sources beyond simply not taking aspirin and Pepto-Bismol. Even our best efforts have not prevented errors by otherwise intelligent and diligent people. For some, the inability to use a beloved product seems heart wrenching and is the most difficult part of their treatment. Other patients would give up anything without a second thought just for the chance to get better.

My first visit with a new patient usually proceeds well while

I take the history, complete my examination, and produce a map displaying the lesions. Then I make a sketch (always on paper towels) as I unfold a story—our version of fibromyalgia. I run through the details of how I began, thanks to an observant man—my tartar flicker. I flit superficially through the metabolism of calcium and phosphate as I believe it relates to fibromyalgia. I dwell a bit longer on the cyclic but progressive nature of the illness and on its genetics. I spend considerable time explaining the role of guaifenesin in reversing our faulty chemistry and the role of the kidneys in the disease. Patients grimace a bit when I get to my description of the reversal process. I explain that it's fully anticipated that they will see great swings in symptoms. They'll cycle quickly or gradually from worse-than-ever to better-than-in-a-long-time hours. Patients handle this information quite well—so far, so good.

I cringe when I even think about the almost certain verbal or facially expressed protest I know will come when I get to the matter of avoiding salicylates, especially in topical beauty products or herbal medications. When it comes to the former, 85 percent of fibromyalgics are women, and the idea of having to replace something they've found that actually works after years of searching for the perfect product is often devastating. We've actually had a few patients dump guaifenesin and us rather than give up some cherished item. One actress actually stated the protocol was "too hard"; she simply failed to appear at her next appointment. Believe it or not, we've also heard: "I'd rather have fibromyalgia than give up my lipstick!" It's sometimes equally difficult to convince patients to part with their all-natural herbal megavitamins, Juice Plus+, or herbal colon cleansings. At this point, we remind patients that had those things worked, they could have saved themselves the expense and time involved with a trip to our office.

Synthetic Salicylates

We'll start the discussion of what you have to avoid with the easiest group of salicylates to identify, the synthetic or pure chemical form. Since salicylate or salicylic acid is exactly what you can't use, obviously that's the first thing you should look for on product labels. The most common salicylate is aspirin or acetylsalicylic acid. It may appear on labels by either name or as ASA (a common designation for acetylsalicylic acid, especially in Canada). Pain medications of many types contain this drug, which releases salicylate when it enters the body. Examples include Anacin, Excedrin, and Fiorinal. (Aspirin Free Excedrin, Excedrin PM, and Fioricet—which don't have acetylsalicylic acid or aspirin listed as an ingredient—are fine to use.)

Ok. for pain

It's slightly more difficult to spot the compound when it's blended into a long chemical name. Sunscreens may list octisalate or homosalate; other examples include Pepto-Bismol (bismuth subsalicylate) or methyl salicylate (Listerine and Ben-Gay). As you would expect, many pain and anti-inflammatory medications include such ingredients—for example, sodium salicylate, choline salicylate, and magnesium salicylate, the actual chemical names. Watch for salsalate, choline magnesium trisalicylate, and salicylsalicylic acid. Notice how easily you can spot *sal* buried within those names?

Acne soaps, dandruff shampoos, and corn-removing products quite regularly include salicylic acid. It's also used to treat psoriasis and seborrheic dermatitis of the face and scalp, as well as to remove calluses. Plantar and common warts are usually attacked with various strengths of salicylic acid. Acne is also often treated with topical solutions. Some names, such as Sal-Clens shampoo and Hydrisalic, are dead giveaways, but names like Clear Away or Freezone provide no clues that they contain salicylates. However, all of the above products in the ingredient portion of the label list salicylic acid 1 or 2 percent. (By contrast, acne medications with benzoyl peroxide are fine to use; that's a different chemical.)

It's easy to see that synthetic blockers are not difficult to avoid, because the term *salicylate, salicylic acid,* or simply the giveaway syllable *sal* is on the label. Overzealous patients sometimes confuse silicate or sulfate and think they're problems, but those are not blockers. Remember that the three telltale letters are *s-a-l.*

Prescription and Over-the-Counter Medications Containing Synthetic Salicylate

Aspirin
Anacin
Bufferin
Disalcid
Doan's Pills
Ecotrin
Excedrin
Excedrin Migraine
Fiorinal
Pepto-Bismol
Triclosan
Trilisate

Common Topical Products Containing Synthetic Salicylates

Buf-Puf Acne Cleansing Bar with Vitamin E
Clearasil Clearstick Maximum
Compound W Gel
Freezone
Gold Bond Triple Action Medicated Body Powder
Occlusal-HP Topical Solution
Oxy Clean Medicated Pads
Sebex-T Tar Shampoo
Salonpas
Stri-Dex Super Scrub Pads
Wart-Off Topical Solution

Natural Salicylates

All plants make salicylates.[2] The appearance of the article proving this, in 1984, was a defining moment for the guaifenesin protocol, a missing piece of the puzzle. What had been hazy and not quite appreciated was suddenly clear. Just as the realization many years before that there was a condition called hypoglycemia had hit like a ton of bricks, this headline was staggering. It took a few more years, some refinements and some missteps, but an important piece of information had suddenly dropped into our laps, and we knew it the minute we read the headline.

It was stunningly logical that if taking aspirin—or acetylsalicylic acid—would block guaifenesin, then so would taking white willow bark, which contains the natural salicylate, salicin. Once past the mouth, these chemicals—because they are identical—fit the same receptors and have the same resulting effect on the body. Only the source was different. But now we suddenly knew that if all plants made salicylates, then *all* herbal medications would block guaifenesin, too, because of their concentration. Medicinal herbs are designed, as are all medications, to get into the bloodstream in sufficient amounts to chemically alter some function of the body.

In the early days of the protocol, herbal medications were not very often used. The supplement market was almost nonexistent except for a few multivitamins. Self-respecting patients back then didn't take alfalfa, borage seed oil, wild Mexican yam, or bioflavonoids. But as time passed, everything old was becoming new again. People who wouldn't dream of taking eight aspirin a day would take white willow bark with a passion, commenting that it was natural and could not hurt them. Women who didn't want to take horse estrogens or synthetic (another nasty word) hormones had no problem with taking black cohosh, yam, or soy that contained other forms of the

no plant name

no medicinal herbs

same chemical—which relieved symptoms by sitting in the same receptors. Exotic juice extracts like nonni and strange herbal names like dong quai were suddenly on the shelf in every market. Asking what was natural about taking grapeseed extract in a concentration that doesn't exist in nature, or taking pills made from seaweed, was suddenly a very politically incorrect question.

The first obvious source of natural salicylates strong enough to block guaifenesin is medicinal herbs. The fact is, those that are most helpful for fibromyalgics, especially the ones known to decrease pain, are exactly the ones highest in natural salicylate. It's not a strange or mystical part of plants that works to relieve aches and pains. It's a single chemical isolated many years ago.

Concerning guaifenesin, it's now obvious to us that you can take no medicinal herbs in any form—pill, capsule, tablet, powder, drops, or tea—without blocking its benefits. Medicinal or concentrated ingredients are easily spotted by looking for a label that reads SUPPLEMENT FACTS. (Foods, by contrast, have a box that says NUTRITIONAL FACTS.) The rule is simple: Any product with a box that says SUPPLEMENT FACTS needs to be checked carefully. Any plant name within that ingredient box demands that you avoid the product. Ginkgo biloba, green tea extract, evening primrose oil, flaxseed oil, and wild yam extract are all examples of what you cannot use. The exact words you are looking for are: *oil, gel,* or *extract* used in combination with a plant name. You must also check this box for *bioflavonoids,* which are concentrated plant pigments and, thus, salicylates. Vitamin pills, supplements, protein powders, and energy drinks all frequently contain medicinal herbal ingredients. All products should be rechecked each time they are purchased to make sure there have been no ingredient changes.

Once you've checked everything that you take as medication, look at products that come in contact with your skin, just as you did when you checked for the chemical form of salicylate. This time instead of the letters *sal,* you're again looking for *oil, gel,* or *extract* coupled with a plant name. For example, no coconut oil, macadamia nut oil, chamomile extract, or aloe gels. Any oil, gel, or extract without a plant name is automatically safe—natural salicylates occur only in plants, not animals or minerals. So mineral oil, vitamin E oil, emu oil, and lanolin oil are all safe to use. The same would apply to an extract such as placenta in a hair conditioner or animal byproducts taken as dietary supplements.

Be sure to gather up everything you use: shampoo, conditioner, bubble bath, body lotions, deodorants, lip balms, face cleansers, bar soap, eye makeup removers, nail polish remover, massage oils, cuticle creams, and so on. Make sure that if it is something that comes in contact with your skin, you know what's in it. We'll make an exception for products like hair color that are only used once every six weeks or so, but if they come with a daily or weekly conditioner, check the contents. Exposure to salicylates is cumulative: a little here, a little there, and eventually you'll have crossed the line and blocked your guaifenesin.

Lipsticks, mouthwashes, suppositories, chewing gums, cortisone creams, nasal sprays, breath mints, toothpastes, razors, as well as shaving creams have the potential to block guaifenesin. Some of these products contain camphor or castor oils; others add natural flavors such as mint, spearmint, peppermint, or wintergreen oils that easily provide enough salicylate to block guaifenesin. There are strips coated with aloe adjacent to the cutting edge of most women's disposable razors. The salicylates in the aloe slide into the tiny cuts made by shaving legs, underarms, or faces and readily block guaifenesin. Hair sprays may also contain plant extracts that you spritz all over your hair, but unfortunately, they also thinly coat the underlying scalp and nearby forehead.

Plant ingredients in most products are not difficult to identify. Rose hips, lavender, rosemary, ginseng, chamomile, and aloe vera are some of the well-known ones. Less commonly known names such as arnica, jojoba, and yucca can be identified with the use of a dictionary or online at www.dictionary.com. Unfortunately, there's a small group of plant names that are more difficult to find in standard reference books. Since the basic ingredients in all cosmetics are similar, manufacturers search for unique-sounding additives that will set their product apart on labels and in advertisements. Rain forests and tropical islands are being raided for cajeput, quillaja, bibia, padauk, and other native plants. These exotic but obscure substances can sometimes be identified only by searching in a specialized source such as Ruth Winter's *A Consumer's Dictionary of Cosmetic Ingredients.* As an alternative, you might use an online search engine such as google.com or contact the manufacturer and, with a bit of luck, you can learn if the funny name on the product label is actually a plant. You should also be aware that there are occasional ingredients that are almost mystical—no one seems to know what they are, or be willing to tell. Sea silt is one of those. It should mean dirt if it's silt, but what else has crept into it? Does it come from the ocean bottom or simply from some beach, and does the collection process simultaneously dredge kelp or other plant debris? There's no way for us to estimate the salicylate content of something like this. Just skip such products and give yourself a fair shake by keeping the odds in your favor.

> "My advice learned from all the digests on the website support group is: Follow the protocol exactly and avoid all salicylates. Don't live in denial and insist on certain gardening habits or hygiene and makeup products. They simply aren't worth giving up recovery."
>
> —*Iris, California*

find

It also bears mentioning that dietary supplements and cosmetics are not required to meet any Food and Drug Administration (FDA) standards; none has been set. In the United States, the quality of supplements is up to the manufacturer, and some aren't particularly meticulous or honorable in their advertising. Batches of herbs are often imported from Third World countries, where they may have been grown and harvested in questionable surroundings or treated with unknown chemicals. Scientific studies done on these herbal supplements consistently show great variability in the potency and content from manufacturer to manufacturer and from batch to batch. Some producers have been indicted for illegally lacing their products with prescription-restricted medications just to make them provide some of the claimed benefits. Without a doubt, cosmetic and herbal packaging claims are always suspect—often they're advertising hype that shades the truth to sell the contents.

Medicinal Products Containing Natural Salicylates

CortiSlim Control Weight Loss Formula (ginseng root extract)
Gas-X (mint oil)
GNC Herbal Plus (saw palmetto)
GNC Vitamin C 2000 (rose hips)
GNC Fast Flex Multi-Action Joint Formula (rosemary, white willow bark extracts)
Health Plus Super Colon Cleanse (fennel, peppermint, papaya, rose hips, and more)
Hydroxycut Fat Loss Support Formula (willow bark, *Garcinia cambogia* extracts)
One-A-Day WeightSmart Vitamins (green tea extract)

Topical Products Containing Natural Salicylates

Absorbine Jr. (calendula, echinacea, wormwood extracts)
Carmex Lip Balm (camphor, menthol)
Colgate 2 in 1 Toothpaste and Mouthwash Icy Blast (mint oil)
Coppertone Sunblock Lotion SPF 30 (aloe, jojoba)
Got2B Foot Polish (mint oil, ruby grapefruit oil)
Herbal Essences Shampoo for Normal Hair (aloe, chamomile extract)
Huggies Supreme Care Baby Wipes (with aloe)
Kleenex Menthol Tissues (menthol)
Paul Mitchell Tea Tree Styling Gel (tea tree oil)
Preparation H Ointment (eucalyptus oil)
Stri-Dex Cooling Foaming Wash (chamomile extract)
Vicks VapoRub Cream (eucalyptus oil)
Zostrix Cream (capsicum, or pepper extract)

Dental Products

What sits in your mouth is really topically applied. Nicorette gum, sublingual nitroglycerin, and orally disintegrating migraine tablets are examples of medications that use this route to get into the bloodstream quickly and effectively. So it is that guaifenesin can be blocked by concentrated salicylates from oral hygiene products. Most oral cleansing agents such as mouthwashes and toothpastes celebrate mint (Fresh mint! Mint blast! Cool mint!) or menthol—the more powerful, the better. But mint oils can also be hidden within the word *flavor.* (When a dental product contains fluoride, it's considered a drug and manufacturers are not required to list the added salicylic acid or methyl salicylate on labels.) All mint is methyl salicylate whether synthetic or extracted from the natural plant and needs to be strictly avoided with guaifenesin. Unless you have keen taste buds, you'll surely get blocked unless you use only what is listed here and on our Web site.

The only toothpastes we know are absolutely safe are Grace Fibro-Smile, Personal Basics by Andrea Rose, and the Tom's of Maine's nonmint flavors (strawberry, orange, grape, apricot, unflavored, or plain fennel). If you can't find any of these in your local store, you should order them from listings in our Resources section.

If you can verify that another brand doesn't contain salicylates, you can use it, but be aware that contents (especially when part of flavors) can be changed without warning. That's the reason we don't suggest using any other brands. Alternatively, you can simply dip your toothbrush in a whitening agent or baking soda, or sprinkle it with hydrogen peroxide to remove tartar. You might want to check with your own dentist for individual suggestions.

Don't forget to check dental floss, breath sprays or strips, cough drops, LifeSavers, gum, and hard candies. You'll need to avoid mint and menthol in any product that sits in your mouth. Other plant oils like clove and eucalyptus when used in the mouth as topical medications need to be avoided, too. Fruit and cinnamon flavors are fine as long as they don't contain mint as well. Dr. Flora Stay, DDS, the dentist and founder of Fibro-Smile, has a number of products and suggestions on her Web site, www.drstay.com. There you will find such products as salicylate-free tooth whiteners, fluoride gel, mouthwashes, and a question-and-answer board for personal assistance.

Dietary Salicylates

It's not necessary to avoid the salicylates contained in foods when taking guaifenesin. Even those foods with higher content, such as berries, fruits, vegetables, cooking herbs, and spices, won't block when they're eaten in normal quantities. The natural salicylates in foods are not concentrated: It is impossible to eat the quantity of garlic reflected in one Garlique tablet taken for cholesterol. In addition to being partially destroyed by the digestive process, they are further neutralized by the liver, which tags on a molecule called glycine.

Salicylate levels can be measured in the blood and in the urine. The average daily intake from foods is in the range of 10 to 20 mg. It was once speculated that the increased ingested salicylates now that fresh fruits and vegetables are more plentiful in our diets might explain the lower incidence of heart attacks witnessed in recent years. That's been refuted by a study that tested urinary salicylate levels using various diets. It supported conventional wisdom that foods add insignificant amounts of salicylate to the urine and, so presumably, to the bloodstream. We've seen no guaifenesin blocking from foods, so we impose no dietary restrictions on patients who have only fibromyalgia.

The salicylate content of many foods has been tested to help those who react adversely to some of their components. Researchers found that not all parts of all plants contain salicylates. Oats are one such plant that people taking guaifenesin may use—for example, in many of the Aveeno products. Although grain kernels (wheat, oats, barley, and rye) contain no salicylates, that's not true for the rest of the plant. Thus, wheat germ and anything that comes from the kernel are okay, but wheatgrass and other parts of the wheat plant aren't. Rice and corn are the two other plants that are not blockers. Articles showing the salicylate content of various foods can be found on the Internet or in medical journals. Bear in mind that salicylate content varies from plant to plant, and crop to crop. Therefore, don't hold reports you find to 100 percent accuracy.[3]

Single chemicals extracted from plants, other than salicylate itself, are acceptable and will not block guaifenesin. For example, alpha hydroxy, or fruit acid, does not contain whole plant parts. Other ingredients in this category are sodium cocyl isethionate, oleoresin, cocamidopropyl, caprylic triglycerides and glycerides, capric acid, beta-carotene, squalene, shea butter, cocoa butter, coconut fatty acids, starch, and sucrose polycottonseedate. In the same way, bromelain, an enzyme isolated from papaya and used to aid digestion, will not block guaifenesin. If it sounds more like a chemical than a plant, or is a single enzyme or chemical isolated from a plant source, it's acceptable for use with guaifenesin. Another way to put it is that what you are avoiding are oils, gels, and extracts—the whole-plant concentrates. Just having a plant name doesn't mean something blocks.

Salicylates and Cosmetics (A Postscript for Brokenhearted Women)

> "These were tough changes for me, but after I realized that *no one* was going to swoop down on a white horse and make me all better . . . after I accepted that I had to do it myself . . . I got better, though I still struggle with apathy."
>
> —*Janet, Canada*

Many women taking guaifenesin lament the loss of some of the products they've come to love. Another common complaint is that they must do without "natural" products. It seems impossible for them to give up items like jojoba oil face masks, almond oil skin creams, or cleansers with aloe, witch hazel, or arnica. In the face of this, it seems futile to point out that minerals are also natural, part of Mother Earth as well. Reminders that plant ingredients and the chemical preservatives required to keep them from spoiling can sometimes be harmful fall on deaf ears when advertisements and cosmetics salespeople have given contrary information for years. Despite this brainwashing by the cosmetics industry, many women have recently started to fear harsh chemicals with unknown action on the body. Breast cancer survivors and those with a family history often decide to use mineral salt deodorants that don't contain aluminum. Mineral lines such as Bare Escentuals are becoming increasingly popular. For guaifenesin users, Ruthie Molloy of Illuminaré Cosmetics offers a liquid mineral makeup line, and Dr. Stay of Grace Fibro-Smile has launched a mineral powder line. Animal oils such as emu and lanolin, as you have read earlier, have been shown to have beneficial effects on our own animal skins. Fish oil also has proven value. With so much help, we may win this battle yet!

It's important to remember that the FDA doesn't regulate cosmetic claims, including the use of words such as *pure* and *natural. Natural* on a label could designate something partly human-made combined with a natural ingredient. It could just as surely indicate an ingredient synthetically extracted from plants using some very potent chemicals through a wholly unnatural process. All-natural toothpastes containing sodium laurel sulfate—a chemical implicated in canker sores—are clear examples of this. Where is the plant named sulfate? It's also important to remember that when plant extracts are used, preservatives must also be added to maintain freshness. These chemicals are often potent allergens and topical irritants. Skin creams containing cucumber extract have a shelf life of several years. How long can a cucumber last in its natural state, even in the refrigerator?

There aren't very many actual moisturizers and humectants, ingredients that seal moisture into the skin. The workhorse ingredients in most products boil down to a very few chemicals whose names you'll see repeated over and over again on labels. Basic soothing ingredients are such things as mineral oil, glycerine, cyclomethicone, dimethicone, petrolatum, and polyethylene glycol. All are laboratory-made and are mainstays in almost every skin cream no matter what else has been added. The most effective moisture-holding agents are glycerine, ceramide, lecithin, hyaluronic acid, sodium hyaluronate, sodium PCA, collagen, elastin, amino acids, cholesterol, glucose, sucrose, fructose, glycogen, and phospholipids—and none is the name of a plant. There are only three ingredients that protect the skin from photoaging and skin cancer: avobenzone, titanium dioxide, and zinc oxide. Cosmetics companies shovel plant material into ordinary moisturizers and makeup to make them seem more exotic and to command higher prices. While some plant ingredients do the job asked of them, none is essential to maintain or protect skin. In fact, it's not uncommon for us to hear from our patients that the quality of their skin improved when they stopped using so many compounds. As many survivors of skin allergies will attest, using products with fewer listed ingredients seems to be easier on the body.

We can all agree that everything that exudes from plants is not beneficial or particularly desirable. Natural poisons will kill just as effectively as synthetic ones. Tobacco comes from a plant; poison ivy, poison oak, hemlock, oleander, and toadstools are all well-known, potentially lethal toxins. Our bodies are not flower beds, and nature didn't intend for us to indiscriminately lather on or ingest everything in sight.

Paula Begoun first published *Don't Go to the Cosmetics Counter Without Me* in 1991. She regularly updates it, and also publishes a newsletter and maintains an informative Web site. Her book reviews literally thousands of products from companies such as Almay, Avon, the Body Shop, Charles of the Ritz, Dior, Coty, Revlon, Estée Lauder, Maybelline, and Vaseline Intensive Care. She reminds us that results are what matter; gouging prices and exotic ingredients don't guarantee a better outcome. Although her book doesn't list ingredients of each reviewed product, it provides an overview and evaluates many cosmetics ingredients, both natural and synthetic, for their effectiveness. She gives her readers an inside look at the way cosmetics are created, manufactured, and marketed that is especially interesting and helpful to patients using guaifenesin. The appendix in her book lists toll-free numbers and Web sites useful for contacting many cosmetics companies.

The first person to step forward and help patients with the task of finding suitable products when they're too sick to read labels was Andrea Rose, one of our patients. Personal Basics by Andrea Rose—as her line is called—offers products that are reliably safe for use by people on our protocol. With her permission, we can report that Andrea suffered severely from fibromyalgia for many years and has been on guaifenesin since July 1996. Like many women, Andrea says that her most challenging task when she started out was to find salicylate-free skin care products and cosmetics. Out of this frustration, her company was born. Her product line can be viewed on her Web site: www.andrearose.com.

The guaifenesin protocol has benefited hugely from another ally: Flora Stay, DDS. Her Grace Fibro-Smile selections range from a full line of dental products to skin care, hair products, soaps, and cosmetics—all of which will always be salicylate-free. Fibro-Smile toothpaste and other offerings benefit from her experience and knowledge as a practicing dentist, as well as her lifelong study of safe, effective ingredients. Her Web site, www.drstay.com, contains information about dental problems and fibromyalgia, and she is the author of *The Fibromyalgia Dental Handbook,* published in 2005.

Paula Begoun, the author of the beauty industry critiques such as the aforementioned *Don't Go to the Cosmetics Counter Without Me*, maintains a salicylate-free selection of products on her Web site: www.paulaschoice.com. Her products are distributed worldwide and can be helpful to patients in Great Britain, Australia, and New Zealand, for example. Inspired by her sister's battle with fibromyalgia, Ruthie Molloy of Illuminaré Cosmetics has a liquid mineral makeup line that can be purchased through spas and the Home Shopping Network. Several other smaller manufacturers of products can be found in the appendix of this book and on our Web site at www.fibromyalgiatreatment.com. Suffice it to say that it is now possible through the above resources to purchase all the products you need without reading a label. As time goes by, we expect more manufacturers to come forward. All it takes is a commitment to check each product and not change formulas. Mary Kay, for example, provides us with yearly updates and maintains a salicylate-free list for its representatives and customers. For accurate information and changes, always check www.fibromyalgiatreatment.com.

One other resource before we leave the subject: The Marina del Rey Pharmacy (www.fibroconnection.com) carries all the above lines and many other products that have been carefully screened for salicylates. If ordering from more than one company, you can save shipping costs as well as being provided with helpful, understanding service. We know of many who have called in, too sick to think, and just asked Kay to send them one of everything essential: deodorant, toothpaste, mouthwash, and soap. Later, when they recovered enough strength to go out, they added lipstick, eye pencil, and sunscreens in travel sizes of their favorite new products!

How do we sum up such an involved chapter? It seems to us that we've repeated only one theme. *Get as far away as possible from anything that might even remotely contain salicylates.* We hope all guaifenesin users will take this to heart, and repeat that sentence like a mantra. Yes, we're terribly sorry that you'll have to pick up dermatology skills at a time when you feel so utterly lousy, but there is no shortcut to expertise, only determined study. Over the years, our patients were the inadvertent human "guinea pigs" whose successes and failures finally produced this chapter. You owe it to yourself and to them to take their hard-earned knowledge to heart.

> "I'm finally having some good days again. I discovered that a vitamin with bioflavonoids and vitamin C with rose hips, was blocking the guaifenesin. Last week, I drove four and a half hours to help my daughter, who was ill. It took a lot of energy to care for her baby and her busy two-year-old, cook, grocery shop, and do laundry. I was amazed at how much energy I had and how little I ached. I could not have done that three months ago."
>
> —*Mary Ellen Stolle,*
> *network leader for the Vulvar Pain Foundation*

Critics say our protocol is difficult when they are being kind, impossible when more strident. We have written this chapter to prove that it is neither, especially when compared with living with fibromyalgia. The time it has taken and still takes us to teach patients how to avoid salicylates has caused us more anguish than any other facet of the treatment. Sorry, but that's the way it is. Luckily, you are not alone. The pages of this book will guide you. The online resources on www.fibromyal giatreatment.com are kept updated, and the support group there will walk you through the process of eliminating salicylates from your products. In-person support groups for the guaifenesin protocol exist nationwide. There are hands outstretched to help you, hands that understand there is nothing harder than being sick every day of your life. Compared with that fate, reading labels when you buy cosmetics or supplements is barely even an inconvenience. We know that when you've had your first good day, you'll agree with us.

FREQUENTLY ASKED QUESTIONS ABOUT SALICYLATES

Which dishwashing liquids are salicylate-free?

Dish soaps are usually okay to use. A few brands may say "New with Aloe" on their labels and should obviously not be used. Those found at health food stores most often contain herbs or seed oils.

I have eliminated all salicylates from my topically applied products and still don't notice any effect from the guaifenesin. What should I do now?

Recheck everything, even your chewing gum and breath mints, for natural mint flavorings such as peppermint, spearmint, or wintergreen. Search your vitamins and supplements for bioflavonoids, rose hips, or other botanical additions. If you find nothing, raise your dose of guaifenesin by one or two tablets. Within the next ten days, you should feel distinctly worse. If you do not, you should be even more suspicious that you are blocking. Check again and ask for help from the online support group at www.fibromyalgiatreatment.com. If you find nothing, you need to go to an even higher dose.

Should I avoid laundry detergents with phosphates?

You do not need to avoid phosphates in anything. Extra phosphates are not a problem. It is impossible to eliminate them from your life, and your body needs a huge amount to form energy. Laundry detergents don't come in contact with the skin because they are rinsed out of your clothes before they are worn. So the answer is no, and no.

I'm a gardener. Is there anything I should be careful about?

You should be very careful doing certain gardening chores. Plant saps are readily absorbed through the skin. For this reason, you should wear gloves if a particular job will expose you to plant juices. The thin gloves worn by surgeons are ideal for delicate tasks, while thicker, plastic (not leather) gloves should be worn when doing heavy work. Plants such as mint, marigold, geranium, and rosemary have higher salicylate contents than others. However, all plants pose the same kind of danger, even if to a lesser degree.

What about smoking?

With everything we know today, it's obvious that you shouldn't smoke, even if you don't have fibromyalgia. For people with fibromyalgia, this is a heightened concern: More than one study has shown that smokers have more pain and circulatory problems than those who do not.

However, the topic of this chapter is salicylates. We're also concerned about the amount of salicylate inhaled through the bronchial lining by smokers, including marijuana users. We don't really know the full impact of smoke, but we've got observant patients who only began satisfactory reversal when they quit smoking though they remained on the same dosage of guaifenesin. We do know from experiments with tobacco plants that the leaves contain methyl salicylates. They're certainly treated, hanged, and dried, but those maneuvers alone would not destroy a chemical. Does the heat or would a filter change that, and if so, by how much? Obviously, menthol filters create a distinct problem.

The possibility is strong that smoking could make guaifenesin partially or totally ineffective. It might merely depend on the crop's potency, but we ask patients to become as pure as possible and avoid any substance they can't *safely* validate—which would include smoking. It's clear that smokeless tobacco avoids destruction by burning and is a blocker.

Chapter 5

Hypoglycemia, Fibroglycemia, and Carbohydrate Intolerance

"The doctor determined that I was hypoglycemic . . . and he also explained that hypoglycemia and fibromyalgia often go hand in hand. There was a name for what I had, an actual medical term! And there were also Web sites with information I could read. I was less than thrilled when he told me about the diet I would be on. . . . Sugar was a no-no, as was caffeine. . . . I gulped as he rattled off the list of the carbohydrates I should avoid, including the 'Big Five' that figured heavily in my diet: pasta (my Italian heart literally broke in two) rice, potatoes, bananas, and corn. . . . The doctor handed me a list of the permissible and said 'Good luck.'

"This diagnosis meant that a morning might come when I could open my eyes and actually feel good to be alive, without fear of pain. Now four months later, I am pleased to say that I've experienced many such mornings. . . . I have more energy, I sleep better, and I'm in a better mood. Friends, family members and coworkers all say they've seen a change in me. . . . Six months ago I would not have thought such a change was possible. But thanks to my own stubbornness . . . and the dedication of my current doctor, I have finally found relief. I guess what my doctor and I have in common is that we refused to give up the search for answers and we chose to ignore people who said there were none. For us both, perseverance has definitely paid off."

—Michelle Fisher, from a published article in
Palos Verdes Peninsula News

HYPOGLYCEMIA AND CARBOHYDRATE INTOLERANCE

In 1964, I was treating a podiatrist who suffered from fibromyalgia. Luckily for me, she had many scientific interests and studied a great deal. At one of her checkups, she brought me a pamphlet describing a host of symptoms that it attributed to low blood sugar. As an endocrinologist, I was certainly familiar with severe hypoglycemia, the kind that made patients faint because of a sudden excess of the hormone insulin, which they were using to control their diabetes. There are a few other quite rare conditions that cause the same catastrophe.

> *Hypoglycemia*—From the Greek meaning "low [*hypo*], sugar [*glyc*] in the blood [*emia*]." The accepted medical criterion for this condition is a blood sugar reading falling below 50 milligrams per deciliter (mg/dl).

As I read through the gauntlet of listed symptoms, I realized that if the information were even 50 percent accurate, I had been missing the chance to help a lot of sick people. The brochure listed fatigue, irritability, nervousness, depression, insomnia, headaches, impaired memory and concentration, anxieties, dizziness, blurred vision, leg cramps, sugar craving, flushing, nausea, gas, bloating, and constipation alternating with diarrhea as the most common symptoms. We soon realized those were the chronic symptoms, which we now segregate from the more dramatic ones we recognize as the acute symptoms of hypoglycemia. The latter pounce quite suddenly: shaking tremors, clamminess or sweating, palpitations, faintness or syncope, confusion, and panic attacks. Of course, these are the easiest ones to spot.

Using gout medications the preceding five years, I had been

fairly successful in resolving fibromyalgia in the majority of patients. But there was a subset of people who weren't doing as well. Though they complained less about former pains and even though I noted improvement by palpating regression of lumps and bumps, they were not getting any perfectly normal days. Something was different about this group and their nonresolving miseries. With a few pertinent facts provided by the brochure, however, the picture was now complete. Enter hypoglycemia.

Suddenly the questions posed by the partially responsive patients were resolved. It became clear that not one but two totally remediable diseases accounted for their multiple complaints. As I gained experience, it became progressively easier for me to separate the two and attack them simultaneously as well as to realize the volume of patients who were affected. Luckily, the treatment for hypoglycemia was already well known and highly effective. No medication is necessary or even

Table 5.1
Hypoglycemia Syndrome*

	Female	Male
1. Total Number of Patients	3,918	305
Percent with no sugar craving or hypoglycemia	71%	40%
2. Number of Lean Patients	2,628	249
a. Percent craving sugar without hypoglycemia	37	45
b. Percent craving sugar with hypoglycemia	39	60
3. Number of Obese Patients	1,290	56
a. Percent craving sugar without hypoglycemia	52	52
b. Percent craving sugar with hypoglycemia	83	75

*NOTE: This chart was compiled from our evaluation of over 2,000 consecutive new patients, both male and female. While it's not a scientific sampling of data, it does show how patterns develop in persons with fibromyalgia and you may find this chart—and the ones like it throughout the book—helpful.

useful. Resolution simply requires eating the proper diet. Patients were deeply relieved to learn that neither illness leaves residual damage. Our mutual frustration vanished as we medically purged fibromyalgia and the diet corrected hypoglycemia.

> "I had just begun to hope that I would finally be able to live without the pain from fibromyalgia. The guaifenesin treatment from Dr. St. Amand gave back my energy and mobility. It was all the more difficult, then, to be disabled by headaches. I was aware that my health was not good, so I ate a vegetarian diet and followed the food pyramid recommendations closely; I ate a diet rich in carbohydrates and low in fat, and the worse I felt, the more carefully I followed these recommendations. Despite this, I was always hungry and faint, and my headaches were steadily worsening.
>
> "Claudia showed me the diet recommended for hypoglycemia and offered me the hope that by following this regimen I could control my headaches. I would have tried anything; I had nothing to lose. In fact, I had a lot to lose: pain, fatigue, and even excess weight. From one day to the next my headaches all but vanished; during the first few weeks my migraines diminished to one or two a week and I had no other headaches, either mild or severe. The improvement was so immediate and so unmistakable that I had no difficulty whatsoever following the diet, even though it was just before Christmas and I was surrounded by sweets."
>
> —*Cynthia C., Michigan*

My education and enlightenment progressed, and I became more familiar with patients who had hypoglycemia as a standalone illness as well as those who suffered from simultaneous fibromyalgia. At the time, I was a spokesman for the Los Angeles County Medical Association. NBC News wanted to present a segment on hypoglycemia, which was at that time becoming the new fad of medicine. Because I was an endocrinologist, I was interviewed and asked to discuss the condition on camera. I was featured along with physicians who were full-time, professorial staff members from two UCLA campuses.

The story was shown on three consecutive evenings as five-minute, serialized segments during the prime-time newscast. Then, due to overwhelming viewer response, the program was shown a few more times in the following months. The Los Angeles County Medical Association, UCLA, and Harbor General Hospital were bombarded with phone calls. Since I was the only interviewed physician in private practice, inquiries were funneled to my office. I was inundated with calls from people with hypoglycemia, as well as the as-yet-unnamed fibromyalgia. Combinations of those two were no longer puzzling to me, but the spectrum of symptoms made patients with other conditions quizzical, and they, too, sought help. Many of those were justified in their suspicions and had been either mislabeled as neurotic or had a properly diagnosed illness with the added onus of fibromyalgia and/or hypoglycemia. My patient base grew rapidly to include people not only from our county, but also from other parts of California and the entire country. The sheer number of these has provided us with a huge database. That's the information we're now sharing with you.

To give you insight into hypoglycemia, you should understand the biochemical sequence that follows eating carbohydrates (sugars and starches). Ancient humans did not find food in overabundance. Lean days far outnumbered their days of plenty. In fact, they might go a day or two without any food at all. When they found sustenance, they devoured it on the spot. Rarely were all of the calories in this delightful repast needed for immediate use. Storage capabilities were necessary to provide energy on the less bountiful days that were sure to follow. In more modern times, however, our storage facilities are kept near overflow because calories are so readily available.

Carbohydrates—Chemicals made up of carbon, hydrogen, and oxygen that provide the body with one of its two main sources of energy (the other is fats). Sugars and starches are carbohydrates. Although we usually read about two types of carbohydrates, simple and complex, there are actually three classifications: monosaccharides (glucose, galactose, fructose), disaccharides (sucrose, lactose, maltose), and polysaccharides (starch, cellulose). Ingested carbohydrates raise the blood sugar, and the pancreas responds with the release of insulin.

Simple carbohydrates—Sugars including table sugar (sucrose), fruit sugar (fructose), honey (maltose), and milk sugar (lactose).

Complex carbohydrates—Starches such as bread, pasta, rice, potatoes, cereals, peas, and beans.

Every meal provides excess that isn't needed for immediate combustion.

Enter insulin—the only hormone that directs excess food (energy-fuel) into storage and attends to the work of conservation even before a meal is completed. It's like an insurance policy that guarantees against starvation, and it's the powerful hormone that kept our ancestors alive in times of famine. It directs cells to store not only glucose, but also fat and amino acids, the building blocks of protein. Insulin sends these stores to the body's energy warehouses, primarily fat cells, but also muscle cells. The liver converts nearly all carbohydrates to the simple sugar glucose. It also jumps to obey insulin's prodding and keeps a bit for itself in a storage form called glycogen. A goodly amount is also dispersed especially to the brain and muscles.

Insulin—A hormone produced by the islets of the pancreas that is released in whatever amounts are needed to clear excess glucose from the bloodstream. It promotes the absorption of glucose into the liver and muscles, where it is stored as glycogen. It also facilitates storage of amino acids and fats, and is known, therefore, as the storage hormone. Without insulin, a person cannot gain weight.

When all of the above gluttons are satiated, the remaining glucose is converted into fatty acids. Those get combined with something called glycerol in a structure we recognize as body fat, or triglyceride. The liver packages these minuscule fat droplets for transport to all tissues, mainly to the storage depots in fat cells. These little packets are what coalesce into the loathsome fat accumulations that are situated where we can pinch far more than we like on ourselves. Fat is nothing more than surplus energy maintained in the form of triglycerides. Our mouths and insulin—the caveman's lifesaving alliance—have become, in today's world of superabundance, enemies that make us fat and ensure we stay that way.

Triglyceride—One of three "blood fats" that are known as lipids. Triglyceride is the principal constituent of body fat. It is manufactured in the liver largely from the sugar and starches that you eat.

Some individuals are unable to process carbohydrates without adverse consequences. We often use the name *hypoglycemia,* low blood sugar, to denote a whole disease. More accurately, this is a metabolic error that is really a syndrome, a cluster of symptoms that keep popping up at the same time. The condition could profit by more descriptive nomenclature, but we're accustomed to using that word and it's easily recognizable—most people have at least heard of it. Patients with this illness suffer a distressing insulin-related conflagration that's regularly ignited by eating certain carbohydrates. (See figure 5.1.)

There are two ways to produce low blood sugar. The most obvious way is by an excess of insulin, but it can also be caused by delayed or inadequate hormonal responses that are supposed to put a brake on a rapidly falling sugar. The latter are known as counter-regulatory hormones because they normally stop the overexuberant attacks of insulin. All kinds of freakish possibilities exist, because a little too much of this or too little of that creates a whole spectrum of stresses. Combinations of various defects viciously strain a variety of cells.

There are four important counter-regulatory hormones, but adrenaline (epinephrine) is the ultimate weapon, and the final safety net. If either insulin or adrenaline is released in delayed, inadequate, or excessive amounts, the other one must decrease or increase its output to avoid hypoglycemia. They dance together, but at opposite ends of the ballroom. It is this bad choreography that causes the distinctive symptoms in susceptible people.

So, you've got the picture. Insulin drives blood sugar down, and adrenaline pushes it up. It's normally quite harmonious. As sugar drops below certain levels, hormones such as glucagon, growth hormone, and cortisol work in unison with smooth orchestration. Normally, we're not aware of the metabolic sounds made by these instruments. In hypoglycemia, however, alarming drops in blood sugar alter the key and discordant notes are sounded. In the overture, sugars and heavy starches are consumed, and this strikes familiar notes in the pancreas. It plays stridently and fast with inappropriate releases

HYPOGLYCEMIA

Chronic Symptoms

- Fatigue, insomnia
- Nervousness, depression, irritability
- Dizziness, faintness
- Blurring of vision
- Ringing ears
- Gas, abdominal cramps, diarrhea
- Numbness/tingling of hands, feet, face
- Flushing/sweating
- Foot/leg cramps
- Bitemporal or frontal headaches
- Impaired memory and concentration

Acute Symptoms

- Heart pounding
- Palpitations or heart irregularities
- Panic attacks
- Nightmares and severe sleep disturbances
- Faintness or syncope
- Acute anxiety
- Hand or inner shaking/tremor
- Sweating
- Frontal headache or pressure

Figure 5.1

of insulin. This threat sets up a chemical counterpoint that like a loud trumpet blast awakens the dozing adrenal glands; they counter with a stupendous release of adrenaline. That's when affected individuals first realize that the customary fine-tuning is errant. One or the other hormone gains the upper hand at different moments, and that makes for unusual syncopation. (See figure 5.2.)

Hypoglycemia's acute symptoms, which are triggered by adrenaline, are truly frightening and generally last from twenty to thirty minutes. They most often strike three to four hours after eating a meal that's heavy in carbohydrates. As we've stressed, this powerful hormone is the ultimate fail-safe weapon that copes with precipitous drops in blood sugar. When it's a bit slow in responding, it makes up for it with a supercharged attack. Unfortunately, this is a good-news-bad-news situation. It prevents fainting and may even save your life. The bad news is that it's responsible for a flock of symptoms that are quite familiar to everyone who has ever been startled or scared. The first sensation is of heart irregularities or pounding, and a feeling of severe anxiety. Shaking hand tremors, drenching sweats, faintness, and frontal pressure headaches complete the picture. Very intense reactions are labeled panic attacks. Nocturnal symptoms are often preceded by the frequent nightmares of hypoglycemia. In turn, sleep disturbances provoke daytime drowsiness and add greatly to the general fatigue.

So now you can understand my level of confusion when I realized I was facing two conditions, often interlocked, for which nothing in my medical training had prepared me. I was forced to treat one ill-defined, misunderstood illness along with another that, in the eyes of my medical profession, might not even exist. This troubled me somewhat, since I didn't much enjoy veering away from the well-accepted and well-researched paths of medicine. In this situation, there was no

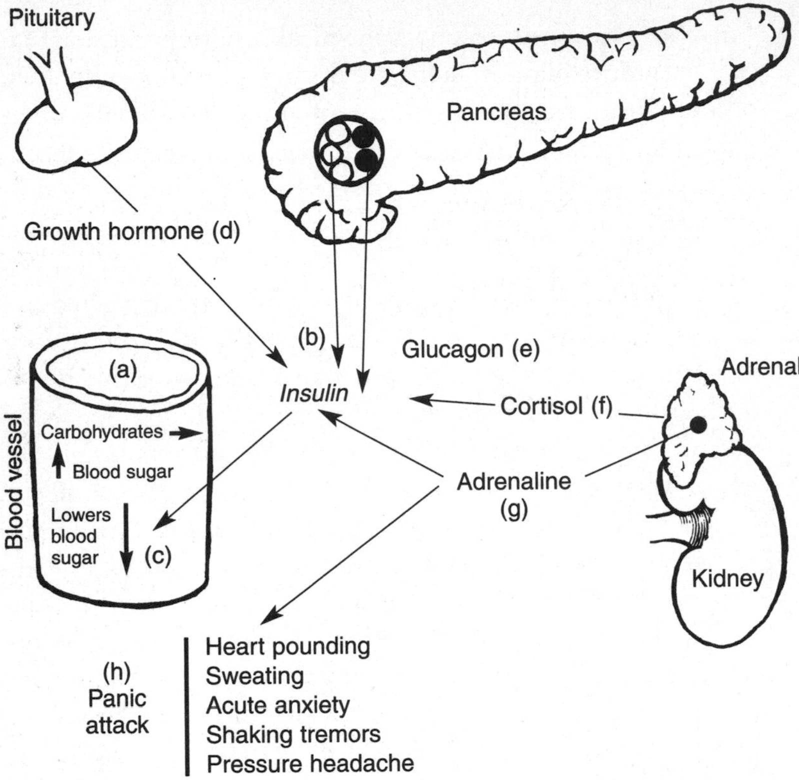

Normal

(a) Eating carbohyrates raises blood sugar.
(b) Bloodstream delivers sugar to the pancreas and releases insulin.
(c) Insulin enters bloodstream and lowers the blood sugar.

Abnormal

Insulin lowers blood sugar too much; the brain reads "hypoglycemia" and stimulates release of:
(d) growth hormone
(e) glucagon
(f) cortisol
(g) Adrenaline, because the hormones can't offset insulin fast enough. Adrenaline can stop the fall of blood sugar in one to two minutes.
(h) Adrenaline penalizes the body and causes acute symptoms.

Figure 5.2

road map to follow; I therefore had no choice but to take, as Robert Frost called it, the road least traveled.

> *Adrenaline* (epinephrine)—A hormone released by the adrenal glands when the body senses imminent danger. It is sometimes called the fight-or-flight hormone. It is designed to increase energy levels in emergencies. When the blood sugar falls in hypoglycemia, the body senses an emergency and releases adrenaline. This release normalizes the blood sugar within one to two minutes.

> *Endocrine system*—This system is made up of glands that produce hormones (chemicals necessary to regulate the body's functions). They regulate or stimulate metabolism, growth, and sexual development and function, as well as maintaining the body in a state of balance (known as homeostasis).

Since patients kept referring others, I was collecting oddball conditions I had not been taught to handle. I had to look somewhere other than the bible of accepted medicine for effective treatments. It's spine-tingling in any field of work to walk over the threshold of uncertainty and come face-to-face with something exciting and entirely new. It was a little intimidating to find that a nameless disease was actually common, and equally astounding to realize that an existing medication could resolve the condition. I had been taught that results are what count. I remember one of my teachers during grand rounds who said emphatically: "Don't just stand there—do something!" I think this was his interpretation of the Hippocratic oath, which could be paraphrased as: "Get the patient well as best you can, but above all, do no harm." What to do seemed simple, safe, and straightforward. I would offer a diet to erase hypoglycemia, prescribe a medication to control rheumatism—or, as it's now known, fibromyalgia—and enjoy my success. It was never to be: Disagreements and arguments in this field persist even though the opposing voices are not quite as loud.

THE DIAGNOSIS OF HYPOGLYCEMIA

> "The glucose tolerance test [is] . . . the worst torture in a lab that can be done to anyone, especially a hypoglycemic. You arrive following a twelve-hour fast and then, while you are half-asleep, a needle is stuck into your arm and blood is drawn. Then you are given a drink called a GLU-Cola, which is basically a cola with half a bottle of Karo syrup poured into it. You have to drink this down fairly quickly without gagging, and then in an hour another needle is stuck in your arm, and blood is drawn again. They do this ten times during the next five hours. In between needle sticks you sit in a chair in a freezing sterile lab . . . and you can't walk around because it will cause you to release adrenaline and lower your blood sugar. And you can't eat anything, and you haven't eaten in seventeen hours by the end of the test. Somewhere around the fourth hour you feel like you are going to die, dizzy, sweating, sick, and then you feel like you are going to pass out. Just when you fall asleep, they wake you up to stick you again. When you finally get home you are horribly sick, and you stay dull-witted and dazed for several days."
>
> —*C.C., California*

The five-hour glucose tolerance test is the standard tool for confirming the diagnosis of hypoglycemia. Patients are given a measured amount of sugar to drink, and blood sugars are drawn periodically to test their response to this glucose load. The party line has always been that if during the course of the test, a blood sugar reading falls below the magic number of 50 milligrams per deciliter (mg/dl), the diagnosis is confirmed. In my earlier days, we subjected every patient with suggestive symptoms to the rigors of this test. To our surprise, many results revealed nothing but normal levels throughout the test. Despite this, the poor patients complained bitterly about a flock of hypoglycemic symptoms they had suffered during and after the experience. Knowing that a spurt of adrenaline can raise blood sugar in one or two minutes, we retaliated by drawing blood more often—every half hour—hoping that added specimens would catch at least one low reading. This worked a little better, but was still far from satisfactory. We quickly learned that adverse symptoms were frequently not synchronous with the rigidly timed blood sampling. In other words, not everyone's blood sugar dropped at exactly the same time after drinking the sugar solution. It was obvious that technicians couldn't insert needles to draw blood fast enough to overcome the rapid effects of adrenaline. No matter how hard lab personnel tried, we all too often missed the glucose nadirs. The hormone was persistently faster than we were.

Finally, because glucose testing failed to confirm our diagnosis about 50 percent of the time, we decided to try a different approach. You can never say we didn't go down trying! We had patients drink the same measured amount of glucose, but omitted blood sampling. Now subjects simply recorded their symptoms during the subsequent five hours. Most of them experienced all of the classic, acute symptoms of hypoglycemia several hours into the test. Others fell asleep, overcome by severe fatigue. Looking at countless diaries, it dawned on me that patients were simply writing down the very same symptoms they had related to me in the office—symptoms that had alerted me to order the test. So why did we need to subject them to the ordeal and the expense? Why make them drink the horrible stuff? Why not just listen attentively to patient complaints, skip unnecessary testing, and simply accept as diagnostic the symptoms they had so eloquently described on their initial visit?

I decided to use the test only if patients were suffering fainting spells or had an abnormally low fasting blood sugar. Either of those two factors should prompt physicians to consider the possibility of an insulin-producing pancreatic tumor. Our new system paid off. It saved patients five hours of testing, multiple needle sticks, a miserable morning, and the sick days that were sure to follow the sugar cocktail. After all, do you really need a blood sugar reading of below 50 mg/dl to tell you what you already know—eating a lot of sugar or starch makes you feel lousy?

In 1994, Drs. Genter and Ipp published some interesting findings that gave us yet another reason to abandon testing.[1] They conducted a simple and elegant experiment that explained why some patients with symptoms don't register the previously considered mandatory drop of blood sugar below 50 mg/dl. These two doctors ordered five-hour glucose tolerance tests on twenty young, healthy subjects who had no symptoms whatsoever of hypoglycemia. A catheter was placed in a vein so that blood could be sampled every ten minutes without repeated needle sticks. Samples were measured for the amounts of various counter-regulatory hormones and the timing of their release following the ingestion of the sugar load.

Surprisingly, during the test about half of the subjects developed varying degrees of the acute symptoms, such as tremors, sweating, heart pounding, anxiety, or pressure headaches. Some had only a few of these effects, but others had all of them. As expected, the battery of tests identified adrenaline release as the cause of these sensations. Very strangely, however, responses were induced with sugar levels quite in the normal range. The lowest was at 58 mg/dl of blood, but most had levels in the 60s, 70s, and one even at 81! This flew in the face of the accepted definition of hypoglycemia, that is, a blood sugar level below 50. This study and a later corroborating paper from France strongly suggest, at least to me, that we each have a set point for blood sugar. If it drops below our own predetermined, daily-changing level, the brain says, *You're in trouble,* and promptly triggers hormonal and nerve impulses to prevent us from passing out.

The problem remains that many physicians are unaware of these studies and persist in ordering fasting blood sugars and tolerance tests when a patient complains of symptoms of hypoglycemia. Normal tests fool physicians into thinking their patients don't have carbohydrate problems. Using purely symptoms for diagnosis, it doesn't much matter what sugar level triggers them. The term *hypoglycemia* should be retained for patients who actually drop below 50 mg/dl. We should accept something that more accurately describes the group we're discussing. The simple designation *carbohydrate intolerance syndrome* wins our vote. Regardless of sugar levels or what name we use, all patients with this symptom complex respond equally well to the same dietary restrictions.

"We're in the process of selling our house and moving because of Jim's job. I've been so busy the past few weekends getting the house ready, I know I couldn't have done it if I hadn't started the HG diet last fall. Before the diet my fatigue was so bad if I got up in the morning and showered and dried my hair and put makeup on I'd be so tired I would have to lie down. But, thanks to the diet the fatigue isn't anywhere near what it was and I've been going from morning to night and sleeping really well. Sometimes I even shower!!"

—*Jo, Canada*

Once I had a better understanding of carbohydrate intolerance, I was much better able to discern the overlapping symptoms of fibromyalgia. (See figure 5.3.) Unless you or your doctor can recognize the distinctive complaints that help separate the two diseases, the second diagnosis might easily be missed. The two diseases share many symptoms: fatigue, irritability, nervousness, depression, insomnia, flushing, impaired memory and concentration. Anxieties are also common to both conditions, as are frontal or bitemporal headaches, dizziness, faintness, and weakness. Each can produce blurred vision, nasal congestion, ringing in the ears (tinnitus), numbness, and tingling of the hands, feet, or face. In addition, nausea, excessive gas, abdominal cramps, and constipation or diarrhea are frequent. Many complain of leg or foot cramps. When hypoglycemia is the cause of these chronic symptoms, they're experienced even in the presence of a normal blood sugar. This is because of the extensive endocrine and metabolic imbalances brought about by months of insulin-induced stress. (Refer to appendix to review the involvement of various endocrine glands.) Even though guaifenesin will correct fibromyalgia, the similarity of symptoms makes it easy to miss the diagnosis of hypoglycemia. Both patient and physician, confused, will think they are seeing only a partial recovery.

There's a certain stiffness of muscles in hypoglycemia, but not the deeper pains induced by the lumps and bumps of fibromyalgia. Much confusion can be avoided by simply using your hands to map swollen areas. This type of examination makes it possible to separate the two illnesses with considerable accuracy. Lumps, bumps, and spastic tissue easily identify fibromyalgia. Fortunately, we also have the acute symptoms of

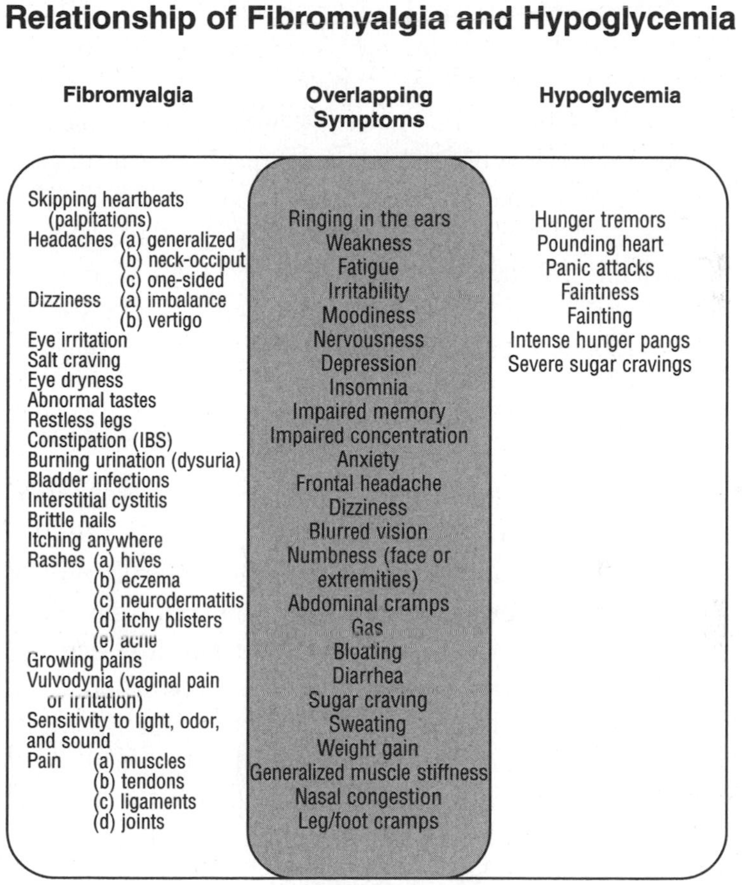
Relationship of Fibromyalgia and Hypoglycemia
Fibromyalgia
Overlapping Symptoms
Hypoglycemia
Skipping heartbeats (palpitations)
Headaches (a) generalized (b) neck-occiput (c) one-sided
Dizziness (a) imbalance (b) vertigo
Eye irritation
Salt craving
Eye dryness
Abnormal tastes
Restless legs
Constipation (IBS)
Burning urination (dysuria)
Bladder infections
Interstitial cystitis
Brittle nails
Itching anywhere
Rashes (a) hives (b) eczema (c) neurodermatitis (d) itchy blisters (e) acne
Growing pains
Vulvodynia (vaginal pain or irritation)
Sensitivity to light, odor, and sound
Pain (a) muscles (b) tendons (c) ligaments (d) joints
Ringing in the ears
Weakness
Fatigue
Irritability
Moodiness
Nervousness
Depression
Insomnia
Impaired memory
Impaired concentration
Anxiety
Frontal headache
Dizziness
Blurred vision
Numbness (face or extremities)
Abdominal cramps
Gas
Bloating
Diarrhea
Sugar craving
Sweating
Weight gain
Generalized muscle stiffness
Nasal congestion
Leg/foot cramps
Hunger tremors
Pounding heart
Panic attacks
Faintness
Fainting
Intense hunger pangs
Severe sugar cravings

Figure 5.3

carbohydrate intolerance to dependably point to blood sugar disturbances. These statements are important. Either disease standing alone requires its own simple approach. A two-pronged attack demands dual and simultaneous treatment.

HYPOGLYCEMIA TREATMENT: PROPER DIET

> "Before I started the diet, I was weak and shaky every few hours. I started eating some nuts for a protein jolt between meals, and eating smaller meals. Having been on the diet for eleven months, I notice I no longer get hungry between meals. My appetite is not as big and I don't get the shakes when I get hungry (unless I don't eventually eat). I don't have headaches all the time now and I don't have the afternoon crash at 2 to 3 PM anymore. It really helps you feel better. I will stick to this diet, because when I've cheated and eaten sugar, I get a headache and feel very sleepy for hours. If you're experiencing a lot of pain, give it a try."
>
> —*Heather, Texas*

Many affected people ask if they should eat more carbohydrates, especially during bouts of hypoglycemia. The answer is an emphatic no! In fact, quite the opposite is true. Actually humans don't need sugars or heavy starches. The body can easily manufacture each and every type it uses in its metabolism. There exist no cases of carbohydrate deficiency for that very reason. However, we should be very clear up front: The required diet for hypoglycemia is not a zero-carbohydrate diet. Both of the diets you will read about in the remainder of this chapter restrict only certain carbohydrates that can be easily replaced by cousin foods—there are many acceptable replacements.

Sugars and starches start raising the blood sugar within five minutes of consumption. Proteins, and to a lesser extent fats, can provide substrates that the liver can convert to glucose, albeit with a fifteen- to twenty-minute delay. Not only that organ but also the kidneys easily convert certain amino acids into glucose. Many people consume carbohydrates in the belief that they'll become superenergized. If some of them aren't adversely affected by eating carbohydrates, we salute their remarkable metabolisms. It's true that healthy people compensate for rises in glucose with perfectly regulated bursts of insulin. In all honesty, however, they, too, probably admit to the late-morning, late-afternoon yawns and fatigue following carbohydrate indulgences. What rises must fall, and insulin action substantiates that axiom. Hypoglycemics have an unfortunate and exaggerated response: Their insulin surges incur overzealous carbohydrate control and induce the symptoms under discussion.

Hypoglycemia can only be controlled with a perfect diet, one that eliminates all of the dangerous carbohydrates. As we previously stated, there's no need to add anything; it's what you remove that guarantees recovery. Patients must not eat table sugar, corn syrup, honey, sucrose, glucose, dextrose, or maltose. Lactose (milk sugar) and fructose (fruit sugar) can be consumed in limited amounts only. Only one piece of fruit should be eaten in a four-hour period. All heavy starches must be avoided, including potatoes, rice, and pasta. Eliminate caffeine. Strangely, it prolongs the action of insulin but paradoxically slows the corrective entry of glucose into cells. The liver extracts energy from alcohol but, a few hours later, stumbles badly from its effects and temporarily loses the ability to convert other food residues to glucose. Sorry, then, but despite everything else we're stealing from your diet, no alcohol. But take heart: This very limited diet doesn't need to be followed forever.

The elimination of all sugars (simple carbohydrates) as well as heavy starches (complex carbohydrates) is mandatory because they cause the body to release so much insulin. If insulin is not released, hypoglycemia will not occur. It's really that simple. In time, each of the affected endocrine glands will recover. In my experience, healing begins with a display of somewhat more energy somewhere between the fifth and tenth day after starting the diet. Some patients feel more fatigue during the first few days as they change their basic energy fuels from carbohydrates to protein and fat. During this initial period, they may also experience headaches from both caffeine and carbohydrate withdrawal. The energy surge that eventually appears may be delayed for those who have been ill for a very long time. Total elimination of sugar and starch may seem like a monumental challenge, but using diligence and willpower, success is rewardingly awesome.

> "I have been able to cautiously—and occasionally incautiously—reintroduce a few carbohydrates into my life, learning what my tolerance level is. But I am not tempted to add many; I have my life back, and compared to that, sweets and starches are a truly insignificant sacrifice."
>
> —*Cynthia C., Michigan*

Let's now look at the specific foods that must be completely eliminated if you are to overcome and maintain control of hypoglycemia.

Forbidden Foods List for Hypoglycemics: Foods to Avoid Strictly

Sugar in any form, including soft drinks
Caffeine from any source, including many soft drinks
Fruit juices and dried fruits
Baked beans
Black-eyed peas (cowpeas)
Garbanzo beans (chickpeas)
Refried beans
Lima beans
Lentils
Potatoes
Corn
Bananas

Barley
Rice
Pasta of any kind
Burritos (flour tortillas)
Tamales
Sweets of any kind
Dextrose, maltose, sucrose, glucose, fructose, honey, corn syrup, molasses, cane or brown rice syrup, and starch (caloric sweeteners and starches)

Our diet for hypoglycemia is divided into two parts: "strict" and "liberal." Both control hypoglycemia equally well. The strict diet was devised for anyone who needs to lose weight; the liberal diet was designed to maintain weight and still offset hypoglycemia. Take note: The above column of Foods to Avoid Strictly is applicable and in fact mandatory for both diets. This can't be ignored in the beginning. *Just a little cheat will do you in!*

Dr. St. Amand's Strict Diet for Hypoglycemia and Weight Reduction

You can eat freely the foods listed below except for the few items given a quantity limit. You can eat whenever you're hungry—there is no need to starve yourself. There is no need to eat on any specific schedule. However, if you don't see something on this list, you simply can't have it. Always check packaged and canned products by carefully studying the list of ingredients. Learn to read labels carefully every time you buy a product. Manufacturers can make changes and issue no warning. Do your homework and don't kid yourself. The very foods that caused you to gain weight are the ones you must give up to lose it. If this appeal to your common sense doesn't succeed, go to the liberal diet. You'll remain heavy but you'll at least control hypoglycemia.

Meats

All meats are allowed, except cold cuts that contain sugar. (*Check labels carefully*. Low-fat or nonfat and turkey cold cuts usually have added dextrose or corn syrup. Bacon and ham are acceptable, although they do list sugar on the labels. This bit cooks off and is not a problem. Hams that are heavily coated should be washed free of sugar.)

All fowl and game, fish, and shellfish are allowed in unlimited quantities.

Dairy Products

Eggs
Any natural cheese (cheese you slice yourself)
Cream (heavy and sour)
Cottage and ricotta cheeses (½ cup limit)
Butter and margarine

Fruits

Fresh coconut
Avocado (limit ½ per day)
Cantaloupe (limit ¼ per day)
Strawberries (limit 6–8 per day)
Lime or lemon juice (limit 2 tsp. per day), for flavoring

Vegetables

Asparagus
Bean sprouts
Broccoli
Okra
Olives
Parsley

Brussels sprouts
Cabbage (limit 1 cup per day)
Cauliflower
Celery
Chard
Chicory
Chinese cabbage (limit 2 cups per day)
Chives
Cucumber
Daikon (long, white radish)
Eggplant
Endive
Escarole
Greens (mustard, beet)
Jicama
Kale
Leeks
Lettuce
Mushrooms
Peppers (red, green, yellow, etc.)
Pickles (dill, sour, limit 1 per day)
Pimiento
Radicchio
Radish
Rhubarb
Salad greens
Sauerkraut
Scallions (green onion)
Snow peas
Spinach
String beans (green or yellow)
Summer squash (crookneck, yellow, and green)
Tomatoes
Water chestnuts
Watercress
Zucchini

Nuts (limit 12 per day)

Almonds
Brazil nuts
Butternuts
Filberts
Hazelnuts
Hickory
Macadamia nuts
Pecans
Pistachios
Sunflower seeds (small handful)
Walnuts

Desserts

Low-carbohydrate products including sugar-free chocolate with sucralose (Splenda) and sugar-free Jell-O
Custard (made with cream and artificial sweetener)

Cheesecake (no-crust or nut crust with cream cheese, sour cream, and artificial sweeteners)
Mousses made with whipping cream and sugar-free syrups or flavored protein powders

Beverages

Artificially sweetened drink mixes like Crystal Light, Country Time, etc.
Club soda, zero-carbohydrate flavored soda waters
Decaffeinated coffee
Mineral or bottled water
Weak or decaffeinated tea
Caffeine-free diet sodas
WonderCocoa, sugar- and caffeine-free
Bourbon, cognac, gin, rum, scotch, vodka, dry wine (after two months on a perfect diet, most hypoglycemics can tolerate a bit of alcohol)

Condiments and Spices

All spices including seeds (fresh or dried), all imitation flavorings, and horseradish
Sugar-free sauces such as hollandaise, mayonnaise, mustard, ketchup, soy sauce, Worcestershire sauce
Sugar-free salad dressings
Oil and vinegar (all types)

Miscellaneous

All fats
Caviar
Tofu and soy protein products that contain no forbidden sweeteners

If cholesterol is a problem, avoid cold cuts except sugar-free turkey. Trim all visible fat off meat. Remove the skin from poultry. Broil or grill foods instead of frying. Avoid full-fat cheese, heavy cream, solid margarine, hollandaise sauce, and macadamia nuts. Use egg whites or Egg Beaters instead of whole eggs. Use liquid margarine only. Nuts should be dry roasted only. Use canola or olive oil.

Dr. St. Amand's Liberal Diet for Hypoglycemia and Weight Maintenance

(Add these foods to the strict diet)

Fruits (limit: 1 piece of fruit every four hours; no fruit juices or dried fruit)

Apples
Apricots
Blackberries (½ cup limit)
Blueberries (½ cup limit)
Boysenberries
Casaba melon (1 wedge limit)
Grapefruit
Honeydew melon (1 wedge limit)
Lemons
Limes
Nectarines
Oranges
Papaya
Peaches
Pears
Plums
Raspberries
Strawberries
Tangerines
Tomato juice (unsweetened)
V8 juice

Vegetables

Artichokes
Beets
Carrots
Onions
Peas
Pumpkin
Squash, winter (such as acorn, butternut, fresh pumpkin, spaghetti, etc.)
Turnips

Nuts (no limit)

Cashews
Peanuts
Soy nuts

Dairy Products

Whole, nonfat, low-fat milk and buttermilk
Yogurt, unsweetened or made with noncaloric sweeteners

Dessert

Sugarless diet pudding (½ cup a day limit)

Breads

Three slices a day of sugar-free white, whole wheat, sourdough, or light rye. No more than two slices at one time or three servings a day of sugar-free flat bread (no more than two servings at a time). Low-carb tortillas—up to three is one serving. Corn tortillas—two are a serving.

Other Food Items

Carob powder
Flour, gluten or soy only
Gravy made with gluten or soy flour only
Wheat germ
Puffed rice, shredded wheat, or other sugar-free cereals
Popped popcorn (1 cup limit)
2 tacos or 2 enchiladas (2 corn tortillas only)

Most of the questions we are asked about the diet stem from confusion regarding the built-in nature of various carbohydrates. Many people have difficulty understanding why they can't eat a tiny bit of potato instead of the daily allowance of sugar-free bread permitted on the liberal diet. Most of these individuals have repeatedly tried calorie-restrictive diets. Here, the number of calories contained in foods are simply added up and, if the total sum is kept low enough, weight loss should begin without regard for the dietary mix. So carbohydrate substitution, gram for gram, would seem logical. Wrong! That type of math won't work with our diets, since not all carbohydrates are created equal. A calorie is a measure of heat: It may take more quantity of meat than of a candy bar to equal the measurement, just as a pound of feathers is larger in size than a pound of lead. But they both weigh the same. A carbohydrate, though, is not the same kind of measure: A gram of dextrose is not equal to a gram of lactose in the amount of insulin they cause the body to release.

> *The glycemic index of foods* (GI)—This index ranks foods on how they affect blood sugar levels in comparison with straight glucose. It is mainly used for evaluation of the metabolism of carbohydrates, since protein and fat do not cause the blood sugar to rise very much unless they are eaten together with those carbohydrates. Initially devised with glucose as 100, it is now more common in America to see white bread set as 100. (In our text, we will use the original scale, with glucose as 100. To convert to the white-bread scale, multiply by 0.7.)

Tables have been devised that permit comparisons of foods by the rise in blood sugar (or the insulin release) they induce. This is called the glycemic index (GI). The base reference is usually sugar (glucose), which is assigned the number 100. Potato consists of glucose molecules strung together and is assigned the GI of 98. On the other hand, fruits contain fructose, which does not raise blood sugar to the same extent and releases far less insulin. A peach, for example, has a glycemic index of 26. Though fructose and glucose are both carbohydrates, you can readily see why we can't substitute them ounce for ounce (gram for gram). In general, you will find that foods with a high glycemic index are excluded from the hypoglycemia diet, foods with a lower one can be consumed in moderation, and the lowest foods can be eaten in unlimited quantities. However, you must bear in mind that the glycemic index is not a perfect indicator. Foods are not eaten alone, and there are other variables in how they affect the body. Many expert studies have been written up showing that this system is less than infallible. Sometimes we appear in error, such as with carrots, which are safe on the liberal diet despite a fairly high index. Their fiber content seems to make a difference.

When we first designed these diets, we had to rely on our patients as test subjects, because the glycemic index had not yet been invented. Any food that induced symptoms of hypoglycemia in even one patient was placed on the forbidden list. This assured that our diet would always resolve the symptoms of carbohydrate intolerance; more than forty years later, this statement still holds. If you're planning to use recipes and foods from other low-carbohydrate diets, beware if you're hypoglycemic. Most of those were primarily devised for weight reduction, and some items don't quite fit the hypoglycemia diet.

In our experience, about two months of perfect dieting are needed to wipe out all the symptoms attributable to carbohydrate intolerance. Consider the dietary process as if you were building a checking account. First, you must make deposits. If you're well disciplined, you can rebuild energy reserves to the highest level allowed by your genetic makeup. Only when your account is full should you begin experimenting with other carbohydrates, and begin making withdrawals on your balance.

Twenty Common Foods and Their Glycemic Index[2]

Fructose	25	Bananas	62
Yogurt	32	Brown rice	66
Milk	34	White bread	69
Tomatoes	38	White rice	72
Apples	39	Wheat bread	72
Pasta	45–50	Cornflakes	80
Peas	53	Honey	87
Sucrose	59	Carrots	92
Sweet corn	59	Baked potato (russet)	98
Corn	59	Glucose	100

You may never be able to indulge in wanton spending. You should be cautious in the beginning. Uncontrolled spending, or too much cheating, produces sequential debits. You may have to push away from the banquet table now and then and take time to replenish your reserves. A negative balance will put you right back into hypoglycemia. If you permit that to happen, brace yourself for the fury of renewed adrenaline surges and panic attacks. Once you've followed the diet for a while, your body is sensitized and responds with a hormonal vehemence that was blunted before by repetition. There's no choice but to go back and restart the process of rebuilding. It's far better to heed whatever early warning signals you get and tighten up on your diet to avoid repeat disasters. That's the key to damage control.

It's in your best interest to become an apt pupil and be as observant as possible. You'll want to learn to recognize the very first symptoms that follow dietary indiscretions. Often, enervating fatigue leads the way, but frontal, pressure-type headaches are almost as likely. After a few setbacks from hit-and-miss dieting, you'll develop an instinct about when to retreat. Times of mental or physical stress, the premenstrual week, and injuries will make you especially vulnerable. Such things will continue to sap your reserves, but if you are careful you can avoid fully submerging deficits. You'll be far less fragile if you can anticipate some of them before major symptoms resurface. In time, you'll properly ration meal contents to match energy expenditures.

No physician or dietitian can predict if you will need permanent dietary restrictions. In the majority of cases, a certain amount of leeway develops when fibromyalgia improves significantly. Remember, as a consequence of this illness, much of your body is working day and night expending huge quantities of energy. As overworked, contracted tissues relax, you may be rewarded by being able to eat almost indiscriminately. Unfortunately, genetics plays a part; some patients will never be able to eat lots of carbohydrates. A family history of diabetes is sufficient warning that you were born with a genetically vulnerable pancreas. If that's the case, adhering to a low-carbohydrate diet is the best thing you can do for yourself.

> "I got on the liberal hypoglycemia diet and have dramatically improved since then. I feel clear-headed with very little muscle pain on most days. . . . If I cheat on my diet more than once or twice a week I pay with nervousness, fatigue, and pain. I had serious withdrawal from refined carbohydrates. It felt like an addiction to me. I now look at foods as nourishment, not a reward or something to soothe me."
>
> —*Heather, Texas*

Fibromyalgia + Hypoglycemia = Fibroglycemia

Our statistics on more than four thousand patients with fibromyalgia are telling. Thirty percent of the females and 15 percent of males have concurrent hypoglycemia. (See figure 5.4.) Most of our patients begin having such attacks later, after the onset of fibromyalgia. Many, many more are intolerant to carbohydrates: that is, they feel worse when they overindulge. This group only rarely exhibits the acute symptoms of the illness, but feels generally more fatigued and experiences increased pain after eating heavy starches or the wrong sugars. We therefore wanted a single name to cover patients who have both conditions. We've chosen *fibroglycemia.*

So what, you ask, is the reason that fibroglycemia is so common in our patients? We've already touched on our mapping system for making the diagnosis of fibromyalgia (see chapter 2). Our hands can easily identify the swollen areas of the body as contracted portions of muscles, ligaments, and tendons. Such areas are puffed up mainly because of accumulated intracellular fluid under high pressure. They're also working tissues, as demonstrated by their spastic, constricted state. These tightened segments are steadily pulling on bones, joints, or adjacent tissues twenty-four hours a day without respite. Though the effort is low grade, these muscles eventually fatigue and begin hurting just as expected from a never-ending workout. We're also aware that, for every lump and bump we draw on our map, there are many other affected structures hidden too deeply for us to feel. They're the invisible accomplices but they also add to the exhaustion. Those who exercise stop when there's too much pain and fatigue. Fibromyalgics don't enjoy that luxury: They can never stop their muscles from working.

Remember that the currency of energy for all cells is ATP. Eighty to 90 percent of the food we eat is converted into this substance. Every bodily function demands huge supplies of this

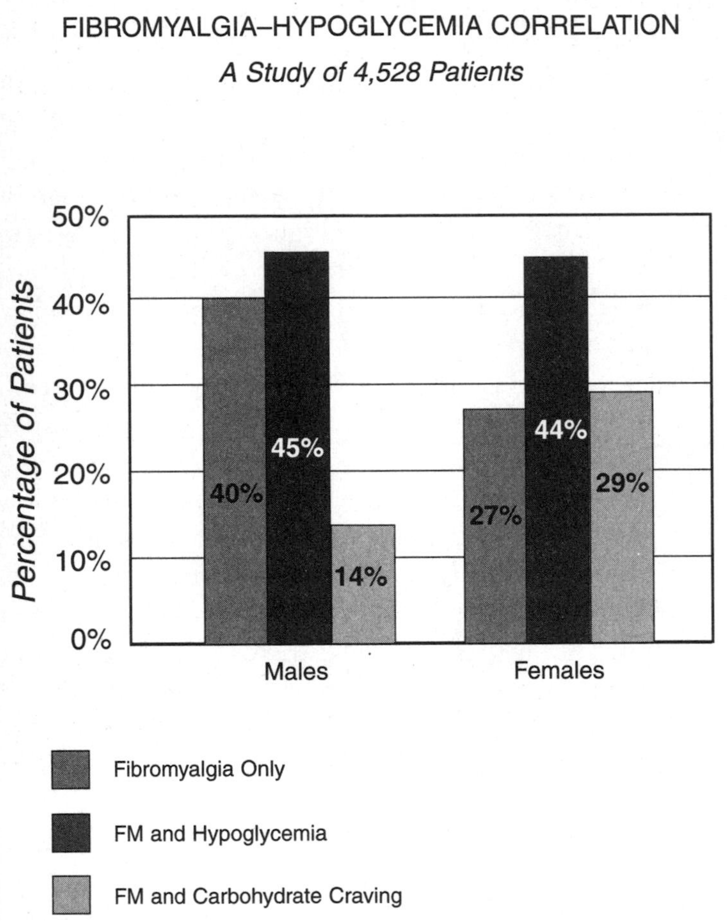
FIBROMYALGIA–HYPOGLYCEMIA CORRELATION
A Study of 4,528 Patients
50%
40%
30%
20%
10%
0%
Percentage of Patients
40%
45%
14%
27%
44%
29%
Males
Females
Fibromyalgia Only
FM and Hypoglycemia
FM and Carbohydrate Craving

Figure 5.4

chemical. We can't even think without using large amounts of ATP for brain activity. Ounce for ounce, the central nervous system—especially the brain—uses more than any other tissue. Fingernail and hair growth, digestion, fat deposition, breathing, urinating, fighting infections, or healing tissue trauma all utilize ATP. The bulk of production and consumption occurs through muscle activity. As overworked tissues fatigue, they use nerves to signal the need for more fuel. The brain receives the message and immediately thinks: *I'm tired. Give me a candy bar.* When ATP production is normal, energy should be available within five minutes of eating such carbohydrates. That's no longer true in fibromyalgia. No amount of eating will totally satisfy the steady or sudden demand for energy.

Most fibromyalgics fall victim to carbohydrate cravings throughout the day in an unconscious attempt to create energy. Those sugars and starches are quickly digested and converted to glucose. Unfortunately, the carbohydrate-craving fibromyalgics quickly saturate their systems with glucose molecules, which force the pancreas to release large amounts of insulin. Such surges rapidly lower the blood sugar by driving it mainly into muscles, but also into fat cells, the liver, the brain, and most other needy areas of the body. These repeated insulin spurts eventually cause hypoglycemia in genetically susceptible individuals. Both the chronic and acute symptoms of that condition are added to those of fibromyalgia. There you have it: fibroglycemia!

These are the sickest of our patients. For them, dietary modification isn't merely a good idea, it's mandatory. They face a huge metabolic chore. They must eat themselves out of hypoglycemia while simultaneously accepting the increased symptoms of fibromyalgia reversal. There can be no compromise for this group. They would continue to feel terrible on a freewheeling diet even when guaifenesin has purged much of the fibromyalgic debris from their tissues. Fibroglycemics must either choose to eat correctly or choose to remain sick!

> "Since being diagnosed with fibromyalgia and hypoglycemia, I've been experimenting with my carbohydrate intake, and I've been able to deduce that my hypoglycemia is pretty severe and is made a lot worse by the fibromyalgia. When I am in a bad fibromyalgia episode, I've found that it is critical that I do not deviate from the strict diet at all. Even one piece of bread can trigger a noticeable increase in all my symptoms. Also, there seems to be a very direct relationship between my carbohydrate intake and my depression. When I am very faithful to the strict diet, my depression quiets down. There have been short periods of time when I experienced real mental peace. If I botch the diet, the first casualty seems to be that sense of peace."
>
> —*Gwen, California*

We've noticed that obesity sometimes offers some protection against hypoglycemia. That's a Trojan horse reenactment. Once fat is overexpressed in the system, chubby cells are gradually provoking a more serious disturbance. The larger a cell gets, the more resistant it becomes to further storage attempts by insulin. It's much more difficult to prod obese cells into opening their transport tunnels when they consider themselves already overstuffed. As a result, fewer amino acids (building blocks for protein) and fatty acids can be inserted into the usual warehouses. The pancreas, ever mindful of the waste-not-want-not principle, presumes its message is not being received. Rather than waste the digested food residues, the pancreatic islets instead increase their output of insulin. That's like hitting deafened fat and muscle cells with a hormonal two-by-four. Reawakened by this louder shouting, they dutifully respond, and storage resumes. Every area of the body willing to accept a bit more fatty acid is ordered to do just that. Overweight becomes heavy and that yields, in turn, to obesity.

Now cells can't as easily become hypoglycemic because they're so profoundly adverse to insulin's instructions. The step beyond simple insulin resistance (as this metabolic state is called) is Type II, or adult-onset diabetes. Cells that are unresponsive to insulin don't absorb glucose as readily as they once did. At this point, the blood sugar no longer drops abruptly; eventually, it doesn't even bother to stoop a little. This is the way obesity sometimes corrects hypoglycemia and dupes patients into thinking they've outgrown their sugar problem. But there's a heavy price to pay down the line. The health ravages of insulin resistance are many, and those of diabetes several times worse. There's a special subset of individuals who have family histories of diabetes in parents and grandparents. They are born with insulin resistance and will invite the same fate for themselves unless they heed our warnings about carbohydrates. We won't explore those hazards any further. Nevertheless, we're adamant in warning you that neither low nor high blood sugar is healthy. We refer interested readers to our book *What Your Doctor May* Not *Tell You About Fibromyalgia Fatigue.*

Many patients crave sugar but haven't yet become hypoglycemic. For those of you who like statistics, here are the numbers. Not counting hypoglycemics, 40 percent of our lean and 60 percent our obese fibromyalgic women crave carbohydrates; men fare better: 35 and 53 percent, respectively. All patients combined, including hypoglycemics, the lip-smacking demand for sugars can be rounded out to 70 percent. Just like the other patients with blood sugar fluctuations, they suffer all of the aches, pains, and fatigue but aren't punished by the sudden adrenaline surges of fibroglycemia. During perverse situations, they can be pushed into that category by heavy sugar binging, alcohol abuse, emotional stress, infections, even the trauma of an accident, extensive dental work, or surgery.

Women are especially susceptible during the premenstrual week. It's as though they're teetering on the edge and only need a nudge to succumb.

Carbohydrate cravers may also feel generalized improvement by sticking to the recommended diet for one or two months. They may get a highly encouraging energy spurt while waiting for guaifenesin reversal benefits. The same often applies to the remaining fibromyalgics who are neither carbohydrate intolerant nor hypoglycemic. Some quick rewards include lifting the fibrofog, better nighttime sleep, and avoiding the drowsiness that regularly follows carbohydrate meals. For nearly everyone, the diet is worth a monthlong experiment. If no improvement is felt, it can be abandoned. We must stress that no specific diet is necessary for those who suffer only from fibromyalgia.

There are other reasons why better controlling insulin should help fibromyalgics as well as fibroglycemics. One of the prime functions of insulin is to drive glucose into cells, but always with some phosphate. Phosphate tags up with glucose and prevents it from escaping back out. That's what keeps it available for local energy needs. Insulin also signals certain kidney cells to reabsorb phosphate that was filtered from the blood and targeted for elimination in the urine. Sucked back into the bloodstream, phosphate ions are transported and then inserted into cells everywhere. Some of these are especially responsive to insulin instructions and soak up much more phosphate than do others. The cells most severely affected by fibromyalgia are the very ones that respond quickest to insulin. Muscles are especially cooperative in this regard. Our theory, you will recall, suggests that an excess amount of phosphate is what eventually slams the brakes on energy formation. The chemistry of fibromyalgia, hypoglycemia, and the combination disease, fibroglycemia, is certainly complex. In simple terms, if you've got the wrong genes,

Substitutions for Adapting Nondiet Recipes to Ingredients for a Strict Low-Carbohydrate Diet

Sugar: DiabetiSweet, SugarTwin, stevia, sucralose (Splenda)
1 tbsp. cornstarch: unflavored gelatin or 2 tbsps. gluten, soy flour, or Atkins bake mix
Whole milk: 1 part cream to 1 part water (add a dash of sweetener, because milk is sweeter than cream)
Buttermilk (1 cup): ½ cup cream, ½ cup water, 1 tbsp. vinegar or lemon juice (let stand 5 minutes, add a tiny amount of sweetener—see above)
Fruit juice: fruit extract and sweetener to taste, Crystal Light orange juice or lemonade
Bread crumbs: sunflower kernels crushed in a blender (unsalted), crushed pork rinds, or soy or egg protein powder
Flour for thickening: Atkins bake mix, soy flour, protein powder, egg protein powder, or water chestnuts mushed to paste in a blender (you may have to add a little of their liquid)

and then uncontrollably yield to carbohydrate cravings, your cells will suffer from more phosphate accumulation.

As if the picture weren't bleak enough, let's make it worse! When either insulin or glucose is added to the fluid surrounding cells, they insist on further company. Obesity, hypertension, and even insulin resistance make the same demand. They all conspire to lure calcium into cells where it remains too long as an unwelcome guest. Please remember that while phosphate is considered the villain, calcium is a sturdy accomplice that unrelentingly goads already exhausted cells into further exertion. The low-carbohydrate diet helps to reduce the excess of calcium and phosphate in the wrong places.

As you would expect, fibroglycemia patients have the same dietary response as do those who are purely hypoglycemic. As we advised earlier, we urge fibroglycemics to adhere to the strict diet if they're overweight and to the liberal diet if they're sufficiently trim. Remember, both versions of the diet control blood sugar swings equally well. The only added benefit of the strict one is weight reduction. It won't heal carbohydrate-induced hypoglycemia any better or any faster.

> "I stopped all my medications cold turkey and went on the hypoglycemia diet. I started guaifenesin and went through some bad cycles. I fell off my diet and suffered for that. But slowly things have gotten much better. I'm down twenty-five pounds in weight, my mind is clearing, my muscle spasms have cleared, and I can sleep. I am not perfectly well but I can make it through the day without having to lie down for most of it. The most important thing is that I now have a life."
>
> —*Gwen, California*

When we begin treating fibroglycemia, we don't wait for the benefits of the diet to kick in before starting guaifenesin. These are very sick people, and we can't think of any reason for delay. After the hypoglycemia portion of the combined disease clears (usually within two months of dedicated dieting), patients may begin adding carbohydrates. Just as we stated in discussing hypoglycemia, people are different. You will have to seek and find your own dietary limitations. There is a spectrum of possibilities ranging from permanent restrictions to none whatsoever.

We know of no modalities other than proper diet and guaifenesin treatment that can reverse the mix of fibromyalgia and hypoglycemia. It takes discipline to avoid all sources of salicylates and adhere to the proper diet, but it's mandatory. As with other chronic conditions such as diabetes, success depends greatly on the tandem efforts of individual and physician. It certainly falls upon the patient to help direct and control her or his recovery. It seems a lot to ask of a person who is already miserable to give up favorite foods and also studiously avoid salicylates. Yet the appearance of the first good hours and days makes it all worthwhile. It's highly exhilarating, especially when contrasted with the preceding and disabling symptoms of these syndromes. Euphoria is the reward.

From the abyss of terrible to the heights of wonderful isn't such a long climb. We've offered you, the patient, a ladder. You'll have to climb it rung by rung—or else not only stay where you are, but also continue your deeper descent into your personal hell. Those of us who've recovered urge you to join us in living.

LIVING LOW-CARB: THE FIBROGLYCEMIA AND HYPOGLYCEMIA DIET

> "Since I have begun treatment with guaifenesin for my fibromyalgia, my carbohydrate cravings have lessened and it is really not so hard to follow the hypoglycemia diet. I would have expected it otherwise—that with the worsening of symptoms, my carb cravings would have become intolerable. But that is not what I have experienced."
>
> —*L. N., Massachusetts*

This used to be a hard section to write. Luckily for us all, it isn't what it used to be. Since the first edition of this book, low-carbohydrate dieting has become very popular. Where once it was difficult, now there are hundreds of choices. Products are well labeled. Fancy restaurants and fast-food joints not only accommodate but actually court low-carb eaters. There are even low-carb stores, Web sites, and cookbooks. Krispy Kreme's stock has fallen, and bakeries are competing for the low-carb bread market. Where once we were a lonely voice in the wilderness begging for foods without starchy sauces or added sugar, we can now find low-carb barbecue sauce, tortillas, and beverages in abundance. And by the time this book is on the shelf, there will be many more additions.

Most people begin their new diet reluctantly and hesitantly, quite afraid of making mistakes. That's the way it should be. Earlier in the chapter, we stressed that a certain reverence must be applied to the required restrictions. Errors are costly, and early on, gains are easily erased. Unlike the sequences necessary to determine guaifenesin dosages for fibromyalgia, the low-carbohydrate diet can be presented in black and white. Your predecessors have done all the work. This you can have and that you can't. Be dedicated and accurate. Don't even consider cheating or getting creative for the first two months.

For most people, breakfast is the most difficult meal. Yet there are plenty of choices. By habit, we tend to define only certain items as being "breakfast foods." But really, it's all the same to your digestive tract. Even if you don't want to consider anything out of the usual, just look around you. On both the strict and liberal diets, eggs can be prepared any style: fried, boiled, or scrambled. Omelets are a bit more work but can be made with any of the usual additions—cheese, bell peppers, sour cream, tomatoes, avocado, and sprinkled herbs. You can eat any kind of meat such as breakfast steaks or pork chops and even sugar-cured bacon, since frying burns off that carbohydrate. (Watch out for sausages, though: Most mulch in some kind of sugar.) Hams frequently have added honey or other sweeteners that should be washed off.

Breakfast drinks can be made with unsweetened protein

powders, egg, or soy. There are even ready-made choices now, and Instant Breakfast! Toss in strawberries unless you want to spare your quota for later in the day if you're on the strict diet. Clever thinking creates other possibilities—say, making a smoothie using fruit, tofu, milk, and sugar-free syrups. There's nothing wrong with a scoop of cottage cheese and a slice of cantaloupe (and sugar-free flat breads if you're on the liberal diet). Smoked salmon and cream cheeses aren't bad choices, either. Egg custards are particularly refreshing, especially on warm, summer days. They can be made in batches using heavy cream, eggs, vanilla extract, and sugar substitutes. The liberal diet permits you to spread peanut butter on toast made with sugar-free bread. A tiny spoonful of sugar-free jelly is a nice addition. On the liberal diet, unsweetened cereal or oatmeal with sugar-free maple syrup is allowed. On both diets, you can find recipes for acceptable French toast, quiches, or breakfast casseroles.

Lunch on the strict diet could include vegetables with or without meat. Deviled eggs make wonderful snacks; they're safe if made with sugar-free mayonnaise and aren't stuffed with sweet relish. Liberal dieters might well get by with sandwiches that use the thinner types of sugar-free breads, tortillas, wraps, or flat breads. When I wanted to lose a few pounds, I used two cabbage leaves as my "bread." Large lettuce leaves can be used to form wraps, and roast beef or cheese can also substitute. Composition salads are great with added bits of beef, chicken, shell- or other fish, cheese, egg, sour cream, and avocado. Taco salads can be made with low-carb tortillas and bean-free chili on the liberal diet. You can inspire yourself by creating your own versions, including variations on the traditional Cobb or Caesar salads, as long as dressings are kept sugar-free. You can always eat hamburgers and cheeseburgers with a fork after tossing out the bun.

Just by custom, we usually conjure a different vision for the components of our evening meal—we're usually less interested in eggs and sandwiches. We also tend to prepare our food somewhat differently, using a lot more grilling, broiling and baking. Fish is less often eaten at lunch but is something we can add to our dinner menu. Vegetables may be marinated, stir-fried, roasted, baked, or grilled along with meats or separately using the same oils and sauces. Steamed vegetables with cheese and nuts are delicious. On the strict diet, it doesn't take much imagination to use al dente cauliflower, daikon cubes, or chunks of summer squash as replacements for potatoes in certain recipes. Celery root or cauliflower can be cooked and whipped into faux mashed potatoes with butter, sour cream, and a little garlic or blue cheese. Artichoke appetizers dress well with butter or sugar-free mayonnaise sauces and shrimp. Slip in curry or hot paprika. Batter is easily made from egg and crushed pork rinds to coat meat such as chicken on the strict diet. Nut flours make delicious piecrusts or coatings for chicken or fish. Your taste buds might like the dramatic change offered by blackened meats. You could stuff large mushroom caps or green peppers with spinach, cheese, or bits of anything you dream up. Spareribs made with sugar-free barbecue sauce or meat loaves that have been stuffed with cheese or topped with sugar-free ketchup make a nice change. Stir-fry shrimp with bell peppers, mushrooms, and scallions; lace scampi with extra butter, garlic, and a few gourmet herbs to avoid menu ennui. Chopped cauliflower or shredded lettuce can serve as a replacement for rice.

There's a world of flavors waiting for your creativity. There are no restrictions on spices; mustard and chili powders; sugar-free sauces; Liquid Smoke; horseradish or garlic paste; or piquant Thai dressings. These ingredients add great zest to whatever you're preparing. The liberal diet certainly provides more variety, but both allow all you can eat! Use unusual items such as spaghetti squash or zucchini ribbons to fake a pasta dish. Toss with any of your favorite (sugar-free) sauces or serve it simply with butter and Parmesan cheese. You gourmet, *fin-bec* people are still permitted favorite escargot preparations and caviars. Several desserts work in nicely on either diet. Whip up egg custards, sugar-free cheesecakes (nut flour shell), and sugar free Jell-Os. There are plenty of other delicious concoctions, even ice creams, now being made with artificial sweeteners such as sucralose (Splenda). Mousse can be easily made with whipping cream and a flavored protein powder. Would you perhaps consider floating ice cream and whipping cream on top of a diet root beer? One patient melted sucralose-treated chocolate bars in her microwave oven and poured it on her strawberries.

Eating out is getting safer as more restaurants are responding to the growing demand for low-carbohydrate fare. Most restaurants readily accommodate their clientele and substitute vegetables in place of rice or potato. Cottage cheese or sliced tomatoes also provide suitable options. Fibroglycemics should bring decaffeinated coffee in packets, get a pot of hot water, and make their own brew because a stressed waiter might mix up coffeepots and serve you the real thing. The main courses are usually as safe as what you would have eaten at home. Ask the waiter if the Caesar or blue cheese dressings are sugar-free. If not, use oil and vinegar with or without a squeeze of lemon juice or a little mustard. Occasionally, restaurants, have flavored olive oil sitting on the table or at least honor your request for some. In Mexican restaurants you can order various fajitas, *ropas viejas, machaca,* or even the chiles rellenos if they're only lightly floured. Italian restaurants usually offer veal or chicken piccata, *bistec,* and assorted seafoods including scampi and calamari. Satisfy your tastes but choose restaurants with cooperative chefs who'll tell you what's in their sauces.

Our book *What Your Doctor May* Not *Tell You About Fibromyalgia Fatigue* also contains many suggestions. We've added these and other helpful references to the Resources section in the back of the book. The Web site www.guaigroup.org has recipe pages that also contain many suggestions for snacks. Included is a complete Thanksgiving Day dinner, all low carb (liberal diet), including faux yams and pumpkin pie or mousse.

It's not within the scope of this book to adequately discuss the merits of fats versus carbohydrates as fuel sources. The battle will rage on for the near future in medicine. However, one fact stands out. Though the hormone cortisol can store belly (visceral) fat, only one hormone can store lipids in all fat cells, and that is insulin. It is released in response to carbohydrates, as we've already discussed. Fats release insignificant amounts and proteins only a bit more unless they're eaten along with carbohydrates. Much larger amounts surge out when they're ingested at the same time. Our strict diet permits weight reduction for three main reasons:

1. It avoids heavy insulin outputs.
2. Protein digestion and storage require more caloric expenditures than that particular food contains.
3. In the absence of surplus carbohydrates, metabolism must burn fats for energy.

For the purpose of this book, we bow to the correct party line and suggest that you avoid large amounts of saturated fats. We're well aware that current statistics show no reduction in heart disease deaths from adhering to recommendations almost universally warning against eating what are actually safe fats. Few are concerned about unsaturated fats contained in vegetable oils and liquid margarines. We'll certainly continue to tell our patients that carbohydrates, both complex and simple, have been erroneously touted as beneficial. We are all witness to the explosion of obesity and adult-onset diabetes a generation of high-carb eating has fostered. Medical doctors such as Richard Bernstein and the late Robert Atkins have made this point and have eloquently defended their positions.[3] The new popular *South Beach Diet* and Suzanne Somers' books are simply variations on the original theme. Many published papers now exist backing the safety of lower-carbohydrate diets and contradicting the idea that fat makes you fat and is the culprit behind the unhealthy Western diet.

> "Several large issues were discussed including my lack of progress with weight loss on Weight Watchers and the zooming rise of my triglycerides on my last four workups at my internist's office. Funny thing is, my rheumatologist said the same thing that Dr. St. Amand said, 'You know what you have to do on both issues.' Back to the strict diet it was. I asked Dr. St. Amand if I went back on the strict would it affect my labs being done three days later and he wasn't too sure I'd see any improvement that fast. I'm here to say my triglycerides went down from 299 to 169, my cholesterol dropped from 184 to 162 and even a couple of my liver tests improved significantly. My appetite is greatly reduced and it takes much less food to satisfy me. Guess I am carb sensitive . . . *duh!*"
>
> —*Marsha, California*

In conclusion, let me say that I've been disturbed by the dietary sermons preached in recent years. What has been handed down is *not* safe eating: The incidence of obesity is rising rapidly, as are its kin, diabetes, high blood pressure, and insulin resistance. Heart disease and hardening of the arteries are also on the rise. These are all killers, and their weapon is excess insulin. Weight reduction can be achieved easily and comfortably with sufficiently low carbohydrate intake. Those who've been unsuccessfully trying to lose weight by adhering to complex-carbohydrate regimens have been seriously duped. It just doesn't work. What you've been eating is what's made you fat, hypoglycemic or diabetic. In deference to my colleagues, I'm not your doctor and can't impose my recommendations over those of your personal physician. But if you have a weight problem, you owe it to yourself to do some research and ask some hard questions. Although my patients don't always follow my advice, they will continue to hear from me on this subject.

I've been on the low-carbohydrate diet for more than forty years. I'm not hypoglycemic, but this diet has been a godsend, first to help me drop the few pounds I wanted to lose, and then to maintain my weight within a three-pound range. I confine myself to the strict diet during the week. That will normally drop my weight one or two pounds below my desired level and allow me to face the weekend in a more liberal mode. I confine my cheating at that time to eating pizza, rice, or bread. That keeps me contented—though it might not be true for you. Each of you will eventually develop your own ritualistic system of dieting and cheating. But first, you must get out of the hypoglycemia part of your fibroglycemia. In that process, if you need to, why not take your weight down to a healthier level? After you've reached that goal, allow yourself only enough cheats to keep you on friendly terms with your bathroom scale.

Chapter 6

The Protocol

"Last winter, I was ready to apply for Social Security disability payments. I only dared to drive my car one or two miles on a 'good day.' I hadn't had a social life for three years. My credit rating was ruined because I was so exhausted I would let bills pile up for months, then try to catch up with them all at once. Nights were torture. I woke up every hour to hour and a half all night long. I had irritable bowel, irritable bladder, and restless legs. In the mornings, my joints ached so much that at times I was forced to get down on my hands and knees and crawl from the bedroom to the bathroom to the kitchen. . . .

"By March, I'd decided I was willing to try guaifenesin. Maybe it wasn't for the faint of heart, but neither was the quality of the life I was living. For the next several weeks I felt miserable most of the time and then, suddenly, I had two days of total reprieve from FMS. Not just 'good' days—extraordinary, amazing days. Then I started into the next cycle. I've had all my old symptoms return in full force. Tomorrow will be two months on guaifenesin and, according to the protocol, I should have reversed one year of symptoms of FMS by now. I can honestly say that I feel better than I did a year ago, and I certainly bounce back from exertion much faster than I used to. So, this isn't easy; it isn't fun; but it works. Follow the protocol to the absolute letter, be ruthless in getting rid of products and foods that aren't good for you, and go for it!"

—Anne, Minnesota

It's time to take a closer look at our protocol. We're going to lay out each step carefully. We've tried to write this chapter as clearly and concisely as we could. We'll skip over some explanations that we've already detailed in previous pages or will outline subsequently. It's very important that you understand and grasp what we say. Please don't allow yourself the seemingly harmless luxury of deviating from the proven path. A few thousand patients have pioneered your way: Take advantage of the trail they've blazed. You're about to benefit both from the success they've had and the mistakes they've made and all that we've learned from them. Please, do it exactly our way.

FIND A DOCTOR TO OBTAIN A DIAGNOSIS

As obvious as it sounds, begin by making sure you have fibromyalgia. This sounds silly, but it's important to rule out more dangerous or potentially lethal conditions. If you haven't been diagnosed, make an appointment with your doctor. If you're seeing a new physician, make sure he or she understands and believes in fibromyalgia. Don't be shy; ask the secretary who makes the schedule. Tell her that you suspect what you have but explain that you want expert confirmation. If you get the wrong vibes, pick another doctor. This may seem harsh, but the road to recovery is difficult enough without having a firm medical alliance. It's too stressful for you at this stage to spend emotional time trying to convince a reluctant partner that you have a real illness.

If you need help finding a doctor, there are several things you can try. First of all, ask your friends. If one of them has a doctor he or she describes as an open-minded good listener, start with that office. Another approach is to call a fibromyalgia support group or the local chapter of The Arthritis Foundation. They usually compile lists of doctors who understand or are sympathetic to patients with FMS. You could also contact your hospital's staff office for suggestions and referrals. Online newsgroups and Web sites are designed to be helpful. Our fibromyalgiatreatment.com actually lists guaifenesin support groups throughout the United States and others based overseas. It displays names of physicians who are at least aware of the illness and cognizant of our treatment. The site will also show you how to connect to an online support group.

You don't necessarily need a specialist to make the correct diagnosis. General practitioners or internists are perfectly qualified to help you. Exactly because they're generalists and not specialists, they'll less likely try to squeeze most of your symptoms into the smaller-size container of their limited specialty. This is no time for preconceived notions that will force you to fail yet another course of worthless treatment. Remember, any physician or other licensed health practitioner will be able to guide you, especially now since guaifenesin is readily available without prescription.

Once you're face-to-face with a doctor, what should you expect? If you've not had recent blood tests, he or she will most likely order some. A basic work-up will scan your body for adverse conditions since any chronic one can cause fatigue and perhaps mild muscular aches. Some tests are altered by recent food intake, so fasting samples should be drawn. Probably included will be a blood count looking for anemia, infection, or inflammation. The chemistry panel will look at your liver and kidneys, screening for lipid abnormalities, diabetes, and the chemical composition of your serum. We should warn you about some results. A normal blood sugar does not exclude hypoglycemia, as we stated in the previous chapter. A low fasting blood sugar demands further investigation, possibly by an endocrinologist.

The ultrasensitive thyroid test of TSH (thyroid-stimulating hormone) is almost mandatory since it's outstandingly accurate for the detection of glandular dysfunction. Far too much confusion exists concerning this single endocrine gland. It's true that 85 percent of fibromyalgics are women. It's also verifiable that 5 to 10 percent of women develop defective thyroid function; the majority of these will be on the low side (hypothyroidism). Expect the two illnesses to overlap, just by chance. It's also a fact that each condition will make the other worse. They're not otherwise linked, though they cause a mutual intensification of symptoms—as you'd surmise from the superimposition of any second disease. Very few illnesses fail to share some symptoms with several other diseases. To conclude this discussion, one simple thyroid test would separate these disparate conditions should they coexist.

If you live in certain areas of the country, your doctor may want to check for Lyme disease or other locally occurring possibilities. If you've traveled extensively, a liver test might be ordered to make sure you don't have any kind of hepatitis. Depending on your family history and age, other possibilities exist.

If you have a lot of aches and pains, your doctor will probably include an arthritis panel in the blood tests. This group will often help uncover the presence of lupus or rheumatoid arthritis. If you're over fifty, a woman and have a particular distribution of pain, testing should be expanded to include the ESR (erythrocyte sedimentation rate). If it's markedly elevated, the diagnosis of polymyalgia rheumatica will be considered. Though it's not related to fibromyalgia, like other adverse conditions it will certainly intensify symptoms. Polymyalgia reaches emergency status because of the threats it poses including blindness and strokes.

At your initial appointment, bring your doctor a list of all of your medications and supplements. This is no time for trying to avoid a professional opinion on the merit of such combinations. Include any over-the-counter products you take, even now and then. Certain herbs and nonprescription items can seriously affect liver enzymes and kidney function. That's why your honesty coupled with appropriate blood tests could well expose problems while they're still minor and correctible. In short, there's nothing ever gained by playing games with your doctor.

We remind you that there are no distinguishing tests for fibromyalgia. The work being ordered on your blood is to reassure you and your physician that something more urgent does not exist co-expressed with fibromyalgia. When such entities are excluded, you and your doctor will feel far safer and can get on with this protocol clearly focused on the problem at hand.

The diagnosis of fibromyalgia is properly made in two parts. The doctor begins by taking a detailed medical history that includes a full systems review. Since fibromyalgia causes fatigue, pain, depression, irritable bowel syndrome, irritable bladder, numbness, leg cramps, headaches, palpitations, and a host of other diverse symptoms, your doctor will explore them, sometimes in detail. Many doctors use check sheets for baselines that itemize symptoms and, later, to track changes. Refresh your memory ahead of time so you can help your professional to establish a chronology of your complaints including their onset and progression. This sequencing will also provide you a rough guide as to when and in which order you should expect reversing symptoms.

After your doctor is satisfied that your symptoms and history suggest fibromyalgia, an examination will surely follow. He or she may not feel comfortable "mapping" as we do, but at the very least will do a hands-on search for the so-called tender points (see the description on page 26). We think physicians should also feel places where you hurt even if they're not included in those predetermined zones. Finally, armed with normal blood tests, a sympathetic ear, and tender-point or mapping results, both of you should feel secure with your diagnosis.

ADDRESS THE CARBOHYDRATE-INTOLERANCE/HYPOGLYCEMIA FACTOR

When you've been officially diagnosed with fibromyalgia, you may have another important item to discuss with your doctor. As we explained in the hypoglycemia chapter, there's no totally reliable blood test. Your experience is really sufficient. You're very well aware of what happens when you eat foods high in sugar, or potatoes, rice, pasta, and other complex carbohydrates. As much as you'd like to deny it, you've actually done the best test over and over again. You ate and you suffered. Tell that to your doctor. Very few will accept a verdict that's based purely on the symptoms you feel. The chances are that he or she may not agree with you, but you can certainly modify your own diet easily following the appropriate chapter in this book. We've described how you do that, so take your own symptom inventory and trust what you feel.

Ideally, what you and your physician should look for is what follows. Remember that symptoms cluster into two fairly separate batches, the chronic and the acute. The latter are the scary ones and generally strike three or four hours after eating and during the night. They're sudden in onset and often violent enough to be labeled "panic attacks." Hand or inner shaking, sudden sweating or clamminess, hunger headaches, heart pounding or skipped beats (flip-flops), severe anxieties, irritability, weakness, dizziness and faintness, and occasionally actual passing out are the others. These unwelcome complaints may not all make an appearance or occur as intensely in everyone. If you have these kinds of symptoms and eating makes them go away, but they reappear when you're hungry, low blood sugar is the most likely culprit.

The chronic symptoms are more generalized. They're with you most of the time no matter the blood or brain sugar levels. They don't appear because of any drastic fall in circulating sugar or surges of counter-regulatory hormones. They're mainly due to the total-body metabolic fatigue from so many fluctuations. Headaches are felt low in the front, suggesting sinus problems, or sometimes they feel like a contracting rubber crown wrapped circumferentially around the head. Fatigue, irritability, nervousness, flushing, impaired memory and concentration, tight muscles, abdominal pain, bloating, excess gas, and diarrhea are part of the not-too-pretty chronic picture. This symptom complex isn't changed much by just eating, unlike the acute ones. Treatment requires a longer and more determined dietary effort.

If you're hypoglycemic, you have no choice but to follow our dietary advice. We discussed carbohydrate intolerance in the hypoglycemia chapter, but it bears repeating. Give the diet a try and see how it makes you feel. Reread chapter 5 and make a couple of copies of the diet. When you're first getting acquainted with its variations, keep one in your wallet and another taped to your refrigerator door. It might be best to slip one into your desk at work or even your car. Before you eat anything, make sure it's on the approved list. You can't afford mistakes. You must follow the diet perfectly for two months before you begin experimenting with off-list foods. Our diet is one of the few that will dependably control hypoglycemia

Remember—if you need to lose weight, you really belong on the strict diet. Your new behavior will provide striking rewards: You reduce weight and simultaneously battle hypoglycemia. Carbohydrate craving starts to ease in about ten to twelve days, and that makes it far easier to stick with it. You may not get all of the things you previously enjoyed, but at least you can eat all you want and never go hungry. Once you've shed the surplus baggage, you're free to add everything on the liberal diet.

If you're a normal-weight hypoglycemic, the liberal diet is for you. The strict diet won't control your blood sugar any faster or better. We repeat—the only reason for the strict diet is the energizing effects of weight loss for those who need it. We also stress that most fibromyalgics feel generally better by observing the carbohydrate restrictions using either diet. There's an inspiring boost in energy beginning about the fourth or fifth day, the brain fog lifts appreciably, and the irritable bowel eases greatly just a bit later. This applies to almost all fibromyalgics if they limit sugars and starches, even if they aren't carbohydrate intolerant or hypoglycemic.

If you're underweight, you may have some difficulty maintaining your precious pounds even on the liberal program. Eat as much volume of the foods that have been added on that diet as you can tolerate if your scale starts dipping into lower numbers. It's tough to correct hypoglycemia and not lose weight. But fruit, nuts, dairy products, sugar-free grains, and the higher-carb vegetables listed on the liberal diet are where you should concentrate. Even for you, dieting is still necessary for a couple of months. Hopefully, after that time you can eat more of the forbidden starches and thereby regain any lost weight.

> "I was experiencing intense GI symptoms which got worse. I couldn't eat and I lost 30–40 pounds, but not in a good way. Last summer after the fun up-this-end and down-that-end tests, my doctor said he felt it was the fibro all along and that other patients of his had experienced this also. I must say, eating the liberal HG diet did help. I have gained some of the weight back and am working on sticking to the diet combined with portion control. (I do better when the portions are smaller and more frequent.)"
>
> —*Sara, South Dakota*

You'll have to plan and brace yourself for your first visit to the grocery store. You're going to need more shopping time. You'll move at a snail's slide from space to space as you pause to read labels. Until you get the hang of the diet, give yourself the luxury of leisure study. In fact, let's do it really right! Carry a magnifying glass and a copy of the diet in your purse. Focus attentively on the "Foods to Avoid Strictly" listings. LOW-CARB on the label isn't enough. SUGAR-FREE isn't always accurate, either, because it may mean no added table sugar only. Lactose-free milk sounds like a good idea until you read the ingredients and realize it's sweetened with corn syrup. Remember, too, that you must avoid caffeine.

You may feel more tired and irritable for the first several days after you start ditching carbohydrates. You've been together for a long time, and they don't let you break the connection easily. It takes about one week before you glimpse a few rewards. Some of your symptoms begin to ease and, crocus-like, a bit of energy pops out through the snowed-under feeling. Within six to eight weeks, assuming you haven't cheated, you'll get most of the benefits the diet can provide.

MAP YOUR LUMPS AND BUMPS

"Mapping" is our term for the manual examination of a patient. It is used to find the lesions, the swollen tissues of fibromyalgia (spastic muscles, tendons, ligaments, and even joints). The findings are drawn on a printed caricature of the body. The size, shape, and location of each abnormality is depicted and shaded according to the degree of hardness. The system is used as a baseline for future, similar drawings to monitor the progress of treatment.

If your physician doesn't feel confident using the novel technique of mapping, you have a few alternatives. Ask for a referral to a physical therapist, chiropractor, or licensed massage therapist whom your doctor considers adept. Copies of your first and subsequent maps can be sent to the medical office for professional monitoring of your progress. Preferably, you'll visit someone who is at least somewhat familiar with fibromyalgia. It will take good hands to feel the lumps and bumps. Make a copy of our mapping system.

It's important that the examiner use the pads of the fingers as though smoothing out wrinkles in muscles and not dig into them, thereby creating ripples of flesh. We draw the size and location of lesions as we find them and press a bit harder or lighten up on the pen to illustrate the hardness of each lump. It's not mandatory for examiners to use our exact system. Variations can be introduced as long as the same examination will be conducted on all subsequent evaluations. It's of prime importance that would-be mapmakers record objective evidence only and illustrate nothing but swellings they can actually palpate. They shouldn't be swayed by subjective expressions of tenderness since dominant pain sites obscure others and therefore vary greatly from day to day. These rapid shifts would be totally unacceptable for making repeated comparisons. Individuals interested in viewing our method can purchase a videotape or DVD from the foundation by going to www.fibro myalgiatreatment.com.

In the unlikely event your doctor has no suggestions of potential mapmakers for you, ask your friends for someone they've used. Most hospitals have a staff of physiotherapists. Your orthopedist will know them or have someone in his or her own office. Most chiropractors now know the diagnosis of fibromyalgia and will either willingly do the job or use a massage therapist on their staffs. Local fibromyalgia support groups almost always keep lists of capable people. You can also post your needs on our Web site, www.fibromyalgiatreatment.com, and ask for help in your particular area. The online guaifenesin support group was created to help solve these and many other problems.

Go to your first appointment with a blank copy of the body map and give it to the professional who will do the examination. You can get it from this book, but it might be better to download it from the Web site so it is full size. You will also want a copy of the blank body map for your examination. This way, the experienced or novice mapper can quickly scan what you need done and make a reasonably similar search of your body. Do your best to obtain this kind of record.

The first map is very important and should be created before you begin guaifenesin. Such a baseline provides a startling reminder of what you were like and helps substantiate progress when comparing subsequent maps. If you've already taken the medication before being examined, mapping is still beneficial to ensure favorable progressions.

All of the professionals we mentioned are quite accomplished in palpating muscles and tendons. They know the feel of tissues and have only to make minor adjustments in their techniques to accurately sense the lumps and bumps of fibromyalgia. We happily allow anyone to copy the caricature we use for mapping purposes.

Now we really need your attention. Be you patient or practitioner, here's an extremely valuable clue—probably the most significant one in this book. Read this paragraph over and over again until you've mastered it. *If you had to choose only one muscle to make the diagnosis of fibromyalgia, you should immediately select the left thigh, the quadriceps muscle.* The name tips you off that it's a four-part muscle. The outside portion is called the vastus lateralis; the front is the rectus femoris. Patients should be checked lying back in the supine position. The examiner will invariably feel spasm (and may evoke considerable tenderness) in 100 percent of adult patients in these sites. We've found this so in more than four thousand consecutive untreated males or females. Equally fascinating, both of the structures clear completely within the first month on the proper guaifenesin dosage if there is no salicylate blockade. The right thigh is barely affected, and only in long-term patients. The difference between the two sides is striking.

When palpated, the lateralis segment is usually the most tender muscle of the body. The rectus is not as smoothly contracted; it's made up of four or five separate bundles of spasm. They feel firmer and progressively more tender going from the top down to just above the knee. There you have it: The diagnosis is easily confirmed by just examining one thigh, and success is assured when it clears.

You may have to take the lead with doctors. If you can only interest them in a minimal examination, plead that they feel the left thigh. Preach a bit if you must, but get them to palpate those muscle bundles to secure the diagnosis and, later, to monitor disease reversal. If the sites clear that first month, the dosage should be correct for the rest of the body as well. The more detailed mapping we recommend produces a very valuable baseline. At the beginning, we do a diligent, bodywide search, and then repeat the same examination on every patient every single visit. We rely on this process to see progress and also for early detection of salicylate blocking. When it comes to mapping: Do your best. Detailed is better by far, but a simple left thigh exam alone will give you valuable information. Once you have found your dose, if you are very careful not to block the guaifenesin, you can make do without remapping.

If someone other than your doctor maps you, make copies to insert into your medical files. Each successive one lets you compare and track the path of your pains. Your mapmaker can focus on the preceding sketch and sensitively palpate for even minor changes. It's highly encouraging for everyone involved to be able to look at serial drawings that visually document clearing. Barring permanent tissue injury, most of those graphic lumps and bumps should become just unpleasant memories. (Figure 6.1 shows a blank map.)

ELIMINATE ALL SOURCES OF SALICYLATES

Before you begin your guaifenesin, there remains one last crucial task. If you don't do it correctly, it will render all the previous steps useless. You must do a thorough search for salicylates in your medications and everything you use on your skin. Be extremely careful and check absolutely everything. Altogether too many physicians suggest that patients try guaifenesin for fibromyalgia and then tell them little or nothing about salicylates. We have repeatedly seen even what seems like minuscule amounts stop all progress dead in its tracks. The blockade caused by this chemical is overwhelmingly the number one reason for treatment failure. If you choose to ignore this warning, don't even attempt the protocol: *It won't work!*

You may want to get a big garbage bag and gather up everything in the house that you use on your body. Set aside some time when you won't be disturbed; sit down with a dictionary, the lists in this book, and carefully do your work. Keep a magnifying glass handy—the type on some packages is impossibly small! You'll end up with three defined piles: products you can continue using and ones you must toss out or bequeath to a grateful recipient. A third pile will contain all the products requiring more information. Those with incomplete descriptions such as "and other ingredients," or that list only "active ingredients," must be researched or dumped in the giveaway pile. Use no product in which you can't identify every ingredient. If you want to rescue any of these, you'll have to get on the Internet, go back to the store and look for complete packaging, or call the manufacturer. You *must* get a complete list of ingredients. Do not rely on the person at the other end of the phone's insistence that the product doesn't have salicylates. Too often you've reached a customer service representative who doesn't know that plants are a problem. Check every list with your own eyes.

You'll also have to go through all your medications. Include prescription and nonprescription medications such as pain relievers, wart removers, first-aid creams, dandruff shampoos, and skin treatments. Check both medications that you take orally and those you apply topically, which include nasal sprays, patches, eyedrops, and suppositories. Make sure none of them contains plant parts and extracts or salicylates by name. Don't skip past over-the-counter or prescription topical preparations such as cortisone, acne, and other dermatologic creams. Vitamins and supplements should invite your scrutiny. All herbal supplements, such as St. John's wort and ginseng, must be discarded. Anything with bioflavonoids needs to be replaced. Don't assume that compounded hormones such as estrogen and progesterone creams, melatonin, DHEA, or other medicinal wonders are clean—in fact, they may contain herbs. If these are topical compounds, you need to know the ingredients that make up the base. "Flavors" abound in many products and may go unlisted—hopefully, you have good taste buds! Mint must absolutely be avoided in any form, natural or synthetic. This includes menthol and camphor. Pharmacists, manufacturers, and Web sites can be very helpful. Here's a powerful hint: Distinguish everything as either vegetable, animal, or mineral. Only the vegetable products (botanicals) are dangerous.

Make sure you've checked every product in your bathroom. Mouthwashes, toothpastes, soaps, shampoos, conditioners, razors, shaving creams, deodorants, nasal sprays, lotions, toners, masks, ointments, suppositories, and acne medications are potential problems. Creams for relief of muscular pains usually contain menthol or methyl salicylate—the identical chemical that flavors both artificial and natural mint. If you've ever used

Patient: ______________________ Date: ______________

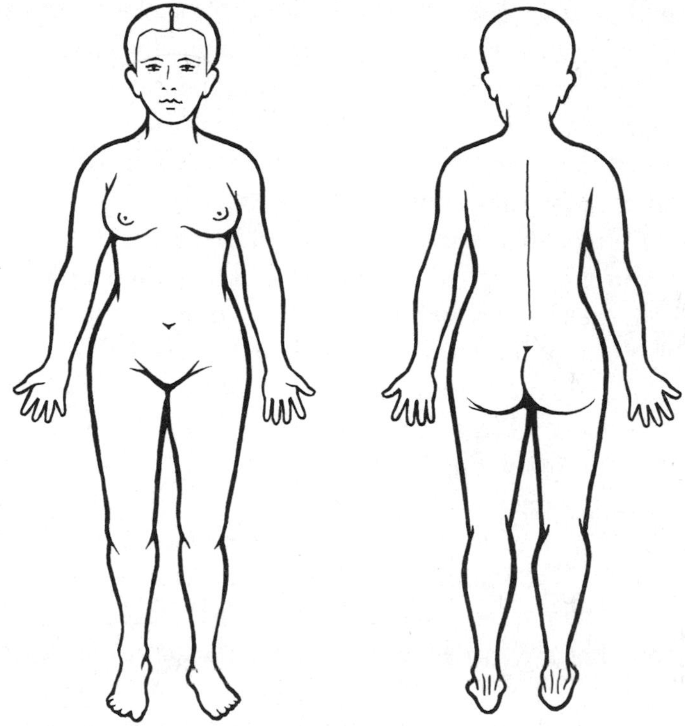

—FATIGUE
—IRRITABILITY
—NERVOUSNESS
—DEPRESSION
—INSOMNIA
—IMPAIRED MEMORY
—IMPAIRED CONCENTRATION
—ANXIETY
—SUGAR CRAVINGS
—SALT CRAVINGS
—SWEATING
—HUNGER TREMORS
—PALPITATIONS
—PANIC ATTACK
—FRONTAL HEADACHES
—OCCIPITAL HEADACHES
—DIZZINESS
—FAINTNESS
—BLURRING VISION
—IRRITATED EYES
—NASAL CONGESTION
—ABNORMAL TASTES
—RINGING EARS
—NUMBNESS
—RESTLESS LEGS
—LEG CRAMPS
—GAS
—BLOATING
—CONSTIPATION
—DIARRHEA
—DYSURIA
—PUNGENT URINE
—BLADDER INFECTIONS
—WEIGHT CHANGES
—BRITTLE NAILS
—ITCHING
—RASHES
—HIVES
—NEURODERMATITIS
—GROWING PAINS
—VULVODYNIA
—PAINS

Figure 6.1

any of them, you'll recall how your skin tingles immediately after application. That's how fast salicylate is sucked into your skin. Imagine how that's speeded up through the thin membranes of the mouth when you use minted (peppermint, spearmint, and wintergreen) mouthwashes, gum, toothpastes, and dental hygiene products. Look even in your first-aid kit for some of the plant derivatives, especially aloe.

Don't forget that your garden is full of natural salicylates. While you can touch their intact surfaces when arranging flowers or the like, be careful when they exude their sticky contents. Let's shout it once more: All plants make salicylates. Year after year, we're on summer alert, since we know that a bunch of our patients will garden. They sometimes forget to wear gloves, or use the wrong kind. Cloth ones are the worst since they become soiled within a few minutes. Salicylates even gradually soak into leather and penetrate your sweaty, open-pored hands. If you dislike working with heavier gloves, try the thin ones doctors use. There are many gardening gloves available now that are made from new materials and that form a tight waterproof seal. Whichever kind you use, make sure they're handy and that you use them every time. Some patients have blocked guaifenesin by simply walking barefoot in grass or wearing sandals that admit tiny blades of grass—effectively grinding salicylate into the receptive dermis.

BEGIN TAKING GUAIFENESIN

As we stated earlier, guaifenesin is no longer a prescription drug. You can get it in various strengths: 200, 300, 400, 600, and 1,200 mg tablets. We've mostly worked with the long-acting 600 mg form, but any kind will do if you take the right amount of a quality product.

Long-acting guaifenesin has a sustained twelve-hour action. We instruct patients to take it twice a day. Short-acting tablets or encapsulated powders are effective for four or five hours. They're more rapidly absorbed, stimulate the kidneys faster, and fade out more quickly, but they're also successful on a twice-daily schedule. Several of our high-dose patients have done well by using a combination of short- and long-acting drugs. The patented release system in the 600 mg tablet by Adams Labs, Mucinex, is a combination fast- and slow-release formula. It's the most expensive as well.

Some short-acting tablets or powders come in poorly sealed capsules or are sold in bulk, so that patients must stuff gelatin capsules as a do-it-yourself money-saving scheme. Based on problems we've seen, we are leery of this process: For good reason, medications are manufactured and stored in carefully climate-controlled factories and labs. Doing it yourself seems a risky proposition, because continued exposure to air will rapidly change the texture and thus can alter the potency of guaifenesin. It's also evident that tablets are only as good as the powder from which they were pressed, so make your best effort to ensure that your guaifenesin is fresh and from a reputable manufacturer.

It's difficult for us to recommend one company over another and ignore perfectly good manufacturers. We have become aware that some formulas contain additives that may be problematic for patients. Hypoglycemics may have trouble with maltodextrin as a filler. Chemically sensitive patients may want to avoid dyes and saccharin. Thus, it may require some checking to find a suitable product. Our Web site, www.fibromyalgiatreatment.com, lists all the formulas we have tested and includes all inactive ingredients for each one.

Powders should be pressed into tablets or inserted and sealed into capsules using well-tested equipment within a few months of production. Once that's been done, the protective outer shells seem highly secure and guarantee nearly full strength for several years. Patient mapping ensures improvement and, obviously, the potency of the drug being used. Our Web site will continue to monitor products and guaifenesin producers using the only laboratory we've got: reports of healing by patients.

Find Your Dose

We urge you to be systematic and hold your dose amount for the specified time, even if you believe that it is not the correct dosage. It will prove much easier for you and your medical adviser if you stick exactly with our outline. Trust us, it's much harder to find a maintenance dosage if you're not initially methodical about establishing your basic requirements. Tempting as it may be to bounce it up and down according to how you feel or you think you should feel, don't do it! You'll otherwise succeed only in confusing yourself and anyone who's trying to help you. You'll soon learn you can't often outguess professionals and other experienced people, especially by adopting tricks like looking at the color of your urine.

Lots of uniformed persons will brashly rush in with suggestions. You may get advice from other patients who think they're expert though they've only handled their first case: their own! Ignore what's contrary to the following paragraphs. We're going to spell it out as we've learned it from the past ten thousand or so patients. In the early reversal period, mapping provides a perfect directional signal. But if you're in solo flight or uncertain about the quality of your mapper and so are winging it alone, following our suggested flight path will lead you to a healthy landing. Keep away from guessing games if you possibly can. This book and the support group at our Web site are there to guide you. Please don't hesitate to consult member-experts who know the protocol and enforce it as written.

When you begin taking guaifenesin, focus your poorly concentrated, fibromyalgic brain as best you can on what's happening. You don't need elaborate paper minutes. Use a calendar and scribble just a couple of words—enough to jog your memory when you need to look back at what you've been through. It's tempting to rate days on a scale of one to ten for all symptoms, especially pain. That seems like a good system in the beginning, but eventually you'll realize that these numbers become progressively more difficult to compare. Keep notations simple: for instance, *bad, good, lousy, horrible,* or *so-so.* In retrospect, you'll be able to decipher patterns etched by *worse, better,* and *good* days. Other possible entries might read: "headache half day," "neck very sore," "more energy AM," "back better," or "shoulder stopped hurting." All of these will help guide a professional if you retain one. Once you're experiencing runs of several good weeks, amnesia sets in. It's difficult to accurately equate today's knee pain with the severity of last year's headaches. Fatigue is still fatigue, but is it less? Down the line, worse days may be considerably better than were the good days before you started treatment. Simple, straightforward entries are best.

As mentioned earlier, guaifenesin is no longer on prescription and is available in many sizes and dosages. We've used 600 mg tablets over the years and still do so with increasing exceptions. Since we begin patients with 300 mg twice daily, our protocol requires breaking tablets in half. Some drug labels caution against doing so, but for our purposes it's perfectly fine. No harm's done if someone prefers less for whatever reason. If you're concerned about your past sensitivity to medications, you can certainly begin with small amounts, but don't waste too much time at such levels. What we've suggested is a very small dosage for guaifenesin. It's regularly prescribed at 1,200 mg twice per day when it's being used for its intended purposes: mucous release and liquefaction. If you're using the 400 mg fast-acting tablets (Pro Health or Solo Guai), you would start at 200 mg twice a day.

You should hold your beginning dosage for just one week. If you become distinctly worse, you've likely found your correct personal dosage; this small amount is sufficient for only 20 percent of patients. Please remember, almost all of you will get recognizably worse when you meet your basic needs. If you're already tired, you may become exhausted; if you ache, you'll hurt more. Symptoms that were mild or barely noticeable may suddenly demand your attention. Briefly symptoms reverse much faster than they set in, so you could sense some entirely new ones. What was gentle could now be harsh; what was soft, hard. Never doubt that there were underlying problems that lurked below your levels of perception. The speed of tissue clearing often accelerates above that level and now races into your awareness.

If you don't feel distinctly worse during this first week, we recommend doubling up to 600 mg twice a day, for a total of 1,200 mg. (With 400 mg tablets, you would go to one and a half tablets twice a day, or 1,200 mg.) If this is your dose, you'll likely notice an exacerbation of symptoms within seven to ten days. Most readers will find this dosage sufficient: 80 percent of patients reverse at this level. In any case, you should hold there for a full month before challenging your dosage. If you still haven't noticed an exacerbation of symptoms, either you're one of the unfortunate 20 percent who needs more, or you're blocking. How do you figure this one out? Do you raise the dose again? Yes, if you're sure there are no blockers, you should proceed to the next step. Assuming that you've been perfect with the protocol, you now start taking 1,800 mg daily. (That's Paul St. Amand's dosage: 1,200 mg in the morning and 600 at night.) You don't have to split the tablet or try to remember a midday dose. You've now reached an amount that guarantees a 90 percent success rate.

If you keep at 1,800 mg a day for another month and nothing changes—you have neither worse nor better days—you've got to suspect blocking. Because success is so high at 1,800 mg, it's time for a thorough search. We ask our patients to "bag their groceries" and bring us all their topicals and supplements for staff inspection. We can only offer faraway people the online support group to guide them through the maze.

If nothing evil turns up and our patients' maps haven't changed, we again raise the dosage. At this point we combine long- and short-acting compounds unless the patient is using Mucinex. For those taking a 600 mg long-acting dose, we add a short-acting 400 mg AM and PM dose. Those on a pure short-acting dose should purchase Mucinex or long-acting compounded guaifenesin to supplement it.

The majority of people find their cycling dosage with relative ease. They get worse and they get better. They forge ahead, whether slowly or quickly, and soon learn the direction of their recovery. By now you've guessed that it's not so simple for everyone. A small number of patients, possibly 5 percent, will have barely perceptible symptoms during reversing. They erroneously think they have to get hammered with pain when they reach healing levels. For them, it's not so. If mapping is not available, this group will probably continue raising their dosages to unnecessary levels in a quest for dramatic reversal symptoms. There is no real downside to this error (except expense), and patients who push up the dose do get well at accelerated rates. We should also mention that a very small group of patients feel better for the first few days after beginning guaifenesin and start to cycle a bit later. That's the reason we hold patients at certain dosages for a designated time. Until a blood test appears for fibromyalgia, mapping is all that we've got to determine the state of affairs. This is why we so highly recommend mapping for anyone who can find talented hands. (See figure 6.2.)

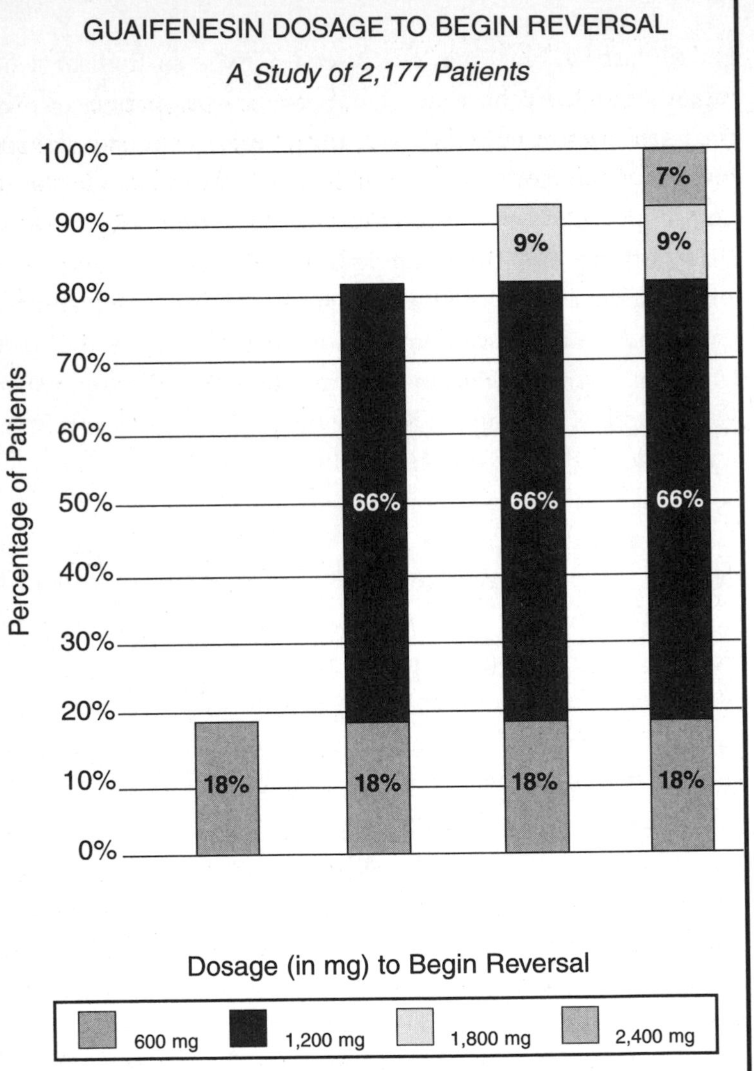
GUAIFENESIN DOSAGE TO BEGIN REVERSAL
A Study of 2,177 Patients
Percentage of Patients
100%
90%
80%
70%
60%
50%
40%
30%
20%
10%
0%
18%
18%
66%
18%
66%
9%
18%
66%
9%
7%
Dosage (in mg) to Begin Reversal
600 mg
1,200 mg
1,800 mg
2,400 mg

Figure 6.2

Remapping on Guaifenesin

When you have your body remapped, it's always best to revisit the same person who did your initial exam and uses the same technique to ensure that the maps are comparable. Certain tissues clear the easiest and soon entirely disappear. At various times during treatment, remapping still remains important since improvement creates changes that become progressively more subtle. When only a few areas remain to be purged, tiny cleansing sites are more difficult to quantify. This especially applies to the late retreat of tendons and ligaments. Because these structures have more marginal blood supplies, the effects of guaifenesin are delayed. The trained hands of a qualified mapper will detect subtleties that others could easily miss.

In our office, we ask returning patients to relate their observations and any untoward symptoms. We map them at every visit. After we've determined their dosage, we stretch out times between appointments to whatever seems appropriate. Lumps and bumps should get progressively smaller, softer, or more mobile. Some of the larger areas, such as those at the hips or tops of the shoulders, may split into one or two smaller areas. We hide all previous maps and refer to them only after completing the new one. This is the best and most objective procedure we can suggest to track fibromyalgia reversal. You and your mapping professional should agree on the frequency of examinations—whatever scheduling makes you both comfortable.

Don't overlook a very important fact: Until very late in the reversal phases, maps may quickly detect salicylate blocking. Once a map shows improvement, any regressions or new lesions are obvious. Eventually, blocked patients are alerted when they start feeling worse, but a map will confirm this early in the process. Their added complaints seem justified when a deteriorating map confronts us. The sooner they report in, the

These maps show results in a 39-year-old woman who has been on guaifenesin 600 mg bid. She was initially seen and mapped on November 7, 1995, but did not begin treatment until May 14, 1996. The results you see, therefore, are the effect of medication over a span of 10 months (from May 14, 1996 to March 11, 1997).

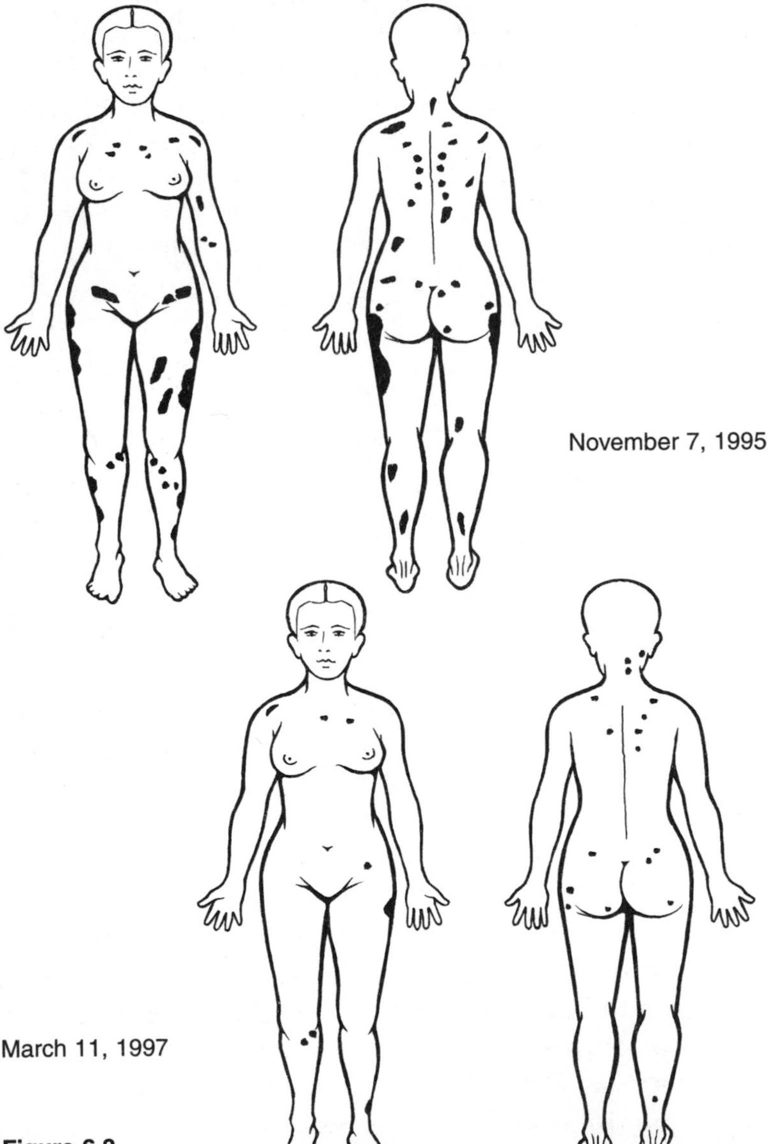

Figure 6.3

quicker we can recheck products and discuss the type of guaifenesin they are taking. We've used this system for many years, and thanks to our astute patients, it's how we've detected most of the more hidden sources of salicylates. (Figure 6.3 shows maps of a patient before and after starting treatment.)

Eventually, most patients ask how long they should continue taking guaifenesin. Once symptoms are gone, many patients are tempted to stop. The answer to this question is simple: Guaifenesin only works while you're using it. The genetic defect that causes the illness is unchanged by taking medication, so your symptoms will return if you stop taking it. The illness probably won't reappear all at once or overnight, but come it will! In time, a better medication will surely be discovered. But for now, rather dependably, the dosage that reversed you may be what you'll need even into the distant future.

If you increased your medication just to speed up the reversal, lowering your intake to the originally effective dosage is proper. But if you try dropping too far, below your therapeutic level, brace yourself for the gradual return of your complaints. There's no harm experimenting if you want to, since the reversing amounts were not all that carefully measured. Maybe now that you're well, you want to try to determine the precise, least amount that will get you by. Remember this: You could take one eighth of a tablet less than your fundamental requirements for the rest of your life and you'll very slowly get worse. Ineffective amounts just aren't enough! If you feel scientifically inclined to use yourself as a living laboratory, remain alert and try to spot the earliest clues that your symptoms are resurfacing. There's no sense in letting the illness gain full ascendancy when it is easily headed off by resuming your proper dosage of guaifenesin.

One patient advises:

> "Just do the protocol. Let time pass and stick it out. Don't worry so much about whether it is working or not working.

Let time pass. Nobody gets well from guaifenesin in a week or even a month. If you have been sick for a long time, which it seems most of us have, then it takes time to get well. Time. Quit watching the clock and live each day to the degree that you can. Try to think of something other than illness. Let the guai work. I was constantly tempted to raise [my dosage]. Did I? No. For me it was better to not think so much. I just tried to live. I concentrated and had faith that if others could get well on this protocol, I could too. . . . It is a path of stealth health. You just wake up one morning, and there you are."

—Gloria, Florida

Part II

Distinguishing the Many Faces of Fibromyalgia

Part I of this book provides a sweeping overview of fibromyalgia. We've given you some of the historical background and experiences that led to our current method of treatment. We touched upon the medications we used in the early years, and explained how we found guaifenesin. We went through the details of the theory behind our approach, explained what we think goes wrong in fibromyalgia, and told you how you can fix it. We hope that in the process we gave you a solid explanation for your symptoms and validated the reason for all of your complaints.

Now we're going to delve into a little more detail. We want to focus on your symptoms, explore the causes, and give you some ideas about how to handle them. In the process, we will cluster them together to structure syndromes simply for convenience and easy reference. We're aware that this creates an artificial set of divisions and suggests a series of different diseases. Please don't be led astray. All you feel is related and fundamentally interconnected. We ask that you keep this in mind when reading through this section. We've also included quotes from other patients who've shared their experiences at various stages of reversal. As you'd expect, we've included mostly favorable statements, but believe us, they're the norm and not the exceptions.

Chapter 7

The Brain Symptoms: Chronic Fatigue and Fibrofog

> "Problems processing things is a huge part of our disease. I had to give up a very lucrative career as an analyst because I just couldn't think the way I needed to. And then I started making all the dumb errors that are so annoying (remote in the fridge, leaving the dog behind on her walk, getting off at the wrong exit, etc.)."
>
> —*Janet, Canada*

THE CEREBRAL CYCLES of fibromyalgia entered medical literature somewhat late in the game. You'll recall that descriptions of the older disease, fibrositis, made no mention of brain involvement. When this term was replaced with the name *fibromyalgia*, problems with gray matter were still overlooked in the official description of the illness. Fairly rapidly, however, academic researchers began connecting the physical pains and brain aberrations as facets of one disease. About that time, a few psychiatrists bravely took a defiant counterstance against their colleagues and flatly stated that the mental disturbances were not psychologically based. In 1996, when Devin Starlanyl wrote her landmark book, *Fibromyalgia and Chronic Myofascial Pain Syndrome: A Survival Manual*, she unhesitatingly described the toll the disease had taken on her energy and cognitive abilities.

The overall change in medical attitude was very refreshing for patients who had been repeatedly embarrassed by past *it's-all-in-your-head* verdicts. Yet it did nothing to help them understand the illness or to offer relief of symptoms. One author summed it up. "Fibromyalgia was often considered to be a manifestation of hysteria and was equated with psychogenic rheumatism in the 1950s and '60s. However, with recent controlled studies it became evident that patients with this syndrome had uniform, stable and reproducible symptoms and signs rather than the bizarre and changeable symptoms of hysteria."[1]

> "I lose trains of thought and action, blank out frequently for brief periods, ride emotional waves of hope and despair, struggle to make my brain function with clarity, suffer memory loss (sometimes total, sometimes recoverable with help), cannot make sense of small print and complex reading, cannot keep my place in following a recipe or shopping list, struggle with almost total frustration trying to organize information/tools/tasks, do not take in what I am reading or almost instantly forget what I have just read, have to proofread what I write several times, and still miss errors, am easily distracted and so on. . . . Certainly stress, overdoing it, too many distractions, and fatigue increase my mental disabilities, just as they increase all of my other FMS symptoms."
>
> —*Virginia, Texas*

There's no longer any doubt that "brain cycles" are disturbingly intense parts of fibromyalgia. Ask anyone who has the disease: They dependably appear when the rest of the body goes under attack. Like any of the other symptoms, they can last for days, weeks, or months, depending on how long you've had the illness. Most of the time, when pain levels ease, the brain clears remarkably well.

The central nervous system symptoms include depression, fatigue, irritability, impaired memory and concentration (scattered mind), apathy, nonrestorative sleep independent from insomnia, nervousness, and the brain-disconnected-from-body sensation. For most of us, the cognitive problems and fatigue are the most overwhelming. They're easily the equal of pain in their negative impact on the quality of life, and many patients consider them distressingly worse.

Table 7.1
Central Nervous System

	Male Patients	% Male	Female Patients	% Female
Number of patients	310		2,176	
Fatigue		95%		97%
Irritability		87%		88%
Nervousness		70%		76%
Depression		79%		86%
Insomnia		83%		89%
Impaired concentration		82%		86%
Impaired memory		84%		90%
Anxiety		70%		75%

CHRONIC FATIGUE SYNDROME—FIBROFATIGUE

"My biggest symptoms are fatigue and exhaustion. It has not been unusual to go to the store and be there for a bit and suddenly feel like a big syringe sucked out all my energy. I would immediately have to sit down or go to the car and lie down. When I had a job sometimes I would close my office and lie down. Sometimes I can feel it coming on but other times suddenly I will just become weak. I don't have a lot of pain like the kind I've heard others describe. For that I am thankful, because I can manage with OTC pain medications. My next set of symptoms come and go but do hamper my life quite a bit. Brain fog, nausea (at times to the point of throwing up), dizziness, and rare panic attacks."

—*Heather, Texas*

Forty-five years ago when I began working with the disease now named fibromyalgia, I was struck by how many people had the same symptoms. Often enough to keep me on my toes, however, there was considerable individual variability. We speak in medicine of the "chief complaint," which is the single worst symptom that brings a patient to us. Many complained bitterly about the intense, widespread pain they were experiencing. Others launched into a series of descriptive words trying to make me grasp how severe was their continuous and numbing fatigue. Yet most of the time, there was that inexorable duet, both pain and exhaustion. In the end, it didn't much matter which of their complaints had brought these people to my office; when I examined them, they all had the same widely scattered, easily palpable lumps and bumps in muscles, tendons, and ligaments. All I had to do was connect those physical findings together with the roster of symptoms patients provided to finally convince me this was a single, big, bad disease!

Nowadays medical literature abounds with well-detailed studies of both fibromyalgia and chronic fatigue syndrome. Many physicians believe they are the same illness. We've treated more than ten thousand patients in these categories, and we can assertively say that we've never seen a case of pure chronic fatigue syndrome. Notwithstanding the variations in history, body mapping reliably ties complaints to physical changes and amply satisfies the criteria of fibromyalgia. Fatigue is the dominant complaint of people with high pain thresholds. Carefully questioned, they relate the symptoms of irritable bowel, bladder or vulvar pain, and musculoskeletal complaints, however minor they may seem. The worst map we ever created was of a woman who swore she had no pain at all, only mild stiffness. Later she admitted that she had dental work and delivered babies without anesthesia. While most patients have a combination of pain and fatigue, some lie at opposite ends of the bell-shaped curve and experience very little else.

Most patients suffer daytime drowsiness that's nevertheless accompanied by nocturnal sleeplessness. Even in healthy people, insomnia results in impaired mental function. Fibromyalgics may or may not get to sleep easily, but most of them awaken frequently throughout the night. That's even more likely to happen with more intense pain cycles. There just aren't enough comfortable spots left on the mattress. When these symptoms occur on sequential nights, patients are sorely tempted to increase their dosage of sleeping medications. Adding hangover effects to an already exhausted body and brain further hinders next-day mental clarity. Sleep deprivation isn't the fundamental cause of fibromyalgia, but it certainly doesn't help.

> "Exhaustion has always been a major problem for me. Especially the past six months or so, I've been in the habit of taking some form of natural energy boosters (ginseng, guarana, etc.) for at least the past 10 years. Since I'm on guaifenesin, I can't do that anymore, so I'm now having a very hard time making it through each day. Sometimes I think I feel good, and then go to the grocery store, and after five minutes feel like I have walked five miles. Sometimes I have to rest my head on my desk or my hands, and take a little 'nap' at work. I have a high tolerance for pain, but also for medications. My body just

laughs at OTC stuff. I even have to take double what most people do for prescription drugs, so I mostly just have to deal with the pain on my own, unless it is so bad I can't walk, write, etc. I think exhaustion is a big part of FMS, and that we all have to endure it. For me it is always there, even when the pain isn't."

Progress report—a few months later:

"As an update, I am so much better it's unreal. I'm on 600 mg/day of guaifenesin now, am working 40 [or more] hours a week, and even take the stairs at work! I still have a bad day now and then (one or two a month), but my progress is so amazing, my doctor has started other patients he has with fibromyalgia on what he calls 'the Tisdale Therapy.' He says I'm his poster child for fibromyalgia. But between the guai and changing all my medications around (I finally got off Prozac after 10 years!), I've lost the bluish color in my hands, I don't sweat all the time now, and overall, I feel pretty normal. My doctor says he's amazed at the difference from when I walked into his office last April."

—*Sherry L., Georgia*

The omnipresent fatigue of fibromyalgia is scary enough, but it becomes terrifying during flare-ups when concentration and memory vanish. Together they create the perfect profile of the early stages of Alzheimer's disease. To say the least, it's a bit difficult to combat this trio, especially when you add to them irritability, nervousness, depression, apathy, and surges of anxiety. If you can indulge yourself with a nap, you can improve a bit, but an intended short doze might easily extend into lifelessness for several hours, which makes it even more difficult to sleep at night. Exhaustion puts you to sleep on the couch despite the blaring TV. Unfortunately, that wreaks further havoc with your internal clock. You might almost hate going to bed early when you know you'll be just as tired the next morning and you are facing the pain of your nightly muscular thrashing.

The good news is that guaifenesin will reverse the fatigue and insomnia of fibromyalgia. They will yield to the same cyclic purging as the rest of your body. Eventually, fewer and fewer days of exhaustion will hound you; the positive rewards are startling. There will be energy to fit your lifestyle and enough left over for your social enjoyment. At first these will appear as isolated hours, half days, and then single days. A glimmer of hope of what lies ahead is enough to keep most people on the protocol. If you are like the rest of us, you will never forget your first energized day.

In the meantime, what can you do about the combination of fatigue and poor sleep patterns that plague fibromyalgics? These are so prevalent that at one time they were thought to be at the very center of the malfunction that causes the disease. There are pharmaceuticals to help you, of course, and those will be discussed later, in chapter 14. But the problem with this solution is that sleeping medications make you tired and diminish mental clarity. Should you use them every night? No. Are they acceptable occasionally when you absolutely need them? Yes. But that doesn't solve the every-night problem.

The first thing that helps sleep is exercise. Getting some during the day will ease stiffness, increase the right kind of fatigue, and even help clear your mind. Endorphin release will cause drowsy, pleasurable feelings, and exercise promotes that. So will pleasant thoughts and peaceful meditation, funny movies or enjoyable activities. Do anything you can to relax your muscles and mind—mild stretching to beautiful music, for example, done early in the evening might help considerably. Comfortable mattresses, dark rooms, and few distractions are also helpful. Some patients derive a great deal of help from sound machines at night. These muffle outside noise and can make your bedroom more peaceful.

Frustrations of Fibrofog

> "These bad periods creep up. You think you are handling everything and then the pain starts to increase and suddenly you are in a panic. . . . When the pain starts, I think I can still continue doing what I have been doing. What creeps up on me is the brain confusion. I get so frustrated trying to sort out the simplest things, until I give up and then I get depressed.
>
> "How do I handle it? Recognizing it for what it is comes first. Then I just have to let go of everything I don't have to do, and keep things very simple, rest a lot, baby myself. Get a massage, physical therapy, pool therapy for pain, or take whatever medications help.
>
> "It is interesting for me to watch this cycle towards depression and see how it is based on brain dysfunction and expectations. The mood swings go with the cycling too. . . . You can't expect too much of yourself when you don't feel well. Your brain is just trying to tell you that."
>
> —*L. N., Massachusetts*

Physicians who treat fibromyalgia regularly hear "I can stand pain, but I need a brain." Someone other than us aptly coined the term *fibrofog.* Combining patient descriptions makes it sound like a deep overcast full of heavy toxins that prevent brain–body interactions. Equally disconcerting, it renders them partially unresponsive to the rest of the world. So bad is short-term memory that it's not uncommon for patients to forget something they've just been told. Sense of place and direction can be sadly disrupted. How many of us have lost our way home and suddenly awakened in a strange location? You forget what you're doing midtask and what you're saying midsentence. Reasoning and deduction may range from difficult to impossible; math becomes a challenge even with calculator in hand. Patients seemingly read without seeing the words—

and why bother anyhow if you can't absorb the material, follow a plot, or remember the characters? Words stumble out of mouths in strange sequences as though letters were glued together. They may be frequently misspelled or look wrong even when they're correctly written. Patients may pick up dictionaries for assistance, but during bad fibrofog, they might have no conception of letter sequences, let alone remembering the alphabet. Names are interchanged and children become each other; *floor* may become *desk*.

Put yourself in the shoes of family members who are forced to play hide-and-seek with various items. Where in blazes are the car keys? For that matter, where's the car? Where did you leave your purse or did you donate it to some charity? Are the groceries out there fermenting in the trunk? The corollary: Patients can't see what they're looking at directly. What's the point of looking for something when you know it won't be there? Patients forget to pay bills, honor appointments, and meet friends; some have even left their kids stranded at school waiting for the delinquent parental chauffeur. Inability to count on your own brain is demoralizing and doesn't do much for irritability, nervousness, anxiety, and sense of isolation. Go through just a few such experiences and you'll understand why we won't even bother to define *fibro-frustration.*

During brain cycles, it's common especially for female patients to express oversensitivity to sounds, lights, odors, and other external stimuli. Women already have more highly tuned senses; now the intensity gets kicked up an octave. Ordinary TV sounds may cause severe discomfort; fluorescent lighting can be intolerable, and even expensive perfume can cause nausea. Not too surprisingly, all the modalities may also induce headaches. These symptom combinations have erroneously led some doctors to look for strange allergies or chemical sensitivities. Many patients go though extensive testing in an attempt to uncover unusual responses to the environment. Patients are quick to tell us, "It's not the chemical I touch; it's the odor that gets me." In our experience, as patients improve, these symptoms usually recede along with all of the other expressions of a totally upset metabolism.

It's up to you, the patient, to learn the skills to cope with fibrofog. Understanding its nature and fundamental cause certainly helps anxiety and, in turn, fibro-frustration. With reversal, cycles of cognitive impairment become more bearable. Still, certain maneuvers provide a little comfort in the meantime. You can ease the fear of forgetting something important and of not being able to rely on your memory.

- Practice being methodical, so that it becomes second nature. Convince yourself to put things in the same place every time. For example, car keys should have their own peg by the door. If you work at always putting them there, eventually you'll do it automatically. Mailbox keys, glasses, unpaid bills, mail needing responses, shopping lists should all have special, designated places. No matter how exhausted you are, every time you hold any of those things, go to the given site and properly hang or file it.

- Post a big calendar in a prominent place—say, on your refrigerator—preferably close to the phone. Write down every appointment the minute you make it. Every morning and every night, be sure to check what's written there. Do it at two specific times: just before you go to bed and when you have your morning coffee. If you're afraid you'll forget something during the day, hang a note where you're sure to see it.

- Make a list of what you have to do. Then train yourself to check the list routinely several times a day. When you get up in the morning, scrutinize it carefully. Each time you complete a task, cross it off immediately—if you wait, you may not remember having completed the chore. Never leave the house without checking your list of things to do. When you go out, take a copy with you; you know how often you forget to do certain errands.

• Keep a pad and a pen near the phone and make sure you leave them there. Don't walk off with them. When you take a message, write it down and do it right now! When the fog is exceptionally bad, you should probably make notes even while you're talking. You may even have to scribble the name of the person to whom you're speaking. Keep the notes concise but meaningful so that you'll grasp what you were trying to recall.

• Post notes somewhere and everywhere. Many patients tell us they can't imagine what they did before Post-its, those little papers with the sticky edges. Some patients hang notes reminding them to turn off lights, lock doors, water plants, remember shopping items, children's school schedules, and even the time when their kids should go to practice dancing, music, or a sport. You might even buy one of those small clipboards that attaches to your dashboard so that you can write memos when you're in your car.

• Make lists to take to appointments. When meeting with a teacher, boss, repairman, or client, prepare notes of pertinent topics. If you have a doctor's appointment, itemize your questions and concerns before you leave home. We usually allocate enough time per patient, but we can get frustrated when, as we try to walk out of the examining room, we're stopped multiple times with an "Oh, Doctor, I forgot . . ." Jot down short phrases to remind you of the answers you've been given. Do the same when you're in meetings at your children's schools or when making arrangements with family and friends. Whenever you speak with someone at a business such as your insurance company, get the name of the person to whom you spoke. These maneuvers will save you embarrassing phone calls and the frustration of trying to find the right person to refresh your faulty memory.

• If you're in a severe fibrofog, limit your driving. Run one errand at a time. Save complicated ones for when you're feeling better. If you drive, turn off the radio to help you concentrate on that single task. It may not seem polite, but plead with your passengers and children to keep as quiet as possible. If your children get noisy and confuse or distract you, pull over and firmly restate the situation. Use surface streets whenever possible. Missing freeway exits and going far out of your way is certain to increase fibro-frustration. And of course, avoid talking on the phone while driving: Clearly, even so-called normal people don't perform that duet too well!

• At home and at work, decrease sensory inputs as much as possible. Many patients find they absolutely can't function well with even minor distractions. For good, fibromyalgic reasons, they lose the ability to tune them out or relegate them to the background. Turn off music while you're working. During a bad cycle, even the most soothing sounds can put some of you into overload after a while. Filter out noise by closing doors of the room where you're working. Allow yourself to concentrate in silence.

• Start working on projects early. Plan on some work taking you twice as long as usual. Don't fight it. In adverse moments, your ability to absorb information is impaired. If the task at hand is impossible for the moment, give it up and try later. Sometimes you have no alternative but to take a break from that clammy little sweat that signals frustration is setting in.

Mood Swings (Fibroflux)

> "There are days like today when I feel as if my ears could explode. Every single noise is so intensified. I have to walk around with either ear plugs or fingers in my ears. My husband

just does not get it. It takes every bit of energy I have to go about the day without going into a nervous breakdown."

—*Tracy, Washington*

The most horrifying facets of brain cycling are the sweeping mood swings. For the most part, patients are acutely aware of them but feel powerless to exercise control. Anger, frustration, fear, depression, and self-pity can attack with great intensity then disappear in a matter of minutes. Unfortunately, their negative effects linger on. How do you retract some of the horrible things you've just said? How will your spouse, friends, or family members retract what they said in response? Female patients often cry buckets with minimal upsets; both sexes can become uncontrollably angry at the slightest provocation.

The best way to cope with your mood swings is to recognize that you have them when you don't. On a calmer, better day, you might want to talk to your spouse and children. Explain that these emotional outbursts are triggered by the stress of being ill. You can tell them that you are sorry for the past times they have been hurt and hope that in the future they will understand when it happens again. Reminding everyone of this every so often isn't a bad idea, either. When you are in the throes of an outburst or pity-party, you may sense that something is off but not be able to admit it. So do your confessing in retrospect when you are more in control.

Meditation and warm showers or baths are other things you can do when you start to feel emotional. Both can take you away from everyday stresses. If it's possible, use the old strategy of counting to ten or taking a walk. Removing yourself from a problem before it starts isn't always feasible, but once you practice the technique it will get easier. When you feel the situation slipping from your grasp, get in the habit of saying, "I will stop now and try to deal with this later." Life will be a lot calmer.

Recognize that all these cognitive impairments and emotional overreactions are a normal part of fibromyalgia, experienced to some degree by all those who suffer from the disease. Be patient and understanding but not too forgiving of yourself. Apologize when you've said something unfortunate in anger or overreacted to minor provocations. We may understand why it happened, but it's not so apparent to the person at whom you directed your fire. Remember to laugh when your fibrofog causes you to do something funny. Everyone agrees that laughter is therapeutic. It also has a way of bringing people together.

> "Your book has probably saved my relationship with my husband from dying a slow death because my husband whom I love dearly started to believe the doctor (the only doctor he went to visit with me) who didn't even examine me but looked at my account of my medical history, appeared amused and pushed a heavy antidepressant at me. My husband being an analytical and fact-based thinker is reading parts of your book and is at last coming around to believing his soulmate once again."
>
> —*Jean, Illinois*

Chapter 8

Musculoskeletal Syndrome

"I am feeling trapped by this new world of pain right now. I feel pain in my hands, arms, feet, ankles, and back. I feel my resistance to pain is especially low and that I feel especially beaten by it. I think to get control of the pain I need to get control of the stress and grief. The medications I have been on are just not working for this low point. I feel in a metaphorical sense that the pain is a prison. It makes the stress worse and the stress makes the pain worse."

—*Camilla, Michigan*

MUSCLES, TENDONS, AND ligaments combine efforts to keep us erect as bipeds, motor us to our destinations, and, not least of all, help us raise food, prepare it, and carry it to our tables. They're also involved in the digestion and elimination of nutrients, and even play a role in reproduction. They're the largest structures of the body and outweigh the skeleton. They're constantly supporting, pulling, yanking—and in fibromyalgia they hurt! Muscles and their cohorts, tendons and ligaments, are dedicated to physical work. They never get the downtime and the relative rest enjoyed by bladders, stomachs, and fingernails. These hardest-working tissues are the first to be affected by fibromyalgia.

Table 8.1
Musculoskeletal System

	Male Patients	% Male	Female Patients	% Female
Number of patients	310		2,176	
Numbness		76%		80%
Restless legs		62%		67%
Leg cramps		59%		70%
Pain		99.7%		99%
Growing pains		41%		47%

If you've had fibromyalgia for a few years, you probably find it hard to believe that there's a distinct muscle type that's first affected. It's also hard to imagine that there's a predictable sequence (though not always perfect) to the order in which the muscles will become involved. Both statements are true. We'll present some supportive evidence in the pediatric chapter, and there's even more detail in our book *What Your Doctor May* Not *Tell You About Fibromyalgia Fatigue*. Let's do a superficial summary here, anyway.

There are two fundamental types of muscle fiber. Careful scrutiny reveals subgroups, but we'll stick with the duo so we don't get bogged down in detail or technicalities. Most animals, including humans, have red (type I) and white meat (type II). The colored strands are most germane to our discussion and the ones mostly distressed in fibromyalgia. Muscles are rarely made up of only one color fiber to the exclusion of the other. Oddly, in the distribution of these fibers, the left side of the body is slightly different from the right. The same muscle on alternate sides may have more type I or II fibers. The differences in composition alter function. Stranger still, handedness makes only a little difference in certain muscle groups. Why do we know all this? It's because of what we said in the previous paragraph. Some muscles are hit much sooner and even one side more often than the other. We'll explore all of this shortly, but let's dwell on fiber types a little longer.

In this discussion, we'll largely ignore white meat. Its fibers are built for speed and designed for short-lived action. They never have sufficient energy for the long haul, but they're great for sprints. Fibromyalgia barely glances at them; it fixates on a far better prospect. Red meat is that color because it has a much richer blood supply. It contains many more mitochondria because it needs to make energy for sustained action. That tells us something—as you'll recall, these little powerhouses convert foodstuff to ATP, or energy. Type I fibers are hard-working muscle components that have to function well to ensure our survival. They are literally our strongest supporters, the hold-you-up and balance muscles. Workaholics, they turn us from side to side and shuffle our arms and legs from uncomfortable to comfortable positions all night long.

Aerobic workouts such as running and distance walking develop red fibers, whereas anaerobic, resistance exercises such as weight lifting produce more white fibers. You can see why pain and fatigue are so prominent in fibromyalgia. It's a disease with red overtones, right smack in the heart of our most productive energy factories. Selected muscles are the first to suffer from ATP deficiencies and, for safety reasons, will linger in a partially contracted state. Calcium promotes this sort of hibernation trance because it can't escape the precise site where it does its duty and keeps goading the muscle to work. There's a pump designed to move calcium out of the inner part of cells, and allow relaxation. You've probably guessed the problem: In fibromyalgia, there's not enough available ATP to work the pump.

We have a very extensive outline depicting what percentage

of the time any given muscle, left and right, will be involved by the time we see a new patient. We gleaned our data from body maps of two hundred adult female patients. This compilation was extracted using some early and some advanced patients to provide us a rough average, somewhere at the mid-course of fibromyalgia. The children's group of 187 maps was equally revealing since we had a few two-year-olds, with the rest scattered up to our cutoff age, sixteen. We learned not only which muscles would most likely be affected at discovery but also which are the first to demonstrate lesions.

We found the left side of the neck, shoulder, and in-between-shoulder-blade muscles swollen in 96 percent of kids; 84 percent on the right. The inside and outside of the elbows were involved in all children we examined. That's where you or a professional should look for fibromyalgic muscles. It's that easy—or is it? Those neck and shoulder (sternomastoid and trapezius) muscles are telltale signs for tots who don't have very many other defective sites. The older they get, the more muscles, tendons, and ligaments will develop swollen segments. These findings are also regularly present in adults, but these tissues are early arrivals and have consequently been sitting there the longest time. The neck, top of the shoulder, and upper back are great places to look for fibromyalgia. Nevertheless, we can present far better ones to confirm the diagnosis in postadolescent fibromyalgics.

We've stressed it elsewhere but because it's so important to us, here we go again. The most significant and diagnostic muscle group in anyone past age sixteen is the left thigh, the quadriceps muscle. It's involved in 100 percent of adults both on the outside and the front. The lateral part is quite regularly very tender even using only moderate digital pressure. It's the portion we call the vastus lateralis. The front of the thigh, the rectus femoris, is less sensitive except in the lower reaches just above the knee; it's not structured to contract in a long, smooth band like the outer thigh and is made up of distinctly separated bundles. Since the left quadriceps is always involved, it's mandatory to check it out on every new patient. You can depend on its being affected. Remember, in follow-up examination, tenderness in the left quadriceps should have completely cleared within one month when taking guaifenesin in proper dosage and completely avoiding salicylates.

Assuming that the history fits snugly with fibromyalgia, can a would-be mapper ignore checking anywhere except the sites we've just described? This notion does offer a tempting shortcut—but once the thigh has reversed, what would remain for follow-up? The answer is simple: More extensive mapping is needed to collect a variety of other, more swollen places. The more thorough the discovery effort, the more tissue will be available for future monitoring. Sequential mapping can then assure ongoing recovery as lumps vanish along with a patient's symptoms.

We can't ignore the many connecting ropes of the body. There are two main types. Tendons blend with partner muscles, and hook onto bones at the other end. Ligaments, on the other hand, connect bone to bone. We find these two structures deeply involved all over the body. They are full partners with affected muscles in causing most of the pains of fibromyalgia. We urge examiners to roll their fingers over the cord-like structures and feel for unusual hardness and, particularly, for swollen segments. Patients respond during this search by noting considerable tenderness.

Let's point out just a few places where those members of the musculoskeletal system are usually ignored or misdiagnosed. Pain from the deltoid tendon on the outside of the shoulder, most often the right, is sometimes attributed to the rotator cuff. Inguinal ligaments connect the front part of the hip bone to the pubic bone. The outer portion is almost always swollen, especially in women. It produces pain across the lowest part of the abdomen by constantly pulling and irritating where it splays across the pubic bone. If doctors fail to put their hands on that ligament and examine it for swelling, they'll erroneously suspect ovarian or bladder problems. The peroneus muscle is on the outside of the lower leg; it begins at the outer knee and goes all the way to the foot. It curls around the ankle and joins another muscle to create a tendon that hooks into the top of the arch. The right one is almost always more affected by fibromyalgia than the left. They both visibly swell just below the ankle bone and make everyone conclude there is water retention. The sole of the foot is more commonly involved than not. Invariably, doctors say the pain is due to "plantar fasciitis" when it's actually due to a swollen tendon. Structural abnormalities described in this paragraph are easily felt and swelling appreciated with just a bit of practice. Simply palpating them and realizing what they're contributing to the pain of fibromyalgia saves a lot of anguish and investigative costs.

FIBROMYALGIA AND OSTEOARTHRITIS

What is generally accepted as fibromyalgia is only the beginning of a long, miserable progression that ultimately leads to osteoarthritis. This isn't the kind that causes crippling deformities, though it can certainly damage joints sufficiently to require knee or hip replacement. Most people accept aches and stiffness as a normal part of growing older, so osteoarthritis is considered "wear-and-tear arthritis" and natural for the elderly. Don't you believe it!

When we see patients for the first time, we take a thorough history and ask about their past. We try to determine if their parents and grandparents had similar symptoms suggesting fibromyalgia, or had known arthritis. If we're lucky, one of these family members accompanies the younger and can speak for him- or herself. When we list the symptoms in order to check them off on our sheet, quite often the older relative will answer also. Most of the time they end by saying "and now I've got osteoarthritis" (*osteo* is from *os*, the Latin word for "bone"). They describe X-ray findings that showed the spurs and degenerative bone changes that are required as part of this diagnosis. (Please remember that we're not alluding to joints damaged in accidents. Known as traumatic arthritis, this issue involves only the areas that were injured.)

It's quite striking how the fibromyalgic body manages to avoid damage to essential organs. There's never cell death or muscular wasting (atrophy) and no accompanying nerve damage. Kidneys perform normally except for the relatively small metabolic error our theory proposes. The liver remains completely functional, and the heart continues pumping blood. The brain thinks, remembers, and still directs traffic, although some cognitive function may be erratic in the presence of fibrofog. Cuts still heal, and the immune system remains capable of fighting disease, though perhaps a little reluctantly. Not so with the joints. The prevailing medical opinion holds that fibromyalgia is a nonarticular (nonjoint) disease, but we strongly differ. They're frequently involved early in the disease, but it takes years before damage becomes perceptible to a radiologist on an X-ray.

The problem is that as fibromyalgia progresses, something has to give. It's logical that as the body accepts punishment from fibromyalgia, it sacrifices less crucial functions. When it becomes necessary to deal with rising levels of phosphate, it's safer to load muscles with metabolic debris than it is to let them circulate in the bloodsteam or end up in more vital tissues. Data collected for our book on pediatric fibromyalgia revealed a pecking order of musculoskeletal involvement that underscored which tissues were most susceptible. It makes sense that there's a benefit in first attacking more expendable structures and preserving activity in more essential areas.

From birth, bones have accepted as much phosphate as their periodic growth status would allow. Once they can accept no more, tendons and ligaments are the next safest place. Even laden with a little excess mineral, they can still perform reasonably well because they are only called upon to perform limited and short contractions. Muscles are next in the reception line and finally step up to help by sharing some of the load. Collectively, they are ultimately distressed and flash messages from the ailing periphery to the brain pleading for relief. The already enfeebled central nervous system in turn capitulates, and energy and cognition vanish. By this point, most patients seek professional help.

The progression of fibromyalgia is not a jerky process where one tissue succumbs first and stops functioning. Instead, the system is fluid, and partial recoveries appear periodically. There are series of failures that eventually recruit more tissues. Meaningful work comes only in spurts, and in emergencies, involved areas may steal energy from others otherwise unaffected parts of the body. So at any given time, 25, 50, or 75 percent of the body may be struggling. A little extra rest or minimal-load exercise might improve percentages, but only briefly.

Muscles and bones, are collectively the largest structures in the body and have accepted much more than their fair share of the load. But when fibromyalgia's effects have exhausted muscles, bones, and other organs, it then targets the joints. Joints become the ultimate repository for calcium phosphate and the lesser amounts of other ions that are also in excess. Realistically, joints have an inexhaustible capacity and, once pressed into full service, will continue accepting deposits the rest of the fibromyalgic's life. Crystals actually form in these areas, whereas in other tissues, calcium and phosphate almost always remain in solution. Even one of these crystals represents an extremely large amount of calcium phosphate compared with the minuscule amount required to seriously disturb a cell's internal metabolism. Aspirated fluid from osteoarthritic joints consistently contains every kind of calcium phosphate crystal known to medicine. Such microscopic rocks abrade and irritate cartilage, ultimately leading to bony overgrowth, spurs, erosions, and irreparable destruction. Now at last, there is tangible and permanent damage to the body that cannot be reversed by guaifenesin. This is just another compelling argument for early diagnosis and treatment.

The fact that the body waits so long before resorting to this damaging scenario illustrates its long-fought and gallant attempt at damage control. Because joints have a huge capacity to accept these ions, the most essential organs such as the heart, brain, kidneys, and liver are forever spared damage from fibromyalgia. If we view the progression of our illness in this light, we're certainly fortunate that joints are so responsive. It's a good solution for a bad condition that still allows patients to stay alive, which, after all, is nature's highest priority. It may be uncomfortable and ultimately disabling, but it at least takes years to happen. By that time, nature assumes we'll have procreated, raised our young to maturity, and are fully expendable in a biological sense.

Our protocol really doesn't address osteoarthritis other than to lay out what we believe is the sequence that leads up to it. It's clear that damage begins with the first small crystals placed in a joint long before there are enough of them to show up on an X-ray. Patients generally complain for a number of years of pain before such a test validates their symptoms. Guaifenesin doesn't have any effect on the bones. It can't change their composition. Once they have been damaged, anti-inflammatory medications are the treatment until the damage becomes so severe that joint replacement surgery is the only option.

Many medications are given for muscle pain: Analgesic pain

pills, muscle relaxants, and nonsteroidal anti-inflammatories (NSAIDs) are the most common. Heat and ice are local modalities that often help, depending on the patient's preference. While most muscle balms (Tiger Balm, Aspercreme, Ben Gay, Zostrix) contain salicylates, lidocaine and patches and creams made with ketoprofen are acceptable. The little heat pads that can be applied directly to painful areas are not blockers. Massage and body work properly done with extreme gentleness may make symptoms manageable. Some studies have shown acupuncture helpful, as well as acupressure. Combining various modalities is generally a good idea until you find a combination that works. In this way, you're less reliant on medications and can avoid the escalation in both doses and side effects that becomes necessary over time.

Most fibromyalgics turn their back on the one thing that has consistently been shown to help musculoskeletal pain and stiffness: exercise. It is inexpensive, it has no enduring side effects, and it has never failed to show beneficial results in the many studies that have been done. Even a small amount can be very helpful. Unfortunately, we know that even this convincing lead-in won't change many minds, but we'll try anyway. Exercise in the form of gentle stretching can help painful muscles, tendons, and ligaments more than anything else. Movement will build more ATP-making power stations, and that will in turn increase energy production and stamina. For those with arthritis or severe back pain, water aerobics combine the cardiovascular benefits of walking with those of resistance or weight training because of the pressure exerted by the water. Exercise causes the body to produce endorphins, our own natural pain-relieving chemical. (It is to endorphin receptors that narcotic pain medications attach.)

With a chronically affected musculoskeleton, it's imperative that any exercise program begin slowly. A simple stretching tape that promotes a gentle workout can be purchased at a low cost. This sort of program can be worked into your schedule at a time that best suits you. Don't expect instant results; still, over time your confidence, strength, and energy will improve. Weakness and lack of stamina are two problems that plague fibromyalgics both while they are ill and when they're on the road to recovery. They are part of the deconditioning process imposed by the preceding period of inactivity. The disease certainly begins because of faulty ATP production, but it is worsened when a person becomes more sedentary, which leads to the destruction of what were once seemingly surplus mitochondria. Just like anyone else, fibromyalgics must exercise to become stronger.

> "There were days that at times turned into a week, when I was cycling so hard I couldn't exercise. Instead of feeling guilty I gave myself a break. Dr. St. Amand says that after two weeks of no exercise you pretty much lose what you've accomplished to that point. So I would discipline myself to do something as soon as I could. Many times I had to start over with very light exercise and build up to where I was before the hard cycling began. The secret is not comparing ourselves to the normal people around us that are exercising. Just do it no matter how insignificant it seems. Be patient. You will eventually see results. I have, and it's great!"
>
> —*Carol H., Texas*

Chapter 9

The Irritable Bowel Syndrome: Fibrogut

"I was never diagnosed with IBS until we arrived at the FMS and HG [hypoglycemia] diagnosis. Everything was a mystery. I had been plagued all my life with inexplicable stomach and intestinal pains, gas and bloating, alternating diarrhea and constipation. The most common medical advice was to 'relax' and take antacids. I have been on the hypoglycemia diet, alternating between strict and liberal versions, for almost a year. It only took a month for my IBS symptoms to improve once I knew how to diet properly."

—*Gwen, California*

SOME FIBROMYALGICS BEGIN their quest for diagnosis looking for an explanation for bothersome bowel symptoms. To them, their other problems are minor annoyances. In cases like these, physicians might understandably have difficulty in assessing a problem deeply hidden within the abdomen unless they're given sufficient patient history. For example, we see individuals who describe dull, steady aching in particular locations and considerable tenderness from just the light pressure of a hand. The small amount of information this provides gives very little evidence as to what's really going on inside. It hardly even tells us what testing might be appropriate. Luckily, patients can usually add a great deal of information when they are questioned properly. By the time we see them, we have the advantage of many past, negative test results that rule out most of the scary scenarios. Let's give you a typical history:

When a patient complains of persistent aching or fairly intense pain in the stomach or abdomen, the primary physician usually does a basic work-up, including an examination, X-rays, and standard blood tests. If pain is present predominantly in the area of the stomach, a special blood test for *Helicobacter pylori,* the bacterium responsible for stomach ulcers, will also be ordered.

If no abnormality is found, the patient is referred to a gastroenterologist. This specialist reviews the lab reports and other findings, and confirms that everything is functionally normal. There may be more tests ordered to eliminate the likelihood of celiac disease, a condition we can't adequately discuss here (it's not related to fibromyalgia). Next comes a manual examination; when that also produces no clue, an ultrasound examination might follow. That usually earns the tag "normal" for liver, pancreas, spleen, and gallbladder. Happy findings indeed, but since the symptoms persist, there's more testing to be done. This usually means an endoscopy of the esophagus, stomach, and upper part of the small intestine. Thoroughness demands a last indignity: a colonoscopy and exoneration of the colon. Our totally tested subject now has a complete, certified list of normal results. Well, so what is wrong? When no "serious" problem is uncovered, the final consultation ends with, "You've got irritable bowel syndrome." Here we go, another *syndrome!*

Ultrasound—High-frequency sound waves are passed by a transducer through the area of the body to be studied, to make an image of solid organs such as the liver. These waves cannot pass through bones or make images of gas.

Endoscopy—This procedure is done with a fiber-optic instrument enabling direct visual examination. A long, narrow tube is inserted through the mouth, down the back of the throat into the esophagus, down into the stomach and into the duodenum, the first part of the small intestine.

Colonoscopy—To examine the colon, a similar but longer endoscope (colonscope) is inserted rectally and passed upward. The doctor then withdraws it slowly, as each part of the intestine and rectum is examined. This procedure is usually done in a doctor's office or hospital "GI lab" with the patient mildly sedated. If only the lower portion of the colon is to be examined, a shorter instrument is used for a sigmoidoscopy.

That's all well and good, but where does that leave our poor patient? Comforting as it is to have a name given to an ailment and a reassuring diagnosis of something that isn't anything deadly, the next step isn't exactly clear. The suggested solutions—eating more fiber, and taking stool softeners and medications that reduce gas and diarrhea or cramping—may help, but what is this irritable bowel, and what can be done to get rid of it forever? What is the underlying cause?

Table 9.1
Irritable Bowel Syndrome

	Male Patients	% Male	Female Patients	% Female
Number of patients	310		2,176	
Nausea		38%		59%
Gas		65%		73%
Bloating		60%		75%
Constipation		47%		67%
Diarrhea		47%		60%

"IBS is one of the overlapping FMS and HG symptoms. I don't think it pays to debate whether it's from FMS alone or HG alone. Where does that get you? And what if you're wrong? If you just do the HG diet perfectly for a couple of weeks, and it helps, that answers your question. If you do the diet perfectly and there is no difference, then it could be just FMS, or it could be a side effect of a medication you're taking."

—*Anne Louise, Minnesota*

Specialists by definition tend to remain in the safety of their field of expertise. Discouraged by too few findings, they may not ask several pertinent questions that could reveal a much broader picture. Patients are often too intimidated or afraid of sounding like a hypochondriac to speak up. What about all of the other, total-body complaints? It's an important part of the process for the patient to speak up and ask questions. You're luckier now than ever before. Given the telltale symptom clues, many more specialists will now suggest that IBS is part of fibromyalgia. Yet too few will offer a healing solution.

Over the years, many other names have been used to describe IBS, including *spastic colon, mucous colitis,* and *functional bowel disease.* Recently, another name has crept into our medical jargon: *leaky gut syndrome.* We consider these simply synonyms for the same condition. Most of the alternative terms describe what physicians inaccurately believe causes the condition. For example, the term *colitis* means "inflammation of the colon." There's no such irritation in IBS. As in the other body tissues, nothing alters the system in a way to produce visible anatomical or measurable biochemical abnormalities. There's no test to confirm the diagnosis, once again; there's simply a collection of symptoms that appear together.

As in all other facets of fibromyalgia, women are affected by IBS in far greater numbers than are men. As you'd expect, just like other symptoms of the disease, intestinal complaints are usually worse premenstrually. The disease may begin at any age but quite surprisingly is very common in children and young adults. It is often the first dramatic symptom of the disease. Many adult patients recall recurring bouts of IBS during their school years.

> "Since my teenage years I have had stomach pain and cramping. . . . My general practitioner would say it was 'a little gastritis.' He would prescribe an antacid and send me home with a pat on the back. I suffered like this for about ten or twelve years. . . . I went to a very eminent gastroenterologist. . . . He pronounced 'irritable bowel syndrome.' When I asked him what I could do for it he said 'Nothing. Just stay away from green vegetables.' . . . I also experienced insomnia and some muscle pain since I was a teen. I had no idea they were all related to FMS. A few years ago the FMS came on with a vengeance, and after seeking a diagnosis for about nine months I finally found a doctor who told me I have FMS with gastroesophageal reflux."
>
> —*Marie, Nevada*

Sixty percent of the fibromyalgics we examine have IBS. As with other facets of our illness, there are many symptoms within the complex, and not all patients have every symptom. There could be intermittent difficulty in swallowing, and acid might reflux back up the esophagus from the stomach. That produces so-called heartburn, which is an acid-induced burning sensation. Such irritation may cause esophageal spasms and produce chest pain closely mimicking angina or a heart attack. We name this gastroesophageal reflux or GER. It is more common in overweight patients and occurs often at night. Waves of nausea sometimes appear out of nowhere. They can last for hours or for only a few seconds but often in frequent, repetitive waves. Gas and bloating are among the most common complaints, but just as high on the patient's list is frequent constipation alternating with diarrhea.

Certain specialists will, when confronted with these symptoms, administer a battery of allergy testing, resulting in a diagnosis of "multiple food sensitivities." The next step might be to confirm reactive skin findings with a series of very expensive blood tests. Though results may be correct in their assessment, very many patients tell us they have no problem when they eat the supposedly offending foods. Hearing this, we encourage them to do an eating test using a small amount of one "abnormal" item at a time and let their gastrointestinal tracts tell them if they really must avoid that food. Each can be tried in sequence; if sensitivity truly exists, symptoms should get decidedly worse. Only if this happens do they really have to stop eating that particular item. This is the true proof of sensitivity, because too often sensitive skin simply overreacts to foreign proteins in allergy tests.

Constipation and diarrhea can take turns in rapid shifts. It's also not unheard of to have one problem for months or years and suddenly have the other one enter the picture. This combination, but particularly recurrent diarrhea, may lead to stool testing for *Candida* (yeast) or parasites. Stool examinations are not for the novice technician. It takes the practiced eye of a skilled expert to avoid being deceived into thinking that certain food residues are cysts or parasites. It's especially difficult to avoid errors since a certain amount of yeast is normal in stool specimens. Repeatedly, patients have undergone many varieties of herbal purges, colonic cleansings, or heavy cathartic "washouts," all in the vain attempt to clean out something that was never there. Still others have spent months or years on antifungal (yeast) medications, such as Diflucan (fluconazole) or Mycostatin (nystatin), without experiencing a change in symptoms.

> "How does it feel physically? I described it to a friend this way: 'Imagine you are just recovering from a bad case of the stomach flu, where you're better but still shaky and not sure how loose your bowels still are. Now imagine you're going to try to carry on a normal life, and pretend you're fine. And imagine every day is like this.' It's hard, it's uncomfortable, and the emotional component is hard too. Cramping, urgency, a feeling of 'looseness,' burning pain in the lower back, nausea, acid reflux, shakiness, and weak knees. These are all symptoms I associate with IBS."
>
> —*R. A., California*

We feel strongly that fibromyalgia is a preeminent cause of IBS, along with undigested carbohydrate. Similar to the cells in the rest of the body, those of the gastrointestinal tract also suffer from energy deprivation. The three smooth muscle layers of the intestinal walls become dysfunctional, just as the skeletal muscle types do. The small intestine has the assigned task of churning and mixing nutritive elements with digestive juices. Such activity begins the breakdown of fats, protein, and carbohydrates into smaller components. Alternate contraction and relaxation of the intestinal wall propels raw materials to the next digestive station, where they submit to the action of various hormones and enzymes. The results are minuscule food particles that may now be assimilated and made ready for bodywide distribution. Quite likely, intestinal glands share in the general problem of fibromyalgia and, along with the musculature, are rendered inadequate for ideal digestive sequences. Nausea, gas, and bloating are disconcerting enough, but the ensuing constipation and diarrhea are more alarming. Like uncontrolled traffic signals, they switch from stop to go in prolonged cycles that greatly interfere with digestion as well as elimination. You can imagine the backing-up effect this has on the entire gastrointestinal tract: a serious malfunction that produces all of the symptoms of irritable bowel syndrome.

Foods are processed, broken down, and absorbed mainly in the small intestine. Here bile from the liver enters the picture and renders fats into microscopic digestible fragments. The pancreas also secretes its enzymes to help the body absorb these tiny fats. The colon (or large intestine) lies downstream, all six feet of it, and it also serves many functions. Its muscles and glands are similarly affected in fibromyalgia and therefore contribute to the irritable bowel syndrome. The main job here is to remove salts and water from what remains, and this process may take several days. For this reason, it's normal for bacteria to take up permanent abode in the colon, whereas the small intestine is normally free of such residents. These organisms use food residues for their own metabolic needs but, in the process, spin off items for our special benefit. As much as 20 percent of ingested carbohydrates reach the large intestine undigested. They're the main nutrition for certain bacteria that obviously thrive when abundantly fed. Unfortunately, they add great amounts of gas as they ferment sugar and starch residues. Gas can cause repetitive, sharp stabs of pain anywhere in the abdomen but mostly in the small intestine. It doesn't

Origins of Abdominal Pain

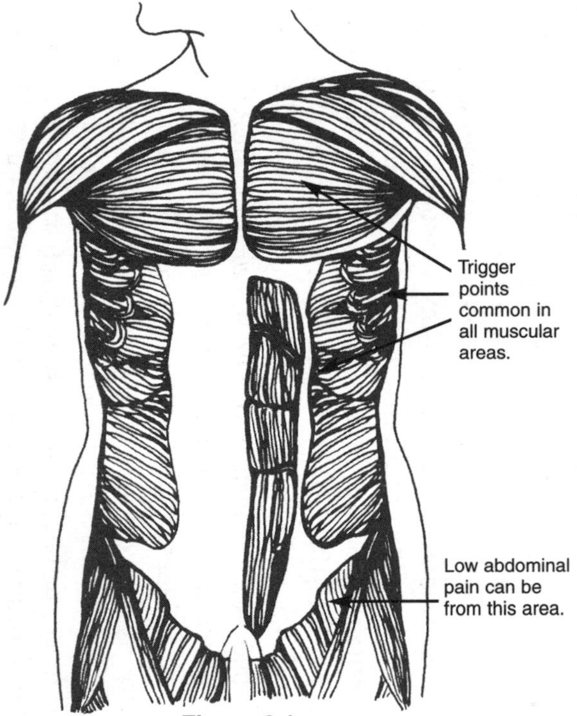
Trigger points common in all muscular areas.
Low abdominal pain can be from this area.

Figure 9.1

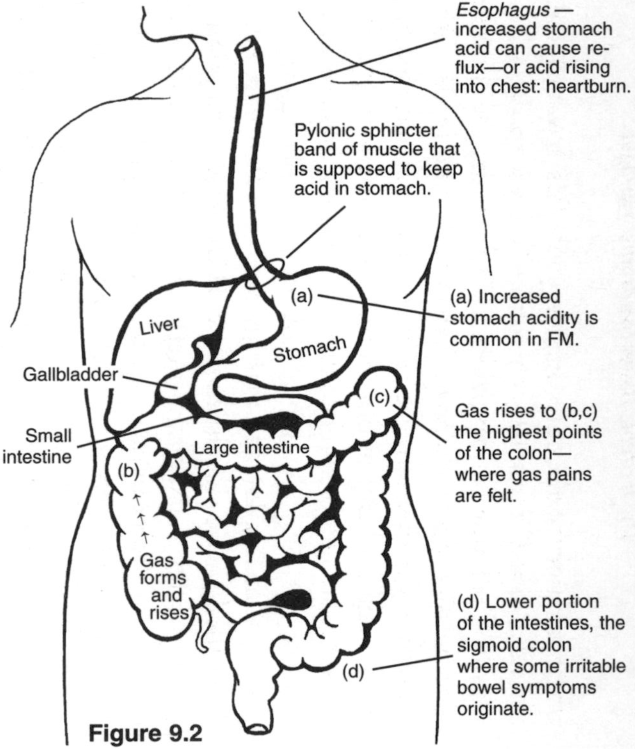
Esophagus — increased stomach acid can cause re-flux—or acid rising into chest: heartburn.
Pylonic sphincter band of muscle that is supposed to keep acid in stomach.
(a)
Liver
Stomach
(a) Increased stomach acidity is common in FM.
Gallbladder
(c)
Gas rises to (b,c) the highest points of the colon—where gas pains are felt.
Small intestine
Large intestine
(b)
Gas forms and rises
(d)
(d) Lower portion of the intestines, the sigmoid colon where some irritable bowel symptoms originate.

Figure 9.2

linger long there since it's quickly propelled forward and expelled into the much larger reception chambers of the colon. There, it encounters forceful contractions of more powerful muscles that shove the now hardening remnants toward the rectum. The large bowel gets distended from improvised collection sites where gas temporarily accumulates. The largest pockets are formed in the upper reaches since air rises to the highest point.

Gas produces an amazing variety of sounds, but it's nothing more than air that's temporarily trapped. Forced to accumulate because of constipation, it further dehydrates stools and makes them rock hard. This cemented food residue plugs up the rectal area and, like a dam, further prevents the elimination of gas. Pressure builds up behind this solid wall, and adds to the existing discomfort of bloating, nausea, and perhaps sour belching (acid reflux). This pressure also induces painful spasms mainly in the lower left side of the abdomen. Glands lining the colon react to surface damage by making slimy mucus just as the nasal and bronchial membranes do in response to irritation. The purpose of this mucus is to make the colon more slippery so that hard stools can slither out without causing further damage to the sigmoid (the lowest segment of the colon) or rectum. At times the longer, stained mucous strings take on the appearance of worms and lead to unnecessary studies. When constipation is bad, the cemented head of the bowel movement is often so hard and so slow to exit that it badly scratches the rectum. This causes bleeding and more pain. If encrusted food particles are embedded on the surface, the laceration may be deep enough to produce what is called in medical parlance a rectal fissure. Higher up, small pockets may extrude outward from the colon. Stool contents can push into them, attract infection, and induce diverticulitis. Rock-like stools can also push rectal veins ahead of them like an ocean wave. They may get inflamed, sandpapered, swollen, and clotted, making them recognizable as hemorrhoids. Any appearance of blood in the stool will also call for more testing to rule out a serious cause.

There are certain predictable sites where gas accumulates because of the way our intestines are structured. These are the areas where pain strikes. First is the lower right abdomen where air blasts out from the small intestine into the colon. Pressure builds in this area, and gas is later driven to the upper right abdomen near the edge of the liver. Cramps cut across the belly from right to left as gas is squeezed toward the highest place in the bowel, the left upper quadrant. A huge air pocket can form under the thin diaphragm muscle that pushes upward toward the heart. Sharp-stabbing or pressure pains reflected into the front of the chest can mimic a heart attack. You may ask, "Why doesn't gas move along with the stools that are forming?" The propulsive efforts of the intestinal muscles are a bit like grabbing a long, sausage-like balloon in the middle. The gas squeezes in both directions but, as soon you let go, it gushes back to the center. The result is repeated pains from the same gas bubble whether it lingers somewhere or rapidly shifts position.

Often, patients suffering from such gastrointestinal conditions are miserable and yearn for "comfort foods," the easily digested sugars and starches. Sixty percent of our fibromyalgics already crave sweets in a vain attempt to make energy, as we've discussed. But excessive carbohydrate consumption only makes things worse, promoting genetic tendencies toward hypoglycemia, weight gain, and diabetes. Repetitive releases of insulin force the liver to convert carbohydrate excesses to fat. Obesity is responsible for many health problems beyond the scope of this chapter, but it also adds to gastrointestinal misery. Heartburn and gastroesophageal reflux occur primarily in overweight patients.

Dull but steady, aching pains arising from the abdominal wall also provide a common diagnostic pitfall for doctor and patient. The ever-diligent physician completes the usually normal examination and testing, surveys the results, and ascribes the discomfort to IBS. Internal pain is not quite the same. It presents as cramping and gas-like, quite different from the surface aching induced by muscular spasm in the abdominal wall. The cause is actually the same contracted tissues of fibromyalgia that we see in other areas of the body. We try to identify this particular problem by asking patients to lie down and raise their heads off the pillow. This maneuver tenses the affected abdominal muscle more than it does normal ones. By comparing one side to the other, we can frequently palpate differences in tension. The feel of such contracted bundles is no different from that of any of the other findings in fibromyalgic tissue.

Another problem area is the inguinal ligaments. We discussed these in the previous chapter, but the subject bears repeating here. These double, parallel cords, one on each side of the groin, run from the pelvic bone in front of the hip to the pubic bone. The abdominal muscles form these ligaments as they curl around each other and make rope-like structures where they attach to the pubic bone. The other end is inserted deeply under the ribs. Together, they give you the leverage to do a sit-up. They're almost always involved in fibromyalgia and easily felt as swollen segments in their outermost halves. Steadily contracted day and night, they exert a steady pull on the muscles. Under the rib cage, spasm causes a constant, dull pain or a more intense charley horse. The innermost portion causes an unrelenting drag on the pubic area that gives the sensation of needing to urinate. However frequently the patient goes to the bathroom, though, nothing much comes out, and the sensation continues. Physicians seem reluctant to probe the groin even though they're not opposed to doing an in-depth, pelvic examination. If you have pelvic pain, ask your doctor to palpate those areas before submitting to an ultrasound or more invasive searches.

IBS symptoms are usually treated with an assortment of medications. Sometimes they help. With almost equal success, patients find partial relief with over-the-counter products such as antacids, cathartics, and gas-reducing agents. Often, especially when patients treat themselves, efforts are misdirected and totally bypass the underlying cause. This can occur because symptoms are confusing and changeable, evoking suspicions about yeast and parasites. Over-the-counter drugs are often added to prescription ones in a "shotgun" approach. Expensive digestive enzymes and cleansing compounds or even colonics are tossed into the mix. Costs rise as patients keep piling one drug on top of another to treat the original symptoms and then develop side effects from these first-line therapies. Adding this fistful of pills to those already used for sleep, nervousness, depression, and pain will help make their pharmacist's monthly car payments but also invites drug interactions.

More often than not, some irritable bowel symptoms are actually side effects of medications taken for other symptoms. Narcotics such as codeine, OxyContin, and morphine as well as muscle relaxants like Flexeril and Soma all cause constipation to some degree in nearly everyone who takes them. Antianxiety drugs such as Klonopin and Valium do the same. Many patients take over-the-counter magnesium because it is touted for fibromyalgia, but excesses may cause diarrhea. Constant use of laxatives is habit forming, and it is difficult to be patient and allow the body to resume normal function when they are stopped. We regularly observe that patients dread eliminating even one of their medications. What little benefit they've obtained from their drug armamentarium can't be risked; they suspect that their entire system will fall apart. Their concern is not ill founded: They're barely coping as is and have no emotional or physical reserves. They can't contemplate how they could survive even one more, however mild, aggravation. The following story is typical.

> "For the last ten years or so I have been diagnosed with everything from colitis to food allergies to systemic *Candida* infec-

tion because I have had so much trouble with diarrhea. Sometimes I would go for days with no bowel function and then out of the blue I'd have diarrhea. . . . I had constant painful intestinal gas that was very embarrassing because I could not control it. I was treated for colitis and then sprue or gluten intolerance. Neither of those treatments helped. Next, an allergist diagnosed me with intestinal yeast infections from antibiotics. He said I had developed food allergies from the yeast and put me on an antifungal drug called nystatin. That helped a little. The next doctor . . . did a two-year series of European allergy shots and gave me an even stronger drug for the yeast. [He] had me injecting myself with allergy shots two to three times a week and taking doses and potions of various things by mouth four times a day. My diet was very restricted, and my weight fell from 118 to 98 pounds. The doctor had me on a high-carbohydrate diet in a failed attempt at weight gain.

In desperation and prayer I turned to the Internet and found Dr. St. Amand's information. After comparing his description of hypoglycemia and IBS to my symptoms, I hoped I had found an answer. I dropped Dr. St. Amand and Claudia an e-mail. Dr. St. Amand assured me I was on the right track. Claudia helped me get started on the diet and told me what to do in the stormy early weeks, as my body fought to adjust to the new fuel. She promised after the first six weeks things would settle down. They did. The gas and diarrhea and other symptoms are gone now as long as I stay on the diet. . . . The good news is I can now eat anything on the HG diet and not have diarrhea or gas. I no longer look like a starved waif, having put on 14 pounds as well."

—*Gretchen, South Carolina*

Patients with irritable bowel syndrome often avoid intimate relationships, just as do those with vulvodynia and bladder dysfunction. All three of these conditions isolate the individual because of the personal nature of the affected areas. Most people suffer in silence and resist explaining their illness to others because it is so vague and embarrassing. The good news is that information services, self-help, and support groups exist. We've listed some of them in the Resources section in the back of this book.

TREATMENT FOR IBS

So how do we treat this irritable bowel syndrome? These are the two simplest paragraphs we've written in this entire chapter. Begin by eliminating all sugars and complex carbohydrates. You'll find the proper diet outlined in the hypoglycemia chapter and on our Web site. The diet is the same as for hypoglycemia except that you do not need to avoid caffeine. These dietary restrictions will be temporary for most of you. The diet alone will quickly eliminate 60 to 70 percent of your symptoms. Once you feel better, add one favorite food at a time beginning with anything but sugar, sweets, and heavy starches such as potatoes and pasta. Unsweetened grains, brown rice, and dairy products such as yogurt or sugar-free ice cream are where you should start this process. Promptly back off when the symptoms return, trusting them as reliable indicators that you've added too much, too fast, or too often. This hunt-and-peck system is really the only way to learn which foods and in what quantity you can tolerate them. The premenstrual week is the riskiest week of the month for resurrecting adverse effects. In time, you'll learn what you need to restrict on a permanent basis, if anything. You'll dependably evolve your own, personal program.

Symptoms may be handled with over-the-counter preparations quite effectively once you are on the diet and need them only occasionally. Phazyme should be used rather than Gas-X, which contains mint oil. Both charcoal and dimethicone products have shown to work quite well. Calcium carbonate antacids such as Rolaids, Mylanta, and Maalox are good choices for an upset stomach (because most women need supplemental calcium)—but only use the fruit flavors. Pepcid (famotidine) and other histamine blockers are now available in over-the-counter strengths and can help with pain from acidy stomachs. Prescription versions are still available if the weaker strengths prove inadequate. Prelief, another calcium formulation, will cut food acid when taken with meals. This is an excellent choice for women who also experience bladder burning when they eat the wrong food. Over-the-counter Imodium can help control cramping and diarrhea if you have a flare-up. Fiber will help with constipation when taken with an adequate amount of liquid, but should be added gradually or it will make things worse.

Be sure to stick with formulas that are sugar-free such as those made by Metamucil, Konsyl, or Citrucel. It's becoming increasing popular to use sugar alcohols such as orbital to ease constipation. This is not a good idea for fibroglycemics, because the actual effect of these sweeteners on blood sugar is unclear and may vary greatly from person to person. Magnesium as a stand-alone supplement can be titrated to help with constipation, and calcium compounds may squelch diarrhea.

Titrate—to determine the proper amount of medication needed for therapeutic action by gradually and systematically raising the dosage until the desired effect has occurred.

If you are taking antibiotics for any reason, you may want to add acidophilus, which can help maintain healthy flora in the digestive tract. It's an inexpensive insurance policy that can save you from an attack of diarrhea. Pressure arising from constipation can be felt in the lower part of the rectum, and can be effectively and safely relieved with inexpensive glycerine suppositories. Hemorrhoids may occur from the impacting stools. Beware of using topical preparations containing witch hazel or other plant extracts. A few days of an over-the-counter anti-inflammatory such as naproxen or ibuprofen may also help. One of the most effective modalities for constipation is good old-fashioned exercise. When you get moving, you'll often find that your bowels follow suit!

There are new prescription drugs on the market for IBS symptoms as well. Hopefully, you will not need to use these for long. Some patients actually get relief from diarrhea and some pain when taking tricyclic antidepressants. Unfortunately, side effects of these include dry mouth, fatigue, and weight gain. In June 2002, the FDA approved Zelnorm for IBS patients with constipation. It is a medication with dangerous side effects and should not be used as first-line therapy. Lotronex is another new drug that is aimed at IBS with diarrhea. It was withdrawn for a while because of questions about its safety. It is now back on the market but reserved only for serious cases and only for those for whom all other therapies have failed.

> "I have been on the HG diet for several years. It has helped me immensely in lots of different ways—however, it never helped my constipation. On average, I had a bowel movement once or twice a week. Obviously, this causes pain and bloating. At the end of a six week period on Zelnorm and ever since, I have almost daily bowel movements. No abdominal pain and no bloating. Zelnorm is designed to re-train the peristaltic reflex—something I don't believe just the HG diet can do for folks who have severe constipation (and a history of years of IBS). I believe that this is something definitely worth discussing with a physician."
>
> —*Judy, Floria*

Many other medications are currently used by physicians. Older tricyclics are often prescribed because of their relaxing effects on intestinal smooth muscles. Anticholinergic drugs also relax such muscles and ease cramping (Bentyl, Levsin). Librax has similar benefits, but contains a benzodiazepine that should be withdrawn only with caution. Serotonin-reuptake inhibitors may be helpful because they keep that neurotransmitter at higher, available levels. One study using one of these, Paxil, showed promise. Whereas 26 percent of patients were greatly improved by simply increasing fiber intake, 63 percent fared equally well by taking a small daily dose of that drug. Peri-Colace is both a stimulant and stool softener, a combination directed toward constipation. GER is sometimes resolved by weight loss, but until that's accomplished, a class of medications called proton pump inhibitors will prove effective. This group includes Protonix, Prevacid, Prilosec, and Nexium. True to their promise, they disable a pumping effect in acid-making cells and potently block production.

The remaining treatment format is equally simple. The steps you should follow are clearly defined in chapter 6. Basically, you must find your guaifenesin dosage and eliminate all blocking sources of salicylates—that's your job, and only you can do it! This entire book has been written for one purpose only: purging fibromyalgia and controlling the hypoglycemia that often accompanies it. Long before you picked up this book, many of you already suspected that interconnected symptoms were being erroneously separated to form so-called syndromes. We strongly advocate the use of only one medication and one diet for a sustainable control of all the symptoms of both those conditions.

WARNING

Irritable bowel syndrome and fibromyalgia do not cause a high fever or severe pain that is persistent. If you are experiencing these symptoms, with or without nausea, diarrhea, or constipation, see a doctor to rule out more dangerous conditions such as appendicitis or diverticulitis.

"I have had cycling IBS pretty bad the last couple of weeks. It has passed now and I am having the most amazing *normal* bowel motions. Sorry to sound gross but it is so wonderful when this happens and to just have one normal bowel motion a day! This happened a few months ago as well so I know I am improving in that department and can't wait for it to go away permanently. I must just say I have been cheating a small bit with chocolate lately and it hasn't made any difference, it would appear, to the IBS, which pleases me greatly."

—Gaye, New Zealand

Chapter 10

Genitourinary Syndrome

"The bladder thing was my most serious symptom and it was guai that allowed me to get off Elmiron, a depressing (literally) medication that controlled the bladder pain. Possibly I would have committed suicide because of bladder pain because it was so bad for years. Within a couple of months on guai I was mostly free. I still have a little blood in my urine sometimes and a tendency to feel bladder irritation but nothing like the intense pain of those years."

—*Hannah*

THE BLADDER, URETHRA, and vaginal tract share in producing some of the most overwhelming symptoms of fibromyalgia. They can induce oppressive feelings that totally overshadow brain, muscular, and intestinal complaints. This intensity leads patients to seek relief from urologists or gynecologists. Unfortunately, while most of these specialists administer local remedies, they fail to recognize the broader picture. In the end, because the underlying disease hasn't been treated, these initially helpful therapies fail. Fibromyalgia is not part of their field of expertise, and patient and physician become increasingly frustrated. Worse still, desperate patients will finally try anything with a ghost of a chance and all too often succumb to damaging topical applications or unrewarding surgeries that fail to live up to their promise and, worse, leave scar tissue behind.

Table 10.1
Genitourinary System

	Male Patients	% Male	Female Patients	% Female
Number of patients	310		2,176	
Dysuria		29%		33%
Pungent urine		38%		48%
Bladder infections		13%		67%
Vulvodynia		N/A		40%

BLADDER

Fifty percent of female fibromyalgics have a medical history that includes three or more bladder infections by the time we first see them. A few women tell us they've had fifty or more documented attacks and repeated episodes of painful urination when no infection was detected. Bladder complaints are quite uncommon in male patients, so a history of bladder infections may be even more significant.

Routine urinalysis, even in healthy individuals, often shows varieties of amorphous calcium crystals in combination with oxalate, phosphate, or carbonates. You'll recall that the entire body participates in trying to get rid of excessive phosphate. These acid particles are secreted through tears, saliva, sweat, vaginal fluids, and bowel excrements. This output is not negligible except when compared with what's excreted in the urine, which is the major dumping system.

Calcium and phosphate don't join together and crystallize inside cells. Instead, the two substances coexist in solution.

This effect is what you see when you drop salt in water: It immediately enters into solution, though the sodium and the chloride are both still there. As long as they're sufficiently diluted, they won't form particles. Phosphates leave the kidney in a dissolved state, but things change in the bladder, which is a reservoir that holds our liquid waste until sufficient volume needs to be voided. While waiting in the bladder, phosphate solidifies in combination with calcium, oxalate, or magnesium. The weight of these microscopic crystals causes them to sink to the base of the bladder and settle around the opening of the urethra. This is rather like the way that sand in a swimming pool gradually migrates to the deepest area around the drain. On urination, these particles are swept out and, like liquid sandpaper, abrade the delicate lining, the mucosa. If the scraping effect is sufficiently injurious, the integrity of the membrane is compromised and, once broken, allows bacterial penetration. The short female urethra—the tube that drains the contents of the bladder from the body—presents only a small distance for infectious agents to travel from where it exits the body, near the anus. Bacteria from the vagina, rectum, and skin find their way up the ureter and into the bladder to cause cystitis, bladder infections. It's for this basic anatomical reason that fibromyalgic women consequently suffer far more problems with their urinary tract than men. (See figure 10.1.)

Cystitis—Infection of the bladder. Symptoms include a constant urge to urinate, pain above the pubic bone, burning, searing urine, and, upon urination, producing only a small amount of urine. Antibiotics are commonly prescribed to treat the infection, as well as local analgesics that work on the urinary tract.

Mechanism of Bladder Infection or Irritation

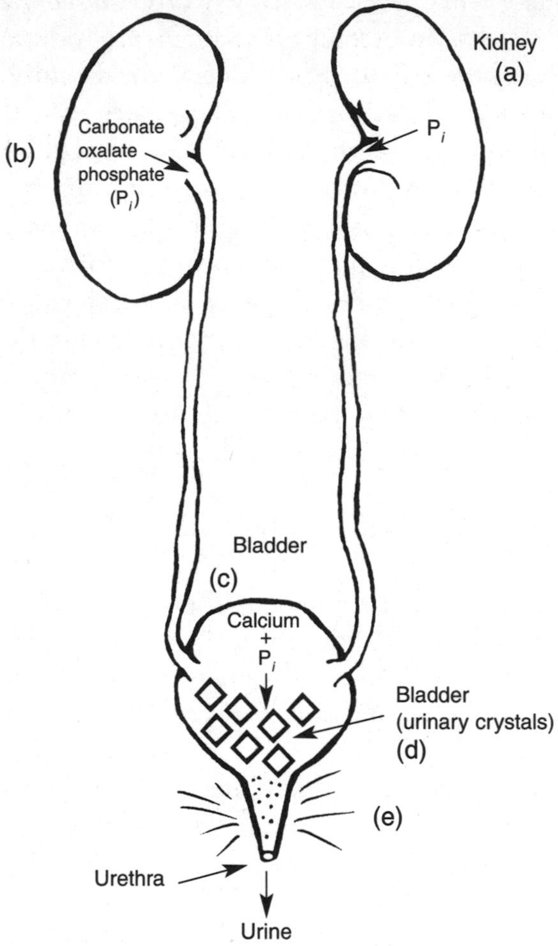

(a) Kidneys retain too much but eliminate some phosphate.
(b) Kidneys release oxalates and carbonates (*anions* that, like phosphates, have two negative charges).
(c) In the bladder the anions combine mostly with calcium (*cations* that, like magnesium, have two positive charges).
(d) The combining of cations and anions forms crystals that settle to the bottom of the bladder.
(e) At the next urination the crystals scrape the bladder neck and the urethra, exposing the lining to infection.

Figure 10.1

Under the same circumstances, intercourse is even more traumatic. Most women know about "honeymoon cystitis," which occurs during periods of heightened sexual activity. Pooled crystals damage the urethral and bladder walls from friction effects of penile strokes. Even the tougher vaginal lining is treated just as harshly and reacts like the bladder, as we'll discuss later when we get to that portion of the anatomy.

When bladder infections are recurrent, patients are sometimes given low-dose antibiotics for an entire year in an attempt to completely eradicate the problem. Sometimes burning urination (dysuria) appears for only a few hours or days and resolves spontaneously. The symptoms of urinary tract irritation with or without infection are frequent and create powerful urges that dribble only scanty amounts of urine without providing relief. If there's an infection, blood or pus is present either to the naked eye or, more often, only microscopically. Without a urine culture, even veteran patients are fooled into believing there's infection where none exists. Since prolonged use of antibiotics can cause diarrhea or vaginal yeast infections, a relatively inexpensive urinalysis is worth doing. It's cost effective in sparing complications from unnecessary antibacterial agents. Recent studies show that antibiotics such as levofloxacin can stamp out infections in shorter order, making them popular choices for faster results. Because infections can travel from the bladder up into the kidneys via the ureters, it's important to treat them promptly.

Eventually, repeated cycles of cystitis invite more thorough investigations by urologists. When multiple urinalyses fail to expose infection, they seek to uncover another villain by looking directly into the bladder (cystoscopy). That search almost always proves futile, so the physician resorts to a biopsy of the bladder wall. Frustration mounts if such specimens appear normal under microscopic scrutiny. Sometimes, small clusters of certain white blood cells are found and, though hardly conclusive, at least point to a possible diagnosis.

> "All my life I've had recurrent vaginitis. When I had a vaginal culture it sometimes came back *no Candida* (I used to wonder if the lab mixed up the cultures) and yet all this irritation and discomfort continued. I used to buy Monistat cream four at a time when they were on sale. My GP even suggested I might be allergic to my own menstrual flow (if you can believe that one) and also said I might be allergic to my husband's sperm (not very helpful). Now, 13 months on guai this pain is taking a bit of a break. I actually have days when I don't have it at all."
>
> —*Vera Lynne, Canada*

Those minimal and inconsequential findings or no abnormal findings earn a commonly offered diagnosis of "interstitial cystitis." There is no definitive test for IC, so the diagnosis is largely based on symptoms. These include steady hurting in pelvic, pubic, or lower abdominal areas and an urgency to urinate so strong that patients might void twenty or more times a day. Urine cultures are routinely negative. Rectal pain may be intensified by hard spasms in muscles lying between the vagina and rectum, the perineum. Decreased bladder capacity and painful intercourse are two other common complaints. A succinct description would be: It's like a ninth-month, never-terminating, pregnant-bladder condition. The diagnosis of interstitial cystitis is rarely offered to males and is often misdiagnosed as nonbacterial prostatitis, prostatodynia, or prostalgia. As of this writing, only about 10 percent of those diagnosed with IC are males. Men can suffer from the same symptoms as women but also may complain of scrotal or penis pain. If you've been diagnosed with IC, you are 10 to 12 percent more likely to have had childhood bladder problems.

Cystoscopy—A procedure done in a doctor's office, in which the urinary tract is viewed through a cystoscope inserted through the urethra and up into the bladder. Through this fiber-optic scope, the doctor can examine the lining and structure of these organs. A patient is usually given a local anesthetic or a mild tranquilizer to help with the discomfort.

Affected individuals have joined in support groups all over the world. It's estimated that some 450,000 are estimated to have interstitial cystitis in the United States, though the number that have actually been given a firm diagnosis is much lower. The average age at diagnosis is forty, about the same as for fibromyalgia. Both of the two large IC organizations, the ICN (the Interstitial Cystitis Network) and the ICA (the Interstitial Cystitis Association), are well aware of coexisting fibromyalgia in a large percent of their members. They now include information on fibromyalgia in their brochures and on their Web sites. From surveys conducted by the groups, fibromyalgia, irritable bowel syndrome, and vulvodynia are very common, concurrent conditions. Both the ICA and the ICN give out dietary suggestions and other hints for controlling symptoms.

The five most common dietary triggers for painful attacks are: cranberry juice, coffee, carbonated beverages, tomatoes, and tobacco. (According to IC researchers, those who continue to smoke after the diagnosis are simply adding to their own misery.) Vitamin C supplements can be a problem because of their acidic composition, even in the most buffered form. For this reason, daily requirements are better achieved through diet, including leafy green vegetables such as broccoli and cabbage. Although we're trained to believe orange juice is the number one source for this nutrient in the diet, the truth is that half a cup of red bell peppers, for example, provides the same amount as an orange. B_6 is another vitamin that may cause increased pain.

> *Insterstitial cystitis*—A disease defined by the absence of a positive test for other bladder conditions, manifested by bladder and pelvic pain and the constant urge to urinate, which produces only a small amount of urine.

Guaifenesin users may continue anesthetic medications such as Pyridium (generic and over-the-counter phenazopyridine hydrochloride) to numb the bladder. This medication is not designed to be used for long-term therapy, as it can build up in the body. It is to be used for acute attacks only. Partial relief can also be attained by neutralizing urine acidity by drinking half a teaspoon of baking soda in six ounces of water three times a day. Tablets are also available. A newer dietary supplement, Prelief (calcium glycerophosphate), achieves the same ends and can add to the daily requirement of calcium. In studies this substance, which is not a drug but a food additive, diminished some symptoms 70 percent. Cranberry juice or tablets are sometimes offered to prevent infection. Since they may actually increase urinary acidity, they should be avoided. However, the active chemical in cranberries that prevents infection, D-Mannose, can now be purchased separately in supplement form, and is safe to use. Other medications such as Urised and Prosed contain phenyl salicylate and are potent blockers of guaifenesin. As always, all medications for pain should be carefully checked for aspirin.

Current therapies for IC include bladder installations: various substances that are inserted into the bladder directly. These include DMSO, heparin, BCG, and the newest, Cystistat and some combination cocktails. Cystistat is a hyaluronic acid and in new studies has been shown to reduce symptoms by as much as 80 percent. The most commonly used oral medication is Elmiron (pentosan polysulfate), which provides a coating on the bladder lining and frequently eases some symptoms of IC without impediment to guaifenesin. Elavil and other tricyclic antidepressants partially cut pain perception and are often useful. No studies have been done on the newer compounds such as Zoloft or Paxil, which may or may not help. The tricylics have an action on smooth muscle that makes them useful for some patients with IC and IBS. Antihistamines are often included in a multipronged attack because they work on mast cells, which in IC release histamines and cause local pain and irritation. Atarax and Vistaril are the two most commonly used, but can cause drowsiness. Over-the-counter versions such as Benadryl at night may not only help sufferers sleep, but also provide the same assistance in subduing mast cells. Antispasmodics are sometimes used for bladder spasm: Ditropan and Levsin are two of these. For overactive bladder complaints, medications such as Detrol may be useful. However, they all have side effects, and the net worth may not amount to very much.

> "When you're having an attack, the constant pain . . . the fear of sex making more pain is debilitating. It weighs down your life, your lightness, destroys spontaneity, makes you standoffish with the man you love because you just don't want to have to explain you're having problems again. That part is bad, but the symptoms that you live with night and day are even worse: never sleeping through a night, having to sleep on the outside of every bed, always worrying whether there will be a bathroom close by, stopping often on car trips, dodging into fast-

food places, hoping they won't catch you not buying anything and telling you the rest room is only for customers."

—*C. C., California*

Guaifenesin eventually clears IC complaints, but they'll get initially worse like all the other symptoms of fibromyalgia. After the first several reversal attacks, future bouts become relatively minor and eventually disappear. It's prudent to fight back at the first signs of IC by drinking extra fluid, and using appropriate medications at the first hint of urinary burning. Prelief may be taken daily as a preventative measure, especially when traveling. Car and airplane rides are notorious triggers. It's far easier to abort an early onslaught than to subdue a well-established attack. Exercise, especially stretching, has also shown to be helpful in the long term. Beginning a fitness regime sooner rather than later, along with taking guaifenesin, will help restore normalcy.

VULVAR PAIN

"As senior gynecologist with special training and expertise in vulvar disease, I have been striving to help women with the enigmatic disorder called vulvodynia, and its most common subset, vulvar vestibulitis. In recent years there has been increasing appreciation of other conditions reported as commonly associated with vulvodynia, such as irritable bowel syndrome, fibromyalgia, and interstitial cystitis. In my own practice at Scripps Clinic and Research Foundation I've discovered that fibromyalgia is at least three times as common in vulvodynia patients as in the general population. I've also noted that vulvodynia tends not to respond to therapy until the underlying fibromyalgia is treated. . . . Dr. St. Amand has done ground-breaking work in the evaluation and treatment of fibromyalgia as opposed to medications that only reduce or help control symptoms. His research, and that of those who follow in his footsteps, will permit fibromyalgia to become merely a painful memory for patients and their spouses. I salute his effort."

—*John Willems, MD, FRCSC, FACOG, head, Division of Ob-Gyn, Scripps Clinic and Research Foundation, La Jolla, California*

Vulvodynia or vulvar pain syndrome—Severe pain, burning, and/or itching in the vulvar area (the vulva is the area of the female's external genitalia). This area is extremely sensitive to touch, and may or may not be red and visibly irritated. Vulvar vestibulitis syndrome (VVS) is less common, and applies to women who have pain only in the vestibule, a smaller area than the vulva.

All too many fibromyalgic women develop extreme sensitivity and irritation of the inner vaginal lips, known as vulvitis. The problem may penetrate deeper into the vaginal opening, where it's labeled vestibulitis, for the vestibule or opening to the vagina. Chronic burning and knife-like pain are often described, as is low abdominal pain. It can be intermittent, localized, or diffuse. In the past six years, we've tabulated the incidence of vulvodynia (or vulvar pain), as these two complaints are collectively known. Out of 3,465 consecutive new female patients, about 40 percent had pelvic complaints. In the early stages, pain may initiate only after intercourse, but later it will occur without apparent provocation. It's important to state here that vulvodynia can appear at any age, including young girls. It is not necessarily a sign of sexual activity. Intermittent bouts are the norm initially but in time become chronic and provoke overwhelming symptoms.

Somewhat like fibromyalgia, vulvodynia is really a diagnosis of exclusion. Some of the conditions that must be ruled out are: infection, yeast overgrowth, genital warts, and herpes. It looks quite different from those conditions because the skin has a normal texture although it may be red like a chemical burn. It usually takes a few visits to different gynecologists and many pelvic exams and failed therapies for yeast before someone suspects the condition. Many times you will also have a vaginal culture to rule out infection. After many delays and painful testing, infectious, nerve, and dermatologic causes are ultimately excluded. A manual exam called a Q-tip test is conducted and reveals exquisite sensitivity in certain areas. Physicians may also wish to do a colposcopy to look at the vulvar tissue more closely. This test is noninvasive; it's simply done with an instrument that provides magnification.

The disease strikes at any age, but on average, the diagnosis is obscure until women are in their forties. It's commonly stated that between 150,000 and 200,000 women in the United States suffer from this facet of fibromyalgia. If there are thirty million women in the United States with fibromyalgia and 40 percent of them have vulvodynia, that's a serious underestimation—and it's clear that too many are going without help. Some specialists in vulvodynia believe that one woman in six suffers from this syndrome at some point in her life. We've treated thousands of patients for fibromyalgia. Of all the clusters of symptoms we encounter, the vulvar pain complex is the most heartbreaking.

As we've pointed out, fibromyalgia regularly affects the inguinal ligaments that connect hip and pubic bones. They, too, cause pain in the pelvic region. We've already mentioned that spasms may occur in the perineum and add to already overwhelming symptoms. In addition, the irritable bowel syndrome with all of its lower abdominal and rectal problems is present in 60 percent of women. Twenty-five percent of those with vulvodynia report recurrent bladder infections and/or IC. Therefore it's not always easy to separate bladder complaints from the vulvodynia complex because of the commonality of symptoms. The same nerves affect all of those areas to cause overlapping symptoms. Because these seemingly separate conditions kept appearing in the same patients, we finally linked them into a single entity. Though we're allocating each a chapter in this section, they're all part of the one big syndrome, fibromyalgia.

> *Oxalate*—A chemical found in the human body as part of the energy production cycle. It is excreted in the urine, and is known as a topical irritant that can cause burning in the tissues. Foods of plant origin, such as fruits and vegetables, are high in oxalates.

Informed professionals agree that fibromyalgia and vulvodynia are often connected but not always in the high percentages we contend. You've already read a statement from John Willems, MD, head of ob-gyn at Scripps Clinic in La Jolla, California. He continues to do pioneering work and has considerable success in easing vulvodynia while acknowledging that those with fibromyalgia must treat that condition as well. As a result, we have many patients in common. Clive Solomons, PhD, in Denver has combined his yeoman efforts with that of the Vulvar Pain Foundation in Graham, North Carolina, to disseminate information about the illness. He, too, has launched innovative treatments and is relentless in his investigations. Also spearheading education is the National Vulvodynia Association of Silver Spring, Maryland. Support is also offered through the two networks above to help spouses of affected patients cope. We refer you to the Resources section of this book for contact information.

For couples, perhaps the most horrible part of all of fibromyalgia is the dyspareunia or painful intercourse that is so common with the vulvar pain syndrome. Women with vulvodynia soon become conditioned to expect excruciating and long-lasting pain during and following intercourse. Soon many become afraid to initiate any contact, even cuddling, for fear that even this bit of intimacy might lead to pelvic disaster. Libido is so dulled and lubricant flow so minimal that just the thought of making love hurts. There's a high incidence of separation and divorce within this subset of fibromyalgia, often due to lack of communication that closes doors. Many women freely admit that they avoid forming new relationships knowing they must eventually perform sexually. A typical story appears below:

> "Prior to the guaifenesin treatments and my proper diagnosis, the most debilitating pain I would experience was the vulvar pain. The muscle pain could be significantly minimized with pain relievers but not the vulvar pain. In 1989 the vulvar pain became extreme and frequent. It was so severe at times that I would miss work. Because of this pain, I avoided intercourse with my husband and rejected the thought of having a baby.
>
> "My only relief from pain was warm baths, but I could not live in the bathtub all the time, so I sought help from my family physician. Even though [he] . . . was aware of my other symptoms (acne, muscle pain, insomnia) he focused on each symptom as a separate medical condition and sent me to a variety of specialists. Since he did not focus on the body as a whole and was ignorant of the existence of fibromyalgia, he did not connect my cycles of muscle pain, and fatigue . . . with my vulvar pain.
>
> "During the first few weeks of taking the guaifenesin I did

> experience vulvar pain an average of about two out of ten days, and the pain was severe. As I continued to take the guaifenesin, both the frequency and the severity of the pain decreased. . . . Since January 1995 I have not missed work due to fibromyalgia or vulvar pain. I am not fearful of sexual intercourse, and maybe one day I will even think about having a baby."
>
> —*Angela, California*

Given these obstacles, it's safe to say that the relationships that endure despite vulvodynia are some of the strongest we've seen. Patient and spouse must both be committed to openness and new ways of expressing emotions.

This blatant and basic assault on these women's fundamental quality of life and the toll it takes on relationships has driven many to embrace drastic "cures." Those who simply purchased miracle creams and lotions were the least harmed by these measures, because for the most part they've suffered only from a wounded purse. Others who may have submitted to repeated injections of synthetic cortisone, alcohol, interferon, and local anesthetics directly into the painful areas may be left with painful scar tissue as a result. Most shocking and horrifying are the reports on file at the Vulvar Pain Foundation describing the unsuccessful and sometimes mutilating and multiple surgeries women have endured. Parts of the labia or vaginal lining were excised in an attempt to eliminate pain-producing tissue. Surgery is too often followed by recurrences and scarring that actually intensify symptoms. In some circles, surgery remains "the thing to do," but prudent gynecologists hesitate and cut as a last resort. As long as there is the hope that another therapy can reverse symptoms and treat the root cause, it should be the preferred course. With guaifenesin, we are offering just that.

Unfortunately, vulvar pain symptoms are often subjected to treatments based on an incorrect diagnosis. It's common for

Internal Female Reproductive Organs

Showing the interweave of muscles and organs responsible for pelvic pain.

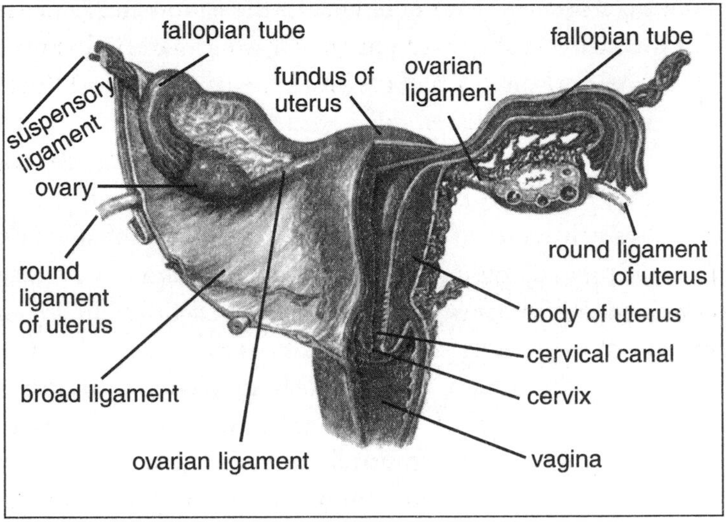

The Vulva

Showing the areas affected by vulvar pain (vulvodynia) and vulvar vestibulitis.

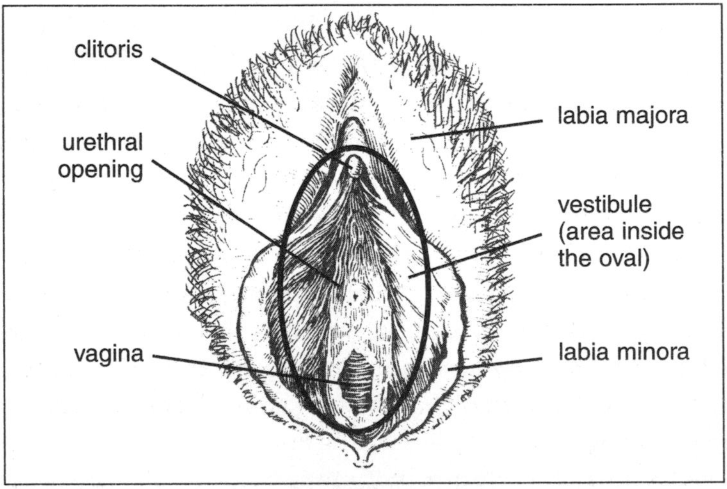

Figure 10.2

women to be told (or think they have) a yeast infection that won't quite go away. It's important to remember that not everything that feels itchy is one of these. If you don't see the distinctive cottage-cheese discharge and your symptoms don't yield to a prescription yeast medication such as oral Diflucan or boric acid capsules inserted vaginally, investigate the cause further. As Dr. Willems says, "If the treatment doesn't work, reconsider the diagnosis." If you're prone to yeast infections, boric acid capsules can be used whenever you suspect a problem. Pharmacists will make them for you, or you can do it yourself using size 0 capsules purchased from a health food store. You can insert them nightly when you have an infection and once a week if you are prone to them. Some women notice a flare-up of yeast activity the premenstrual week. If you do, you can use boric acid monthly to avoid this.

Dr. Willems has developed a treatment protocol that includes several therapies with refreshingly effective results. He outspokenly condemns surgery done without clear indications or done before all else has failed. He has discovered that some compounds ease symptoms and others even repair damage. Expert biofeedback and pelvic massage or pelvic floor therapy can make pain bearable and are highly recommended. His protocol is usually initiated using topical estrogen (estradiol) to rebuild often thinned vulvar tissue.[1] Fibromyalgic women should insist on hormones mixed with plant-free emollients to avoid undermining guaifenesin effects. There are safe commercial preparations, and compounding pharmacists can easily create them if necessary in a base of such substances as vitamin E—which has also been shown to help in a standalone treatment. A few cooperating pharmacies and Scripps Clinic are listed in our Resources section. When it comes to topical estrogen, Dr. Willems uses Estrace cream as his compound of choice. He has said that Premarin or conjugated estrogen cream can achieve the same goal, but at a significantly slower pace. It is important to stress that vaginal estrogen creams are used in very small, pea-size amounts and do not significantly alter estrogen levels in the body. In this day of worry about the effects of hormone replacement therapies, topical compounds are not a concern. Once healing has occurred, the maintenance therapy requires lower doses still.

Emu oil is a natural anti-inflammatory that also has the ability to rebuild thinning, damaged tissue due to its content of fatty acids. For patients already using hormones, it can be used as an adjunct to that therapy. Sources are also included in the back of this book. It should be noted that both the topical compounds that rebuild tissue take some time to work. They may increase pain and itching at first, which may feel like a mild yeast infection. The process itself is the same as the itching you feel when scar tissue heals. Some patience is required. Lidocaine in a 2.5 percent solution, and its chemical cousin Xylocaine, can be used to actually deaden pain. Newer combinations of local anesthetics called EMLA or ELA-Max may also be used. For some, these are irritating and should not be continued. Unlike the estrogen compounds, these are only for treating symptoms and are of no therapeutic value to the tissue.

Women who have had a history of vulvodynia at any time in their lives or have extremely fair or sensitive skin should talk to their physician as they approach menopause. Because the body's estrogen levels plummet at that time, this sensitive tissue is the most vulnerable. Pain will not be evident until tissue damage has occurred, and then it takes time to build it back. It's for this reason that prophylactic therapy should be considered. Especially for those who have done well on guaifenesin and no longer have symptoms, it's heartbreaking to have them recur when simple prevention is so effective.

Prelief, the calcium supplement suggested earlier for interstitial cystitis, is also helpful for vaginal burning. When used

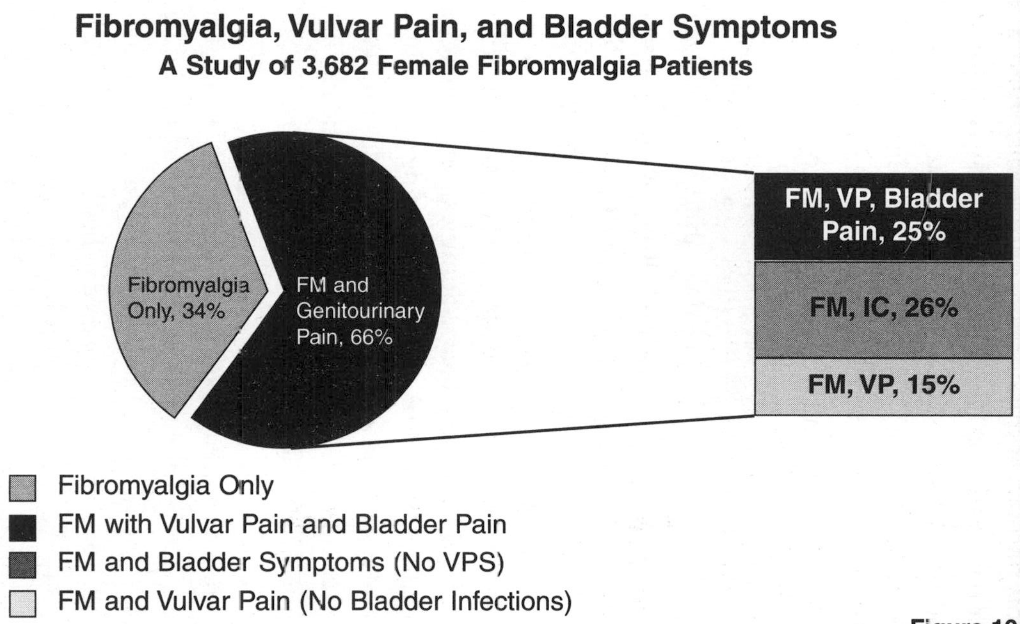
Fibromyalgia, Vulvar Pain, and Bladder Symptoms
A Study of 3,682 Female Fibromyalgia Patients
Fibromyalgia Only, 34%
FM and Genitourinary Pain, 66%
FM, VP, Bladder Pain, 25%
FM, IC, 26%
FM, VP, 15%
Fibromyalgia Only
FM with Vulvar Pain and Bladder Pain
FM and Bladder Symptoms (No VPS)
FM and Vulvar Pain (No Bladder Infections)

Figure 10.3

for this purpose, it can be taken with meals. It is also available in a powder form to be sprinkled directly on food. It can be found in drugstores in the section with digestive aids such as antacids. If you can't find it locally, prelief.com has a list of pharmacies that do, and it can also be ordered online. Calcium is known to be helpful for the symptoms of vulvodynia, so this may be beneficial in several ways.

As with interstitial cystitis, mast cells are involved in the vulvar pain complex. To hinder their ability to disgorge their irritating contents, both prescription and over-the-counter antihistamines can be used. Because it's often difficult for women with this type of pain to sleep through the night, the over-the-counter formulas for insomnia can be used to solve two problems at once. Benadryl is the active ingredient in formulas such as Simply Sleep, Sominex, and generic drugstore sleep aids. This can be taken only during a flare-up of symptoms or nightly. It is not habit forming; it's safe for pregnant and nursing women. Effective doses vary greatly. If morning grogginess is a problem, simply lower the dose.

> "I know the feeling about going for a GYN exam. They told me it hurt because I was tense. I wasn't tense until it hurt. My first exam was when I was very young, a teen. It did not hurt at all. That is how it is supposed to be. Then came the FM and so came the pain there. Every person I have had do these exams has basically blamed me. One physician's assistant used a smaller device on me, which helped a little. Ask them to use the kids' one. I think this problem should improve on guai. I do believe it is the FM. You are still young so hopefully the guai will help before marriage. Most husbands are patient with us, or ask for divorce. It is a real sad thing either way."
>
> —*Karen B., Massachusetts*

When these simple measures don't control the pain adequately for comfort, prescription medications may be used. As always, we view these as stopgap measures that should be used only as long as needed. Once guaifenesin has done its job of clearing fibromyalgia, they should no longer be necessary. Antidepressants are often the first drugs of choice, as they are with other forms of chronic pain of unknown etiology. As with IBS, the older tricyclics such as amitriptyline (Elavil) have been shown to be the most effective because of their action on smooth muscle. Effective doses vary greatly, from 10 to 50 mg a day. It is also possible that these drugs are beneficial because they have some anticholinergic effect.

Not all patients experience benefits, and if that's the case there's no reason to continue therapy. That's true for all the medications we'll mention here, because they are merely prescribed to make you comfortable and don't actually help cure the condition. Trazodone (Desyrel) may be the drug of choice if sleep is a problem. Ativan (lorazepam) and Klonopin (clonazepam) may also be prescribed, although they should be used with extreme caution because they are addictive. Recently, gabapentin (Neurontin) has been added to the arsenal of medications for vulvodynia. Newer variations on this drug are in the pipeline and will soon be available. Neurontin is an antiseizure drug with many side effects, but it can help especially with nerve pain. Once again, there is a huge variation in effective doses, from 300 to 3,600 mg.

Dr. Clive Solomons, who was mentioned earlier in this chapter, is a research biochemist who has devoted much of his time to studying vulvodynia. He constantly improves his recommendations as he hones his skills combining dietary restrictions and using various over-the-counter supplements. His use of calcium citrate and other innovative products has documented benefits. Dr. Solomons measures oxalate excretion in timed urine specimens to evolve treatment schedules. We have also seen excesses of this compound excreted in urine, especially after we introduce guaifenesin. He has taught patients to counter this with timed doses of supplements, including calcium citrate and glucosamine. Patients are instructed to follow a low-oxalate diet. The Vulvar Pain Foundation has borne the cost of analyzing foods and has published a comprehensive cookbook, listed in our Resources section. Foods to avoid include tea, coffee, chocolate, cranberries, eggplant, soy sauce, and peanuts. Some of the same supplements that cause bladder burning are also best avoided in vulvodynia. Vitamin C, for example, should not be taken in amounts over 250 mg a day.

There are other things you can do to help your symptoms. Women soon learn to avoid tight jeans, nylon underwear, or pantyhose. Seams press into the vagina and severely irritate or chafe vulnerable tissues. Using unscented white toilet paper and wearing clothes that are loose in the crotch area are two obvious things. Some women are too sensitive for toilet paper and do better with a little spritz bottle of cool distilled water (to avoid chlorine) and a soft cloth to blot the area. Acid urine burns and increases injury as it spills over the irritated vulva. If this is a problem, try a simple solution: Pour distilled water over the area as you urinate to wash the tissue and dilute the urine as you void. It's important not to use bubble bath or scented soaps, and make sure underwear is rinsed twice. Tampax are quite problematic. Instead, white, unscented (even cotton such as GladRags) menstrual pads should be used. When you are well enough to attempt intercourse, only water-soluble lubricants such as Astroglide are nonirritating. Bike riding and sitting for long periods without moving will always make symptoms worse. While exercise and stretching may be painful at first, with time they will prove two very helpful approaches. Scantihose (stockings with no ridges) and other such items may also be useful.

> "I have suffered from vulvar pain since 1990. I went everywhere for help. I even flew to Michigan for laser surgery from a now infamous doctor. I hooked up with the Vulvar Pain Foundation and found out about the low-oxalate diet and citrate. I began this treatment and got a little better. I added Estrace cream per Dr. Willems at Scripps Clinic in La Jolla, CA. . . . I found out about Dr. St. Amand from the VP Foundation and read up on him. I firmly believed that I did not have FMS because I didn't have the body aches and pains. But as I read through the symptoms of FMS I was astounded. I was reading my life's history. I began the guaifenesin, and the first thing that left me was the vulvar pain. Now I do indeed have the general aches and pains (but that's due to the cycling). I also realize that I have a high pain tolerance and just tolerated the aches. I cycled fairly quickly. Dr. St. Amand recently mapped me, and I'm almost cleared out!"
>
> —*Mary B., Alabama*

We have usually seen guaifenesin eradicate the above symptoms given sufficient time. Patience and gentle management are required for healing the damaged tissue of vulvodynia. Some maintenance measures may be required for life, but none is particularly intrusive or demanding. Certain patients who are extremely sensitive might wish to avoid the FDA-approved 600 mg guaifenesin tablet, Mucinex, because one side is colored with bright blue dye. For those patients, Grace Fibro-Smile and Pro Health Guaifenisen FA would be better choices. Despite the difficult and embarrassing nature of vulvodynia symptoms, support and help are out there.

Chapter 11

Dermatologic Symptoms

WE'VE DEVOTED ENTIRE chapters describing the fibromyalgic assault on susceptible systems. Long before we wrote the first edition of this book, most experts in the field had realized that the musculoskeletal and central nervous systems were both victims of the same illness. Some are now becoming aware of the extent of gastrointestinal tract involvement. Newer studies are emerging connecting genitourinary tract problems with fibromyalgia. Almost none speak or write about the accompanying eye, ear, nose, and throat symptoms that most patients suffer. We'll describe that cluster in the next chapter. Meanwhile, we have clearly seen that FMS certainly affects the skin, nails, and hair—yet we know of no researchers or authors who are working on this connection. This chapter is dedicated to our observations on this subject.

SKIN

"I have had this consistently since I got sick; my first symptoms being fatigue, itching rashes, and hives. I have been a notorious complainer about pins and needles, tingling, and painful burning of the skin. The itching intensified when I started the guai in November 1996. I used to use Benadryl almost every night for this. I also tried Caladryl, Benadryl cream, cortisone cream,

Table 11.1
Dermatologic System

	Male Patients	% Male	Female Patients	% Female
Number of patients	310		2,176	
Skin sensitivity		36%		45%
Itching		65%		74.%
Rashes		52%		59%
Brittle nails		37%		73%
Bruising		23%		78%
Salt craving		45%		46%
Sugar craving		33%		70%
Sweating		58%		65%

etc. I have found several things that help: (1) Dry brushing with a bath brush before a shower. (2) Using a bath brush in a bath with Epsom salts, sea salts, and baking soda (1 cup each). Take a shower afterwards to wash off the salt. (3) Lac-Hydrin or Aquaphor lotion. (4) Benadryl or prescription medications for itching or sleep at night. It has started to get better for me after a year and three months on guai."

—*Heather, Texas*

The skin is the largest organ of the body in terms of area. Average adults have about two square yards of skin, and it performs many functions. It protects against invaders, produces vitamin D when exposed to the sun, and contains millions of tiny nerve endings that relay messages to our brains. We tend to forget that the hair and nails are specialized offshoots of the dermis and are technically part of this same system.

The skin is made up of two layers, the dermis and the epidermis, with a layer of subcutaneous fat directly beneath. The epidermis is a thin layer that's constantly active. Cells are created there, and as newer ones are made, they push older ones up toward the top, where they flatten and become squamous cells. Finally they are moved higher still to make up the stratum corneum and are sloughed off. The average life expectancy of a skin cell is one month. The dermis has large amounts of collagen that serve as supportive tissue. Obviously, the skin contains blood, nerve, lymph, and muscle cells along with hair follicles and sebaceous glands. As you might imagine, it takes a lot of energy to keep this huge system running properly. And we all know that fibromyalgics are energy-challenged everywhere!

All types of rashes, including eczema, nonpustular acne, seborrhea, hives, rosacea, large red patches, tiny red bumps, scaly and dry areas, and small, blistered eruptions, occur in fibromyalgics. Diagnoses such as dermatitis and psoriasis are common, too, as are mysterious skin eruptions that are never quite given a name. Nails crack, chip, or peel and often become ridged. Cuticles shred and tear. Hair is usually of poor quality, dry and short lived, with premature falling out. It's all related and it's all easily explained.

In 1998, a scientific paper reported mast cell involvement in fibromyalgia. These are highly specialized white blood cells that produce more than thirty identified chemicals and proteins. The twenty-two women in this study underwent skin biopsies that showed these cells disgorging themselves of their contents. Their stockpile includes histamine, a strong perpetrator of allergic reactions, including itching, hives, and other rashes. These cells are involved in the immune response, and those with hay fever are well aware of histamine's handiwork: swelling, itchy eyes and nose, excessive tearing, sneezing, congested sinuses, wheezing lungs, and runny nose. Other studies have also found higher-than-normal blood and tissue levels of histamine in fibromyalgic individuals. This compound works through the lining of bronchial tubes, the lungs (asthma), bladder wall (interstitial cystitis), and vaginal tissues (vulvodynia). Mast cells are also implicated in facial flushing, cramps, and diarrhea. Sound familiar? These findings have been documented system by system and merely lack the unifying theory that fibromyalgia provides. It's estimated that about 20 percent of the population has suffered from hives at one time or another.

Interesting but disconcerting is the tiny foot of immunoglobulin G that suddenly protrudes through the wall of a stimulated mast cell. It sticks onto a willing receptor in the deepest layer of the skin, the epidermis. Immunoglobulin G is a known stimulator of autoimmune reactions. Do you wonder that, in combination with histamine, the skin can be supersensitive, on fire, itch, and explode with strange sensations? We now know that mast cells are also activated by a brain factor called CRF (corticotropin releasing factor) secreted into the bloodstream under stress conditions. It's all starting to make sense, isn't it? The body activates most of its cells, including the brain, to respond to anything irritating, injurious, or deemed as foreign to its tissues.[1]

Only in recent years have we realized the variety and extent of skin symptoms in fibromyalgia. Now we rather expect patients to tell us about tingling sensations in their fingers and toes or in scattered areas such as the face and lips. All kinds of other weird effects appear. Crawling feelings anywhere on the skin feel like errant hairs or insects that are never there. Burning can be felt anywhere on the surface of the body, commonly on the back of the neck, arms, or thighs. Fibromyalgics ritualistically cut irritating tags off their clothes before putting them on for the first time. Fiery hot, itchy soles and palms are relentless. So intense is this burning sensation that I would thrust my feet from under covers even on a winter night. My hands were best quenched by holding bagged ice wrapped in a washcloth. I'm certainly not the only one who has made such improvisations.

> "Sensitive skin is something many of us feel. Just a breeze on my skin feels like knife blades cutting me. Just a touch on my skin is painful like a blow. I'm always having traveling pains and shooting pains. Weather changes make it worse. I can't stand extra weight on my skin so I sleep with light covers. Heavy ones hurt. I can't tolerate synthetic fiber clothing at all. So I wear 100 percent cotton everything. I have to wear my underwear inside out so the seams don't hurt. I put all my clothes through about four extra rinse cycles because any detergent left over will irritate my skin. I cycle rashes."
>
> —*Ron C., California*

Nearly all fibromyalgics experience itching. It's almost always worse at night. Warmth generated under blankets sets it off and spreads it more universally than at any other time. Humid weather is also a trigger. I soon learned not to scratch. Even gentle rubbing seemed to set in motion a seven-year itch that didn't stop even when my skin was bloody from scratching it. When itching began in the evening, I knew I was in for a particularly sleepless night. It signaled another distressing cycle of fibromyalgia.

Generalized hives are among the worst of the rashes. A woman flight attendant was the first to show us how intensely those could affect a person. For many years, she suffered bouts of a strange type of giant hives that oddly involved only her face and neck. Each patch was accompanied by an underlying redness and an unusual amount of swelling. She described herself as looking "like a gargoyle." We finally saw her during one of those cycles and had to compliment her on the accuracy of her description. On hives days, she had to call in sick to cancel her flights. She'd undergone exhaustive testing for allergies and autoimmune diseases. At that time, we had never thought there might be a connection between hives and fibromyalgia. Under treatment, the mystery gradually unraveled.

She was the first to realize that hives always appeared during her pain cycles. In between attacks, her skin was clear. As you'd expect from the story, there's a happy ending. She's now almost totally free of fibromyalgia attacks, and in her rare and mild reversal cycles she no longer has to deal with the unwelcome skin intrusions. Less fortunate as of this writing, we have another, more severely affected patient who is covered from head to toe with never totally remitting hives (urticaria). She, too, is distinctly worse during her more intense cycles of fibromyalgia. We wish we could predict the outcome of her treatment.

Cortisone or topical steroid creams are often suggested for hives, but this generally is not very effective. The reason is that hives are caused by dilation of the capillaries, which allows fluid to leak into the surrounding tissue, or epidermis. Angioedema is the result of a similar but deeper process in which the fluid goes deeper into the lowest layer, the dermis or subcutaneous tissue. Since no cream can penetrate this deeply, they only improve the appearance of upper layers. Neither cortisone creams nor topical antihistamines like Benadryl cream are blockers if no plant derivatives such as aloe have been added.

Hives can be acute (episodic) or chronic. Chronic hives are those that have appeared at least twice a week for longer than six weeks, although that number is somewhat arbitrary. In 75 percent of patients, hives have lasted longer than one year; 50 percent, for longer than five years. In 70 percent of these cases, no cause is ever identified. Sometimes a thyroid condition may have developed, but there isn't much testing physicians can do after they've checked that gland and for a few autoimmune conditions. Skin testing shows little benefit for the simple reason that most people who have hives react to every substance that's applied to their skin.

Chronic hives are much harder to treat; antihistamines need to be taken regularly until they are controlled. These work by blocking the release of histamines, and once they have been released these medications have no effect. Some anti-anxiety drugs have been used with some success in a few patients, but due to the very common side effect of fatigue they are rarely used for long. As an alternative, the histamine-2 blockers—drugs primarily taken to block histamines in the gut where they induce stomach acid—may be used. Pepcid and Zantac are two examples of these. Of the tricyclic antidepressants, doxepin powerfully blocks histamine release, so it is often used in patients with allergic skin eruptions. Short courses of oral steroids may be given if hives are very bad but should never be used for long periods because of harmful side effects such as skin and bone thinning and immune system depression. Some newer topical lotions such as DesOwen may work well with fewer problems. Ephedrine is another substance that is a powerful histamine blocker, but because it raises blood pressure and speeds up the heart, it is only used for short periods. Occasionally, a certain type of blood pressure medication, a beta-blocker such as propranolol, is given.

About 16 percent of patients with chronic hives can identify a physical stimulus as a trigger. If exercise is a trigger for histamine release, anticholingeric drugs are sometimes prescribed. For a small number of people, cold, sun, heat, and water may cause attacks. Topical doxepin, already mentioned as having a potent histamine-blocking effect, is marketed as Zonalon, and will not stand in the way of guaifenesin therapy.

"I just got over the itching. It lasted for three weeks. All the Benadryl and prescriptions for itching didn't help it much at all. What helped me was just plain Tylenol or Advil. Heat seemed to make it worse but ice did help. I was also given a prescription for a lotion to use that would keep the skin from looking too bad from all of the scratching. It was Aquaphor ointment. After my itching was finally over, I did go into a pain cycle and am now coming out of it. In fact today I feel pretty good. Yay Guai!

—Katy, Arkansas

Most of our fibromyalgia patients have already visited dermatologists who have diagnosed their scattered, dry, and scaly patches of skin as eczema or neurodermatitis. The worst case we've ever seen was in a young attorney. All of his skin was affected, but his main problem was the appearance of his hands. They were cracked, often bleeding, and covered with small scabs. He was so embarrassed that he had stopped offering clients a handshake and was so overwhelmed by his other symptoms that he was virtually ignoring his muscular aches, fatigue, and minor cognitive difficulties. Upon examination, we found the telltale lumps and bumps of fibromyalgia. While we could at least reassure him about their response to treatment, we couldn't promise resolution of his skin issues. However, his rash became worse during each of the early reversing cycles of guaifenesin—which, of course, was a good sign. Finally the rash has completely cleared. This is one person who'll never give up guaifenesin!

In my own case, patches of seborrheic dermatitis tormented me. Despite the superficial scaling, they felt raw and burning. They were concentrated in my scalp, my eyebrows, and the sides of my nose. I also got intensely itchy, little blisters on my fingers. I would deliberately burst them since I much preferred the burning of the denuded base I'd left behind. Our patients have described the same eruptions on other body surfaces. People with psoriasis notice worse outbreaks during attacks of fibromyalgia. Psoriasis is characterized by small areas of red-pink raised patches that are flaky, itchy, and sting. These occur primarily on the scalp, elbows, knees, and lower back. It's not contagious and very common. Once again, dry skin, stress, alcohol, changes in climate, and lack of exposure to sun make symptoms worse. A commonly used medication, Dovonex, a vitamin D derivative, is not a problem with guaifenesin. Coal tar preparations in cleansers, shampoos, and baths are also safe to use.

One night I was speaking to members of a support group and found it hard to avoid staring at one woman's face. She had already been diagnosed with rosacea. This is another skin problem related to histamine release that stings and burns but doesn't itch. Eyelids and skin around the eyes may be the worst hit. It produces a distinctly red color, but hers was a deep magenta. Red bumps and pimples may emerge, and thread-like blood vessels may become visible over time. As we began treating her, this woman soon observed that the severe display cycled in step with her fibromyalgia. She's now symptom-free, and the rosacea has cleared. Rosacea currently has no known cause, but things that make you flush, such as extremes of heat and cold, rubbing or scrubbing, spicy foods, and alcohol, may make it worse. If symptoms are bad, dermatologists often prescribe metronidazole cream; this will not block guaifenesin. Some patients keep a diary to help identify triggers but always notice that the number one trigger is a flare of fibromyalgic symptoms.

In most patients, a much less dramatic, selective or generalized flushing on the face and upper torso may appear only during adverse cycles. Using a fingernail or blunt instrument, we can sometimes write on a patient's skin, a condition called dermatographia. It's caused by ballooning capillaries that hold excess blood and fluid in a thin line that maintains the inscription for several minutes.

> "Approximately 18 to 24 months before I was diagnosed with FMS, I was diagnosed with rosacea. I was devastated. Now looking back on it I see that a lot of things were going wrong back then, but it was the symptoms on my face that got me to the doctors originally. I took tetracycline daily for 3 years. I hated it, but if I stopped I broke out so bad, and my skin would peel away, and I was red!!! Within a few weeks of starting the Guai I gave up the tetracycline as an experiment. I have not used it since. The symptoms have been manageable, although stress will trigger it again. Right now I am in a bit of a flare over a new job, but not enough to send me back to the tetracycline. My eyelashes grew back, and fell out, and grew back. I am very confident that the longer I am on the Guai the scare of rosacea will be behind me."
>
> —*Dawn, California*

Many fibromyalgia patients suddenly experience an outbreak of acne. It's not uncommon to hear, "I must be in my second childhood," or "I never even had pimples in high school." Acne, whiteheads, and blackheads are caused by blocked pores, which, in fibromyalgia, may occur because of the general inefficiency of the skin's processes. On the other hand, hormonal fluctuations of menopause can also have a hand in this development. Acne can be treated effectively by using a mild antibacterial cleanser and, if necessary, a spot treatment. Benzoyl peroxide or triclosan will not block guaifenesin. Acne products should be carefully screened for salicylic acid, which is commonly used in soaps, washes, cleansers, toners, scrubs, and other products for this condition.

The most beneficial way to ease the symptoms that arise from the dermal system is to use common sense. Expensive preparations are rarely needed and usually not helpful. The release of histamines from mast cells is responsible for the bulk of the annoying symptoms. Itchy eyes, facial flushing, or flushing of the upper torso and rosacea are outward manifestations of this single process. The treatment of choice is to avoid triggers, many of which are environmental. These include: sun exposure, heat, alcohol, spicy foods, hot drinks, and hot baths. Skin should be cleansed with lukewarm water only and patted, not rubbed, dry. Skin care products should be screened for dyes, fragrances, and other irritating ingredients such as alcohol and botanicals like the mint family and citrus extracts—which, luckily, you will no longer be using with guaifenesin. It is no joke but a serious observation that many women who begin guaifenesin report that their skin has become much better in tone and texture simply by using products with a fewer number of ingredients, and all of them simple and basic.

For very dry flaky skin, an alpha hydoxy acid cream or lotion is a great solution if used regularly. My coauthor Claudia Marek advocates AmLactin (or Lac-Hydrin), which is the most potent of these compounds on the market. It has the benefit of having lactic acid, our skin's natural alpha hydroxy, as the active ingredient. Dry skin should also be babied with the avoidance of extreme hot and cold, and gentle moisturizing. Some newer creams on the market contain wax compounds as well to seal in moisture. Elta is one company that manufactures several of these; Surgeon's Skin Secret is another such company. Prescription retinoids are also okay with guaifenesin: Both Retin-A and Renova will also help with acne breakouts, as will triclosan and benzoyl peroxide compounds.

FINGERNAILS

"Nearly everyone in my support group can identify with having bad fingernails that break. Lots of us have dry fingertips that are always cracking. My nails finally got so weak that I could not even wear acrylic nails because my nails would bend

> and break underneath them. It took several years on guai, but now my nails are much stronger. I know they will never be glamorous, but at least they are normal and look presentable."
>
> —*Janeen, Idaho*

We have a checklist of symptoms we ask patients about during their first visit. We include each of them because we so often get a positive answer. Patients have already answered some of them before we ask as they recite the story of their fibromyalgia. The state of their fingernails is one of these questions. Many times it's impossible to ascertain the truth that lies beneath acrylic nails.

Chipping and breaking are so common that we're a bit surprised if nails are perfectly normal. Sometimes bad nails don't break but easily peel in sheets like mica. Early in FMS, nails grow fairly well because they have alternating good and bad layers, but quite suddenly four or five of them shatter all at once. In long-standing fibromyalgia, they finally remain broken all the time. You can understand the cause of this phenomenon if you compare nails to the concentric rings of a tree. During untreated fibromyalgic cycles, there's an abnormal concentration of debris in the bloodstream. These minute excesses visit all parts of the body, as you've seen in earlier chapters. Tiny clusters of calcium phosphate hunker down in the nail root as fragile and unstructured sediments. Outward growth over the next eight to ten months brings a very brittle, horizontal ring to the nail tip. All it takes is minuscule pressure to chip it away like so much dried mortar from the next, healthier layer. Even during successful treatment, nails keep doing the same thing. It's from the same fundamental mechanism. When debris pulls out of muscles and other sinews, it sails into the bloodstream destined for renal excretion. Kidneys are a bit slow responding, as we've theorized. Delayed urinary extraction permits bloodborne calcium phosphate to linger long enough to repeat past performances at the nail bed. The difference now is that nails stay solid for ever-longer periods of time until they become as strong as your genetic makeup allows them to be.

Hangnails are common because the softened fingernail easily tears at its edges. I also remember dry, thick, cracked skin around my nails and knuckles before I treated myself. It was hard to explain since the problem lingered throughout the seasons regardless of weather. Cuticles may get dry, get irritated, and shred. Bleeding and cracking are very common. Vitamin E, lanolin, or emu oil rubbed directly into them can be helpful. Hand treatments of pure paraffin also will not block guaifenesin.

Some fibromyalgics have problems with nail fungus. It's not really related to fibromyalgia except that the immune system might not be quite up to par. Drugstores sell topical compounds that should be checked for salicylates; the prescription drug Penlac is compatible with guaifenesin. Oral medications for fungus need to be taken for a long time, once again, because nails grow so slowly. For those already taking multiple medications, this may not be desirable, and it's certainly safer to use topical products directly on the nail.

Fingernails grow slowly, and it will take some time for them to change. In the meantime, massaging the nail, the fingertip, and the cuticle with gentle oil such as emu or vitamin E will help. Artificial nails, while tempting alternatives, do damage the nail underneath and cause it to be weaker. Once they are removed, the nail will ultimately come in stronger, but once again, it's a slow process. Remember that it takes twelve to eighteen months for your toenails to grow from the root to the free edge, and eight to ten months for fingernails. Certain paint-on nail strengtheners have fibers that help hold the nail together. They are often first-line treatments that provide protection against painful, low-down breaks. It should be remembered that, like hair, the part of the nail to which you can apply expensive treatments is dead. Although such treatments may be marketed with extravagant claims, these tissues have no blood flow and cannot be altered, except in surface appearance.

HAIR

> "You will notice [after beginning guaifenesin] your hair is getting back to normal, actually better. Mine used to be dry, but got to where I could go a few days before I had to wash it (when I was sick, I didn't wash it for three days and it wasn't greasy). My hair is very healthy now. Just give it some time. I am taking 3600 mg of guaifenesin a day, and have been totally pain free for about three months."
>
> —*M. B. F.*

Fibromyalgic hair is frequently defective. It has split ends, is limp, and grows slowly. From the preceding, you'd surely expect just that. Cyclically, it can fall out in what seems like a lot of hair loss at one time. That's frightening enough, but it commonly gets worse in the fourth or fifth month of guaifenesin treatment. You'll recall that reversal of fibromyalgia takes much less time than it took to generate sequences of the untreated disease. Hair loss is also accelerated, but only the bad comes out; the good stuff stays intact. It's a sound rule that mostly sick tissue participates in the cleansing process. We've mostly given up referring to dermatologists unless someone needs that reassuring consultation. Abnormal results and scalp pathology rarely show up. Luckily, hairdressers are our expert allies. They're used to telling clients about periodic hair loss even if it's not usually so flagrant. Since healthier new growth is fairly easy to spot, they are able to reassure patients and inspire them not to panic.

There are many compounds that are advertised to help hair growth, but in reality, for hair loss caused by fibromyalgia, patience is the best medicine. Gentle shampoos, conditioners, and a good stylist are the best weapons, along with time. Minoxidil (Rogaine) is the only product approved for female hair loss. It needs to be applied daily and is not really useful for people who are too tired to deal with that effort. In younger women, hair loss can be helped by avoiding contraceptives with any androgenic activity. Other compounds that might stimulate male pattern baldness are testosterone or androgen precursors such as DHEA.

It should also be mentioned that hair loss with aging is to be expected in some two thirds of women and an even higher percentage of men. It's not realistic to expect guaifenesin to give you a full head of lustrous hair if that isn't something your own genetic makeup allows. Reversal of fibromyalgia will help your hair to improve and be the best hair you can have, but it won't make miracles happen. When reading advertisements for miracles, remember that except for the root, your hair is dead. Nothing will improve anything more than the surface appearance, and many products in all price ranges can effectively accomplish that.

Most dermatological symptoms, with the exception of chronic hives, are not constantly troubling. Many of them can be managed with a gentle cleaning system, the use of lukewarm water instead of hot, a little very light scrubbing, and an appropriate topical compound. There are many new dermatological compounds on the market these days. Some of them may be helpful in controlling the strange skin rashes and eruptions of fibromyalgia. Over time, guaifenesin will render all this attention unnecessary; in the meantime, there is no evidence that expensive topical compounds or procedures have any benefits over simpler ones.

> "I have been losing a lot of hair. The part that I minded most is all of the little hairs that are coming in. I walked in the snow the other day, and when I got home there was all of this fuzzy dandelion fuzz sticking out—my hair is very curly-frizzy. Then I went to the hairdresser and she was pleased that I had so much healthy new hair coming in. I didn't know that it was new hair growth and that I am on my way to healthier stuff."
>
> *—Jan, Kentucky*

Chapter 12

Head, Eye, Ear, Nose, and Throat Syndrome

YEARS AGO IN medicine, there was a specialty in head, eye, ear, nose, and throat. Then eyes became too complicated to remain a subset and became a stand-alone discipline. Perhaps as a reflection of my years in medicine, this chapter will deal with the all-inclusive cluster of symptoms that affect all of HEENT (head, eye, ear, nose, and throat). Most fibromyalgics find at least a few problems in their heads (the outer structures). Very few physicians in this limited field are able at this point to connect them to the underlying disease. That's one of the reasons we've added this chapter—so that you can!

Table 12.1
Head, Eye, Ear, Nose, Throat

	Male Patients	% Male	Female Patients	% Female
Number of patients	310		2,176	
Frontal headaches		50%		69%
Occipital headaches		41%		57%
General headaches		38%		31%
Dizziness		80%		84%
Vertigo		19%		37%

	Male Patients	% Male	Female Patients	% Female
Imbalance		75%		77%
Faintness		18%		25%
Blurred vision		49%		64%
Eye irritation		64%		72%
Nasal congestion		73%		75%
Abnormal tastes		50%		63%
Bad tastes		40%		54%
Metallic tastes		35%		48%
Ringing ears		62%		63%
Sensitivities		16%		28%
Chemical		2%		4%
Light		16%		23%
Odor		15%		31%
Sounds		6%		16%

EYES

"I could always tell when my younger son, Sean, was in a cycle, although he did not complain much of pain. When I would wake him up for school in the morning, his eyes would be almost glued shut with gooky stuff. I would have to put a wet washcloth over his eyes and let it sit for a while to soak this off. The clumps in his eyelashes were stiff and incredibly hard to get out. Those were the days when he would wake up irritable and tired, and have the most trouble in school."

—C. C., California

Most fibromyalgics have problems with the so-called inner skin, the mucosa that lines every moist membrane in the body. All these areas are subject to the irritating effects of fibromyalgia. The primary reason for this is that the watery secretions that keep them wet become acidic and create surface burning. Eyes react with excessive tearing that dries during the night. Water evaporates, leaving behind mucus and calcium phosphate. This forms the sticky and sometimes gritty "sand" we notice in the corners of our eyelids in the morning. It's a mistake trying to rub it away, since lids get scratched and remain irritated for the next few days. It's better to dissolve and wash it out with cool water on a washcloth.

It's tough not to keep fingering itchy lids. Imperceptible soapy residuals get wiped on and forced into already damaged tissue. This further removes protective mucus, however; the eyeball shares the irritation, and vision blurs. Even dim light from TV screens makes patients wince, and brighter sources are downright painful. Contact lenses are extremely irritating at these times, getting cloudy and needing constant cleaning. Light sensitivity is high, and patients instinctively shove sunglasses into place immediately before facing sunlight. Ophthalmic-safe creams help the lids, and artificial tears provide a protective corneal cover. It's soothing to hold something cool in place, but insert such things as chilled cloths into plastic bags to keep water from further marinating the lids. It is not safe to use ice directly on this sensitive tissue; it must be wrapped inside a cloth. Tissues are burned by something that is too cold.

Blurred vision can have other causes as well. There are four eye muscles attached to each eyeball. They're hooked into the orbits to maintain coordination in eye movements. Any of the eight can be affected with fibromyalgia. In my early years with the disease, I could feel swelling, spasm, and tenderness in any one of them at various times. Blurred vision results when these fibromyalgic muscles tire from trying to maintain focus because they can no longer synchronize with the others.

The lens of the eye is a live, gel-like structure. It participates in fluid shifts and admits nutritive substances through its membranes. All the blood's chemicals move in and out under tight control. Just as glucose can enter to excess, so can calcium phosphate. Any ion intrusion has to be accompanied by water to guarantee safe dilutions. Extra water loads thicken the lens and alter the focal point to induce temporary nearsightedness. When they're eventually sucked out, the lens flattens to a more farsighted state. Ever-changing lens thickness causes blurring, and fibromyalgics periodically fight to maintain focus. Remember that reversal cycles reproduce symptoms, so blurring occurs whether the disease is getting better or worse.

At other times, both eyes get dry and red, what in medicine we call injected. Tears don't stream out adequately; even the mucous channels are dammed up. The inner eyelids get dry, and patients blink excessively. It doesn't help: No lubricants pour out to coat the eyeballs or lids. This ocular upset may also involve tiny eyelid muscles. Their responses are automatic spasms that cause uncontrollable blinking at various tempos. It looks to all the world like a nervous tic. The only way to stop this performance is by holding light finger pressure on the offending lid. Dryness may help provoke this scenario, and in that case, artificial tears will help ease it. There are many over-the-counter brands as well as prescription formulas such as Bion Tears, GenTeal, Lacri-Lube, and others. None contains salicylates.

"I am 47 and have had dry eyes for what seems forever. I recently had to go to the doctor it got so bad. My left eye first turned so red I thought I had an infection. Then because the antibiotic dried it even more than normal I scratched my eye with my own eyelid. That was corrected, but the dryness continued. My doctor gave me a prescription for an eye drop. This I use in the AM and PM. In between for lubrication I use Bausch & Lomb artificial tears. My eyes still get 'glued' in the AM, but not as bad. So it has gotten somewhat better, just not cured. I do believe it is the fibro. I always had dry eyes, just not as bad. They will probably start to get better at times and worse at times."

—*Christine*

EARS

"I too have noise sensitivity that comes and goes. Some days I cannot tolerate the sound of the TV or radio. I cannot tolerate noisy neighbors who play the radio with the bass blaring into my home. It drives me crazy and I have been known to tell some of them off for it. Sometimes I cannot tolerate the noise in restaurants of people talking, kitchen clattery, etc. Other days noise does not bother me. I can say now that after these years on guai it is getting better. But I was raised on a farm where there was no noise and to this day, I miss it."

—*Char, California*

Women have more acute senses than men, and there's no doubt that they're kicked up an octave during bad cycles or flares of fibromyalgia. All fibromyalgics, regardless of sex, have heightened sensitivities to light, sounds, and odors; it's just that females are more sensitive to begin with. Any of the three can trigger headaches and, oddly enough, nausea. For some reason, the noise of the television can be unbearable at times, especially when the shows have a laugh track. Anyone with a fibromyalgic spouse is familiar with an anguished shout from the next room: "Turn the TV down!"

Like the start of some forgotten melody comes sudden ringing in the ears. It's almost always brief, but occasionally it persists for hours. If that sound is steady and unchanging, it's usually not due to fibromyalgia. Less frequently there's a buzzing or the sensation of flapping insect wings deep in the auditory canal.

Hearing is at times dulled, and momentary deafness may follow. Many years ago, I lost my hearing in one ear for two days. I was in my thirties, and the sudden onset was frightening. A colleague looked into the canal and found nothing. My premature deafness cleared as quickly as it appeared and never returned.

Externally, the ears may have symptoms as well. Ears may glow a deep red like a Christmas tree ornament that's suddenly plugged into a light socket. They feel burned and, at times, actually hurt when touched even lightly. Earrings are unbearable at these times. The canals can itch and invite a Q-tip misadventure that temporarily satisfies, but usually resurrects discomfort within a few hours. If flakiness and dry skin are visible, a gentle oil may be applied. Emu oil, because of its anti-inflammatory properties, is commonly used.

Generally, the symptoms arising from the ears need little intervention because they come and go so rapidly. During a period when you are experiencing tinnitus, it can be most annoying at night when you are trying to sleep. When it's quiet, the funny noises your ears make can make you miserable. At this time, a noise machine or quiet music will help make it less audible.

> "Someone recommended the book to me *Too Loud, Too Bright, Too Fast, Too Tight: What to Do if You Are Sensory Defective in an Overstimulating World,* by Sharon Heller, PhD. Whether my sensory defectiveness came along with the FMS I am not sure, but this book sure helped me understand these things better. It also helped explain things to my nine-year-old son."
>
> —*Kathy, Florida*

NOSE

> "My sinuses have cleared up considerably—I used to have a tissue in my hand 24 hours a day. Now I'm not even taking Allegra except during ragweed season. I used to get colds or sinus infections 3 to 4 times a year. I haven't been sick since I started guai."
>
> —*Karen, Texas*

The membranes of the nose are not immune to fibromyalgia. They express their discomfort with mucous outpourings due to histamine release, as we have already mentioned. The majority of patients report classic symptoms of this: chronic nasal congestion or postnasal drip. Waking hours are spent sniffing, blowing noses, or clearing throats. Mucus is usually clear, but the appearance of yellow or green phlegm indicates a superimposed infection, which must be treated appropriately. Occasionally, because of the excess mucous production, affected individuals mistakenly blame the "sinuses" for their frontal fibromyalgic headaches. Antihistamines, both over the counter and prescription are quite effective, and generally the newer nondrowsy formulas are better tolerated. Allergy medications are the least likely compounds to contain natural salicylates because reactions are so commonly induced by exposure to plants.

We've already mentioned that the bodily secretions of fibromyalgia are acidic. Nasal membranes are delicate and easily burned by surges of watery mucus. Inopportune bursts of sneezing are triggered by the irritation and represent nature's effort to blast out some particulate offender. Itching is provoked out of nowhere; relief is scant, even with rigorous rubbing of the nasal tip.

Facial rosacea also attacks the nose, causing it to light up and swell a bit. It's slightly suggestive of Rudolph's dilemma and requires a lot of powdering to dim the glow. Patchy areas of pimples and irritation can occur anywhere on the body but can be most annoying on the face. For dry skin inside the nose that causes cracking or easy bleeding, skin oil such as mineral oil, vitamin E, or plain Vaseline can help soothe, coat, and protect the area from the repeated assault of Kleenex. If your skin is very sensitive, you may wish to use a soft cloth handkerchief.

Some odors are amazingly oppressive. Sensitive patients must avoid all scented lotions, colognes, and perfumes. It often takes some effort to find household cleaning products that don't irritate them, or set off their symptoms. Headaches spring up after only a brief exposure, and nausea is not uncommon under the same circumstances. What makes these symptoms difficult is the prevalence of fragrances and heavy perfumes in public places. Many patients are seriously disabled by their inability to be around others unless it has been requested in advance that everyone abstain from using strong chemicals.

THROAT

> "I've . . . found that sinus problems and IBS can both cause bad breath. For at least 10 years I finish brushing my teeth by brushing my tongue and brush way to the back (I have no gag reflex). My daughter commented how I don't have bad breath anymore as I used to have from time to time. I don't have the chronic sinus drainage that I used to have before Guai, nor the allergies and such either. IBS is fading, too. Guai is changing my life one step at a time . . . or is that one pill a day."
>
> —*Sandy, California*

The throat begins in the mouth. The entire surface is lined with almost equally sensitive membranes. Salivary glands are involved in trying to rid the body of unwanted phosphate (phosphoric acid). Their acidic secretions scald, leaving a burned sensation, as if you'd taken a big sip of an excessively hot cup of coffee. The same sources can be blamed for sour or metallic sensations emanating from taste buds. Saliva leaks out during sleep and causes rashes around the corners of the mouth. (This is more often visible in those with fair skin and small children.) More distant membranes aren't impervious to the acid wash, which can cause a sore throat or dry, hacking cough. Menthol-free cough drops, such as Fruit Breezers, Halls Vitamin C drops, or old-fashioned Luden's are some that won't block guaifenesin. Herbal lozenges and any that contain mint and menthol, of course, need to be avoided.

Let's not forget dental calculus. We discussed the nature of tartar crystals very early in this book. You may remember that it's made up of calcium phosphate, the components of the salivary outflow. These small crystals wedge between the teeth and invade surrounding tissues to cause gingivitis. Salivary glands may occasionally swell slightly, ache, and become tender, irritated by their own acid secretions. It's not uncommon for gums to bleed when brushed, especially in the early stages of reversal.

The tongue shares the same bathwater. It sports the largest of the oral taste buds. Like any other muscle, the tongue may become tender or feel as though it were cut. Sometimes only the borders are affected, feeling as if they've been abraded by an emery board and unduly sensitive when rubbed against the teeth. Foods may seem altered, tasteless, or distressingly foul. It's also common to see mouth sores typical of those caused by outbreaks of the herpes virus during fibromyalgia flares. Smaller sores can be touched with an inexpensive (and old-fashioned) styptic pencil. For cold sores, various compounds will shorten them: Abreva, acyclovir, and zinc lip balms.

> "As a dentist who treats patients with fibromyalgia, I often get complains of constant battles with bad breath. There are many reasons why this occurs including medication, oral hygiene habits, the foods you're eating, the dental products you use and

> old, defective fillings, crowns (caps) or dentures. Many medications have a side effect which leaves the mouth dry. This is a major contributor to bad breath. In general, bad breath is caused by sulfur gases that are given off by bacteria. If you clean your mouth thoroughly: flossing, brushing the gums and cleaning the tongue, bad breath will be history."
>
> —*Flora Stay, DDS*

Another very common complaint in fibromyalgia is a dry mouth. Sometimes this may be caused by the illness itself, but just as often it is a side effect of a medication. Antidepressants, sleeping pills, and muscle relaxants can all cause it. Treatments include using toothpaste designed for dry mouth—Tom's of Maine apricot for dry mouth, or Grace Fibro-Smile Original. Hard candies made with xylitol will help also, as long as they are not mint flavored. Strong flavors such as cinnamon may also be irritating, but citrus flavors will actually help by increasing salivation. Drinking plenty of fluids and using a mouth spray designed for this condition, such as Salivart, will also help. If your mouth is overly dry due to medications, you could talk to your doctor about lowering your dosage. Flora Stay, DDS, has written a book about dental complaints and fibromyalgia titled *The Fibromyalgia Dental Handbook* listed in our Resources section.

Sensitive teeth are also a problem for many patients, especially after they have had a chemical bleaching done. Topical fluoride gels that are painted on are the most potent treatment for this. Be sure to get a nonmint flavor such as those marketed by Grace Products (www.fibrosmile.com).

The sore throat of fibromyalgia is usually unlike that of an impending infection. It's more superficial and often accompanied by frequent swallowing. Clearing the throat doesn't help much, and coughing doesn't raise anything but the usual clear mucus. At other times, spastic midneck muscles may impinge on nerves and cause an intense sore throat indistinguishable from a strep infection. Only an examination and the lack of swollen glands can differentiate between the two. Swallowing is sometimes downright painful, as though a foreign body were locked in some deep recess. Patients sometimes think that a pill has become embedded in the tissue. However, this sensation can last for months and doesn't give rise to other tissue problems.

> "My ENT says my larynx is swollen but other than that couldn't find anything wrong. I've been really hoarse all this time and the left side of my throat is also swollen. (He saw that it was swollen also when he did the scope on my throat.) He is sending me to a voice specialist in Salt Lake. I've had throat problems a lot in my past. I'm 56 years old. My tongue has had sores on the left side and on front that come and go. I have been diagnosed with fibromyalgia and my regular doctor says this is all part of it, maybe from a swollen tendon in my neck."
>
> —*Elaine, Utah*

We need to review the fate of all of these various symptoms. Remember that all your symptoms appeared off and on while you were developing the illness. They will also resurge when you're clearing on guaifenesin. When so many things keep popping up, how do you tell whether you're going forward or backward? Like the other components of fibromyalgia, the only way you'll know without mapping is by surveying the systemic effects of treatment to date. Progressively more good days should grace your life as you get better.

MISCELLANEOUS SYMPTOMS

> "Profuse sweating—I'm 35 now, this started when I was around 23. I thought it was peri-peri-menopause. It wasn't. I

always felt like I was burning up inside from the inside out. I would be dripping with sweat. It was very embarrassing."

—*Chantal, Michigan*

Every time we write a paper or book, we have leftovers, symptoms that don't fit into any category. They reflect the overall metabolic problems facing the body. Let's take a moment to look at them here.

Table 12.2
Miscellaneous Symptoms

	Male Patients	% Male	Female Patients	% Female
Number of patients	310		2,176	
Weight changes		33%		55%
Allergies		26%		29%
Palpitations		45%		56%

Weight Gain

Most fibromyalgia patients gain some weight, and about 35 percent put on twenty or more pounds. We mentioned the loss of mitochondria that occurs in sedentary people. Muscle biopsies have shown up to 80 percent fewer mitochondria when compared with well-toned athletes. Lacking a full complement, we're left with many fewer food-burning stations to eat up calories. Insulin to the rescue: If you don't burn it, store it. And fat cells are very accommodating.

The easiest way to lose weight when you have fibromyalgia is on a low-carbohydrate diet, the one we detailed in chapter 5 of this book, on hypoglycemia. Low-calorie diets actually cause the metabolism to slow down, because the body fears starvation. A low-carbohydrate diet, in contrast—because it is high in protein and fat—doesn't have the same effect. We also touched upon the other reasons why this diet will make most people feel better. Losing weight will certainly improve your self-image and mobility. Once you can, creating more mitochondria through exercise will help replenish your energy stores and stamina. It's too easy when you're sick to rationalize your inability to take these two important steps, but without them guaifenesin cannot do a perfect job.

Temperature Regulation Problems

Patients complain of low-grade fevers, and some push the thermometer up over one hundred degrees. The majority of fibromyalgics sweat excessively any time of day. Even minor fevers break at night and interrupt sleep by drenching bedclothes. Hot flashes are common in both sexes—I often joke that I went through menopause at age thirty-two. The body's thermostat malfunctions in various ways, and you may feel comfortable only in a very narrow range of temperatures. It's common to feel too hot or too cold. Layering clothes that are easy to take on and off is about the only way to deal with this annoyance. Be sure to always have a jacket or shawl in your car or locker at work.

Water Retention

We've previously discussed water retention, so we won't review the physiology here. The body holds on to what only seems like excess water. It has to retain two or three pounds during attacks to facilitate the ionic shifts of calcium, sodium, phosphate, chloride, potassium, and magnesium as well as larger-size compounds. Water accumulation will happen both ways, with depositing attacks or during reversal. It's the same chemistry going forward or backward. During cycles, fibromyalgics are accustomed to swollen eyelids upon awakening and rings that temporarily don't fit anymore. During the day, gravity takes hold and fluid leaves the torso, piling up in the legs. Suddenly in the late afternoon, your shoes may not fit well. Even if swelling is not obvious, the skin is stretched from within. This tugs on the millions of tiny nerve endings and causes the restless leg syndrome. This, along with foot and leg cramps, can make nights miserable. For cramps, vitamin E (800 mg) or magnesium at bedtime may ameliorate symptoms. If not, ask your doctor to offer an old remedy that now requires a prescription, quinine sulfate. Walking around and stretching before bed may diminish the misery of restless leg syndrome. Sometimes medications are used for this condition, but they should be considered second-line therapy because of side effects including fatigue and mental fogginess.

Each reader could probably add to this list. You've likely had that sudden leg kick or arm jerk just as you're falling asleep; intermittent nightmares; boil-like tenderness of your scalp; sudden toothaches though nothing's wrong; sharp stabs that run through your ears; unexplained shivers or total-body chilling; vibrations that come out of nowhere; electric currents that zigzag down your extremities. They're all real and not figments of your imagination. Just remember that we believe—and our theory supports the notion—that every cell in the body is affected by fibromyalgia.

> "It used to be that I read all the time. Then I stopped reading. Oh I could see the words, I knew what they meant. But I couldn't get from understanding the words to the thought converted by the words. By the time I'd turn the page I had no idea what I was reading on the previous page. I thought there was something wrong with my eyes, or, perhaps the optic nerve, but the ophthalmologist just looked at me with a glazed expression. During the past year I read three or four books though I thought I'd never read a book again. It's amazing."
>
> —*Claudia, Arizona*

Chapter 13

Pediatric Fibromyalgia

"When I was growing up, my nickname was 'Slow as molasses in January.' As I grew older, the sense that I was not like other children deepened; I could not stand still and hold my arms out to have my clothes fitted; I needed more sleep but could not seem to get it; I had little energy and took refuge reading, lying down, on a window seat instead of playing outside. Burying myself in books, I felt the pain and difference of my childhood less acutely, but the guilt was always there; I felt that I was failing everyone around me by not being like them, by not being able to do what they did so effortlessly. My parents, after taking me to the doctor for thyroid tests, concluded that my tiredness was a character trait and not an illness, and I grew up believing them, never having heard anyone say otherwise."

—*Cynthia C., Michigan*

FACING THE PROBLEM: DID I GIVE MY CHILD FIBROMYALGIA?

As we learn more about fibromyalgia and think about how it's affected our lives, we become aware of similar symptoms in those around us. Sometimes others will confide that they have the illness by name; other times we realize it when we listen to their complaints. And since fibromyalgia runs in families, it's inevitable that this will happen close to home.

During the process of guaifenesin reversal, for most of us it's inevitable that at some point we come face-to-face with the child we once were—the pain we had in our side, unexplained headaches, irritable bowel syndrome that baffled doctors, growing pains centered on the knees that woke us up in the night, charley horses the day after gym class, days on end with fatigue and a horrible, drifting mind that kept us from concentrating in school. This process can be healing because it gives us a chance to see ourselves more clearly and be forgiving of what we may have previously perceived as weakness or hypochondria. At the same time, during the process, we may also realize that one or more of our children have been going through the same struggles. Nearly every day, we are asked by at least one patient, "My daughter has bladder infections and growing pains—it is possible she has fibromyalgia, too?" "My son used to love sports, but now he doesn't even want to dress for PE. Something's always bothering him—could he have fibromyalgia like I do?" We are asked about lethargy, headaches, former A students who suddenly don't achieve in school—all in the same anxious tones. None of us wants our children to suffer as we have, but deep inside we may be terrified that they have the same problems we do. Before our questions have even been put into words, we know our suspicions are more than suspicions, and I can tell you that most parents are not wrong.

Older children with fibromyalgia have slowly learned they're not like other kids although they may not really know why. Why can't they do schoolwork when it was so easy yesterday? Why is it that they're still tired after sleeping twelve hours? Why do they have so little stamina at times when their friends can go and go and still have lots of energy? How can they solve these puzzles when grown-ups, including doctors, flounder about for solutions? Lacking comprehension, they soon become adept at making seemingly valid excuses. By the time they're teenagers, many have really good reasons as to why they hurt or why they no longer want to participate in activities they once enjoyed. But when you look closely, you know those reasons don't really quite hold up.

For younger children, it's different. They have never really felt any other way and may think it's normal, and everyone else feels like they do. As a result, it often sticks in their minds that they are just weaker or less determined because they cannot do what others seem able to do effortlessly. Since they don't know that their physical symptoms aren't what everyone else feels, they may conclude that their problems are just due to a lack of fortitude.

We know one little girl who began painful cycles at the age of two. She would wake up during the night crying from leg pains. Her parents soon learned how to handle her complaints. They'd soak her in a tubful of warm water, dry her off, and then massage her. That was the only way to save them all from another painful and sleepless night. This family of six—mother, father, and four children—all have fibromyalgia. Having two parents with the illness has made it genetically inescapable for their offspring. The youngest three began having appreciable symptoms by the age of four. The only difference was the extent and severity of their complaints and physical findings.

Becky, the eldest, was severely affected by the time we first saw her at age eleven. Already suffering from unrelenting symptoms, she had seen chiropractors, physiotherapists, and physicians. No one could explain why, and few would believe that she sometimes crawled on the ground as the only way to get home from school. Leg pains and weakness were so bad that she couldn't keep walking or even stand. We also had trouble with that one. We had never encountered a crawling fibromyalgic or one so young with such intense symptoms. We began to suspect she was highly neurotic and using her illness for some emotional gain. Yet there were sobering balances to redress our thinking. Becky was a straight-A student and strikingly intelligent. She knew when she could study effectively and rested when she had no other choice. She took pain medications and antidepressants as prescribed by her family physician, but even in her sedated state, she continued to excel. Her mother was unwaveringly supportive and staunchly insisted that Becky was truly as ill as she described herself. Yet she continued to try to give Becky as normal an upbringing as possible. Becky attended public school and even in her back brace lived as normally as her symptoms allowed. She was never allowed to withdraw from life and, with full family support, fought through pain and fatigue with singular success.

Time, Mom, and Becky taught us about how severe symptoms could be in children. But it was a slow process for sure. Her response to guaifenesin demanded precise adjustments. She simply couldn't tolerate much worsening of symptoms. Because of this, she improved very slowly. Tiny increments in dosage would set off such intense reversal that she couldn't make it to school. Even had she struggled to get there, it wouldn't have been worth the painful effort: She couldn't possibly sit for even the first hour of classes. Becky's personal war against fibromyalgia continued for more than three years, but each tiny advance was a major battle won. Our first edition of this book reported that she was an A student completing her senior year in high school. She's now a college graduate enjoying life as a wife and full-time mother. We see her once a year for her checkups, and it's wonderful to hear how well she's doing.

> "When my younger son, Sean, was small, his father took him to a pediatric rheumatologist who diagnosed him with a 'pain syndrome.' The doctor hesitated to make the diagnosis of fibromyalgia, he said, because Sean did not seem to have a

sleep disorder. This doctor, who admitted he had never heard of guaifenesin, was willing to write a prescription on the spot for Elavil and Flexeril—for a seven-year-old child who was far from being in intractable pain. I could not believe this. He did not even know what was wrong with my son except that he was in pain, and admitted it, yet he was willing to change the chemistry of a seven-year-old child's brain."

—*C. C., California*

Becky's story is heartwarming, but there are also very sad ones. Too many children have ended up invalids because of bungled treatment. Some parents become defeated and crumble at the sight of their children's suffering. They keep them out of school at the slightest provocation. They accept the child's mounting inactivity and the loss of friends. The entire family eventually revolves around the child's symptoms. The search is soon narrowed down to immediate relief and not long-term results. The work it would take to get better seems impossibly difficult to them. Before too long, the "usual" medications don't help. As drug tolerance mounts and even powerful ones fail, there seems to be no solution but to turn to narcotics and sleep prescriptions. The child progressively withdraws, and eventually nothing seems to work. Heavier narcotics such as morphine pumps may be added in teenage years, sometimes coupled with powerful stimulants—drugs normally reserved for ADD, such as Ritalin and Provigil.

We don't have to belabor the fact that school absenteeism destroys a child's academic edge. The new information age grants little mercy in today's fierce competition for college. Slowly, the fibromyalgic youngster loses his or her perpetual catch-up race. Though determined parents may manage to wrench home-schooling tutors out of their budget-conscious school districts, it doesn't compensate for the well-rounding effects of extracurricular activities. Only social interactions with peers can provide certain skills during teenage years. The self-esteem and confidence we desire for our children is hard to come by when successes are isolated and they've been taught to believe they are too ill to compete.

Time is oddly suspended in the present for these families. There are few discussions about the future. What happens when Mom and Dad can't continue as caretakers? Adulthood doesn't end drug dependency or social isolationism. All too quickly parents share their home with an introverted adult who has few skills. At a certain age, nonstudent offspring can no longer be carried on the family medical insurance plan. It's impossible to qualify for substantial disability when you've never worked.

Recounting these stories brings to mind a little boy I remember vividly. When we met, Joe was sick, and he was afraid of both doctors and having more pain. Bravely he undertook our protocol and gradually reversed most of his complaints, although his mother was tentative and thought it might be too difficult for him. As time progressed, I learned to appreciate his good qualities. We became friends. One day he brought a poem of gratitude he had composed especially for me. I hung it on my office wall and saw him glow as he looked up at his masterpiece.

Joe and his family moved away. When he came back a few years later for a checkup, he wasn't Joe anymore. He was sadly changed. He wasn't following the protocol and had been off his guaifenesin for some time. Because of severe headaches, his mother and his new doctors had put him on narcotic pain medications. These were the very drugs I had steadfastly refused to prescribe because I did not want to sap his already low energy. I wasn't even sure they were safe for growing children. But now, narcotics were Joe's new friends that made him feel better about his life. They certainly gave partial relief for the headaches and much faster than the gradual improvement I could offer if he chose to resume guaifenesin. I argued in vain with his mother. I don't know what happened to him after his last visit. I don't think Joe ever fulfilled his boyhood dreams of playing college basketball.

These two are contrasting stories at very opposite ends of a spectrum. Becky's story always makes us smile but it only partially offsets Joe's failure. She owes a great deal to her mother, a strong and supportive parent who didn't shy away from a rather long road to health. She never gave Becky the option to quit, deny her illness, or stop her medication. She wasn't afraid to be a parent. Joe's mother was motivated by the same love and determination for her child, but she made different choices. She didn't feel it was right to make her child work through his problems, and this allowed them to take over his life.

Both these stories appeared, minus the updates, in our previous edition. It seems hopeful to add another one. Recently, we were presented with a talented young man whose life was becoming increasingly circumscribed by the prescription medications given to him to control his considerable pain. As a result, he also was suffering from depression. Both he and his parents were quite aware that his future wasn't very bright, and that he was descending into a cycle of stronger and stronger drugs that were working less and less well. They all came to see us and spent the afternoon listening to what we do and how we do it. Even before guaifenesin lessened Jason's symptoms, it gave him hope. And when he started to respond as we predicted he would, for the first time in a long time, Jason dared to dream.

Luckily, Jason proved to be a low-dose responder. Because he is a dancer, despite his heavy narcotics he was aware of his body and able to feel it changing. And we are overjoyed to announce that he is now in college out of state, having been accepted into an exclusive and demanding ensemble at a wonderful university. A tour of Europe is in his immediate future. As he improved, he cut back on some very difficult pain medications, including morphine. With courage, determination, and hope, he has begun this process. So not every foray into these substances ends up a disaster. Odds are against kids like Jason, but they do exist, and hope under any circumstances is a powerful ally. Another is strong, compassionate parents who keep the faith even when frightened themselves. Jason's dad is a member of our online support group, and now he tells his son's story and offers a helping hand to others.

It's imperative for physicians and parents to make an early diagnosis of fibromyalgia and attack the cause, not cover the symptoms. It will take persistence to accomplish this, but the stakes are high. Our children really don't have many formative years, and it's never too early to show them how to accomplish things by determination and hard work. In general, children haven't lived long enough to see impact on many tissues, so there's less disease to reverse. Recovery is much faster than in adults.

Perhaps the only reward for fibromyalgic parents is the bonus of recognizing themselves when they were in the early stages of their own illness. Once parents know there's a genetic trait lurking in the family tree, they should start paying attention. We don't think kids fake many complaints—it's unusual for them not to want to participate in pleasurable activities. Missing a math test is one thing, but missing a homecoming dance is quite another. We should accept and collect the few signals children give us and offer our understanding and support. Children do not need us to feel sorry for them and let them fail. As parents, we can show them how to fight and triumph over what can really be a minor problem if it is handled properly.

"I do not remember a time when I did not have headaches. Since my mother had always suffered from migraines, my headaches seemed to be part of my destiny. The pain in my head was, at least, taken to be real by my family. Not so by the outside world, in which, during my adolescence, I would often hear: just relax, lie down in a dark room for a few minutes, and take an aspirin. Fasting glucose tests, an electroencephalogram, an electrocardiogram, and other tests at the university clinic showed nothing. I had migraines, and not much could be done beyond living with them. Expensive shiatsu and acupuncture gave me sporadic relief but no more than that. I lived my life around my pain, as frustrated as my doctors. I hid my pain as best I could, but I could not hide it from those closest to me. By the time my daughter was three, every week I was taking a bottle of naproxen sodium and Tylenol, and as much sumatriptan as I could get my doctors and medical plan to provide, and yet I was still helplessly spending my afternoons on the couch. I had severe headaches every day, and most of them were migraines. I felt isolated by my pain, unable to even begin to communicate to anyone what my life was like, and increasingly devastated and guilty from the effect my pain was having on my family."

—*Cynthia C., Michigan*

THE FIBROMYALGIC CHILD

"I remember clearly the moment I knew my son had fibromyalgia. And it was not his complaints of pains or nervousness that tipped me off. I didn't know that children do not normally complain of headaches, because I had them all my life. I didn't know there was no such thing as growing pains. His aches and pains did not disrupt his life, and I did not think much about them either. But one day I was standing in the doorway watching his trumpet lesson, and I heard his trumpet teacher say: 'At this point I shouldn't have to tell you how to play a B note.' And I looked at my son's face, and I knew that at that moment he had no more idea how to play a B on a trumpet than I did, although he did know. All the times in my childhood when I was yelled at, told I knew things I could not bring out of my mind because my mind just wouldn't always work to produce them on demand, came flooding back. I knew then and there Malcolm had fibromyalgia too, and I would have to get him help."

—*Claudia Craig Marek*

If you or anyone in your family has fibromyalgia and you are concerned, the first thing to do is to look as objectively as possible at your child. No doctor on earth will ever know that little person as well as you. What should you look for? We've mentioned that kids don't fake pain very often, and when they do it's usually to get out of doing something obvious. They're not seasoned actors, so the put-on is fairly transparent. Not well coached in the role they're playing, they can be easily distracted. The challenge is that they may be fairly inarticulate on nondescriptive and won't say much more than "it hurts" or "I got a headache." Younger children, or those who have had the disease for a long time, won't even recall times without this or that symptom, so they don't identify them as something unusual or abnormal. If they've always had poor stamina, it's normal for them to simply think that they're weaker or less tough than the kids around them. They may not understand—because they have no reference point to tell them—that it isn't usual for legs to hurt every night or to have a headache a few hours after breakfast.

So where does that leave you, as a parent on the outside trying to look in? Well, it leaves you with some questions. Are your children exhausted some mornings even though they've had a substantial amount of sleep the night before? Have you ever seen them leave off playing with friends or siblings and lie down for a rest or for a nap? Can you spot intermittent difficulties with memory or concentration? You might notice that they easily complete tasks one day but badly fumble them on the next try. Do they have abdominal pain, constipation, and diarrhea? Does your daughter have bladder infections, painful urination, or vaginal irritation? Do they complain of leg and knee pains by day and seemingly more vicious ones by night? We've even wondered about a colic connection in babies who draw up their knees while bellowing, possibly reacting to abdominal pain. There are no follow-up studies on these children as they age, or on the prevalence of fibromyalgia in their parents.

Children with FMS may start adverse cycling from an early age, even during preschool years. We've had the opportunity to diagnose and treat four two-year olds and fifteen four-year-olds. In each of these cases, a parent with the disease was first to suspect the illness and bring the child to us for confirmation. The youngest kids can't articulate where they hurt, but cyclic whining, crying, and irritability are all too eloquent. Slightly older children can at least alert their parents about pains in their knees and adjacent structures. These are often dismissed as "growing pains," especially if grandparents are consulted. Since they're often the earliest recognizable symptoms of fibromyalgia, we record them to pinpoint the onset of the disease. Depending on pain thresholds, don't forget that for other children fatigue, irritable bowel, or bladder symptoms may be the first clue. We even know of some girls for whom vulvar pain was the earliest complaint.

Most children begin hurting between the ages of seven and ten, but sometimes as early as five years old. Pains come and go without rhyme or reason and may recur over a few months or several years. These early attacks are sporadic and totally unrelated to growth periods. About 50 percent of the fibromyalgic adults we question recall having pains in their legs when they were young. Remember, there are no such things as growing pains! The term is actually a misnomer because the hurting begins well before the enormous growth spurt of puberty. Growth is not painful. A baby triples his or her size in the first year of life and doesn't seem to experience any discomfort in the process.

An interesting fact is that before puberty, boys and girls and boys are equally affected. When we wrote the first edition of this book, we were just beginning to assemble statistics on our pediatric cases. Since that date, of course, many more families have come in to be examined. While working on our book *What Your Doctor May* Not *Tell You About Pediatric Fibromyalgia*, a chance observation by my coauthor that we see as many boys as girls struck me as odd. But when we pulled the records from our charts, we were able to document that indeed the sexes were evenly divided. We've since found that other physicians have made this same discovery, and statistics from pediatric pain and rheumatology clinics have made their way into press. Most adult patients are female, but that's not so before puberty. What changes at that time to skew the incidence to 85 percent women? We finally realized that adolescent muscles and bones soak up great quantities of phosphate. Though both sexes get more massive at that time, boys get much bigger and will have to sustain that size for most of their lives. They may be taking in more phosphate than they can excrete, but suddenly their bodies can use every bit of it. Later in life, pain and fatigue may resurface to become the male percentage of fibromyalgics, about 15 percent.

The disease regenerates in the later teenage years or well beyond that time. Many factors determine how soon the disease resurfaces. We don't have space to outline them here. At first, symptoms may only nag during the premenstrual week. Severe menstrual cramps, PMS, and headaches often of migraine intensity strike regularly. Near that time, physical deficiencies surface. It becomes impossible to keep step with peers in gym activities or on playing fields. Formerly promising athletes begin tiring far too soon and lag behind less capable prospects. Just the thought of expending energy terrorizes these children, who know that muscular pains will surely follow within twenty-four hours. Most kids with fibromyalgia barely comply with compulsory physical education requirements, but that's as far as it goes.

Older children gradually realize that they're different. They know they don't have the same stamina as their friends. They're fully aware of brain-haze days when their textbooks might as well have been written in hieroglyphics. For no apparent reason, they are suddenly faced with dizziness and exhaustion. It's not possible to get enough sleep, and their backpacks seem to weigh a ton. Eyes go in and out of focus, and countenances get that glassy look teachers interpret as deliberate inattention. Everyone is too quick to assume that these symptoms are due to attention deficit disorder (ADD) or to being a normal but lazy teenager. What a rotten conclusion! And then suddenly everyone is baffled when the symptoms wane and everything seems much better for a time.

These days, we treat more and more children under the age of sixteen, but we've both had other firsthand experience with pediatric fibromyalgia. My three daughters suffered their first cycles at ages eleven, thirteen, and sixteen. My grandson, Nick, in the next generation was found to have fibromyalgia at age twelve. My coauthor Claudia's sons were both quite obviously affected and required treatment by age seven. Her younger son, Sean, a gifted athlete, had a high pain threshold and complained of only minor aches, but we soon realized he had irritable bowel symptoms that we thought might be manifestations of fibromyalgia. I examined him and easily located the telltale body lumps and bumps that clinched the diagnosis. When guaifenesin rapidly reversed his symptoms, we were elated. The elder of the two, Malcolm, my guaifenesin guinea pig, was fully articulate (seemingly from birth) and able to express himself very forcefully. He had the usual mess of symptoms, including those that affected his brain, musculoskeletal system, and gastrointestinal tract. He posed no diagnostic dilemma! In the case of grandchildren, nieces, and nephews, you can certainly hand information to the parents if they notice problems or seem receptive. How much you accomplish certainly depends on the nature of your relationship with them. Cynthia Craig, who has written so eloquently above, has since realized her own daughter also has fibromyalgia—although interestingly, her daughter's initial symptoms were quite different from her own. Instead, like her aunt, my coauthor Claudia, Camilla was suffering from repeated bladder complaints at a young age. But Aunt Claudia stepped in firmly. Now in middle school, Camilla only needs guaifenesin; no more bladder medications are necessary!

Physicians must depend on parents for crucial information and observations. Until more doctors are willing to recognize the early intrusions of pediatric fibromyalgia, and understand that there is an effective solution to treat it, as parents we are on the firing line. We must trust our instincts and our reliable, long-term observations. We've said it before: No one knows your child like you do. We cannot sit back and watch our children suffer because most of the medical professionals we encounter don't understand the problem. It's up to us to find solutions as part of our greater responsibility as parents. Luckily, because most of us have suffered so much, we are determined to save our children, and it comes naturally to us to do so.

TREATING CHILDREN

"I think I had FMS for about 20 years. Looking back into my childhood, I can now see the very first symptoms beginning around age nine or ten. . . . My daughter Jill is sixteen years old. Since my diagnosis, I realized that she had some of the symptoms of FMS. The symptoms became more and more pronounced and I finally realized about two years ago that she also had it. At that point I was unwilling to tell her this. How could I tell a fourteen-year-old adolescent that she was going to be in as much pain as her mother . . . without any knowledge of a cure? At that point in my illness, I was in excruciating pain, cried every day and didn't know what to do for myself.

I started guaifenesin under Dr. St. Amand's guidance in October 1996. He was incredibly gentle, helpful, sincere, but most of all he gave me hope. Once I realized that guaifenesin worked, I finally had the courage to tell my daughter what I suspected . . . that she also had FMS. I confirmed her diagnosis with a doctor and we agreed that she would start the guaifenesin once school was over in June.

"No matter how much pain I am in, it does not compare to the emotional pain of seeing my daughter in pain with FMS. Even worse is that I know what her pain feels like . . . because I have it too. I now realize that Jill has probably had FMS for about 5 or 6 years . . . we just didn't know it at the time."

—Aileen, New York

Someone sent us a paper written in 1928 by a family practitioner. He described children with growing pains, "great mental and body fatigue," "cold extremities," and "feeble digestion." He listed so many other symptoms that the diagnosis of fibromyalgia is obvious in retrospect. He successfully treated his small patients using a tree bark extract called guaiacum. Fifty years ago, that compound was purified to guaiacolate and became an ingredient in some cough preparations. Five years later, it was synthesized as guaifenesin for another brand of cough syrup. Twenty-five years ago, it was pressed into tablet form and has been marketed in this long-acting formulation ever since. Sadly, its use to relieve some miserable symptoms for children was lost to time.[1]

There's no need to go into great detail about treating children, since it's not much different from adults. As we've stated, guaifenesin is an over-the-counter medication and available in various strengths. Younger children may need a liquid form. These are formulated in two strengths: 100 mg and 200 mg per teaspoon. Slightly older kids may be able to swallow small tablets or capsules, which are slippery. Those can be found in 200, 300, and 400 mg concentrations. Tablets may be broken to create smaller doses. Crushing is not advisable—without a capsule, guaifenesin lands directly in the stomach in a large dose, and nausea could well be a problem.

All guaifenesin is bitter, so it takes a bit of ingenuity to hide the taste. Liquids can be disguised in juice, applesauce, or pudding. You may have to delay treatment until children can swallow tablets because the liquid is so bitter. Long term, it is very difficult to make them swallow it in the quantity that's required to treat fibromyalgia. We start children at 300 mg every twelve hours and gradually raise their dose until subsequent mapping shows reversal. If that technique is not locally available, parents have to wing it and make conclusions based on complaints and behavior. Simple notations about fatigue and pain levels on a desk calendar are really sufficient to monitor progress in most cases.

Unless the situation is desperate, it's sometimes wiser to initiate treatment at the beginning of summer vacation or the long winter break. This allows more time for rest and avoids simultaneously struggling with reversal cycles, school, and homework. Within a few weeks, most children demonstrate noticeable improvement before classes resume. Parents should not hesitate to begin guaifenesin in a student who is failing because of impaired memory and concentration. It may be helpful at first to cancel music or dance lessons for a month or two, depending on the severity of the illness and individual stamina. It may be counterproductive to remove just-for-fun activities so that a child feels left out or different. If a temporary break is necessary, assure your child that he or she is getting well and will soon resume a normal routine. It is also wise to consider resuming activities one by one without waiting for a complete response. Most children can cope just fine even when they've only partially purged. Getting back with friends prompts confidence, takes the focus off the illness, and convinces them that they're not really different from their peers.

It's tough to watch an ailing child, especially if you're the one who transmitted the defective gene(s). The first few reversal cycles are disturbing, but you should use all of your parental skills to make them tolerable. The preschooler can rest and take warm baths; those of most ages can swallow liquid or solid Tylenol (acetaminophen), Advil (ibuprofen), or the likes for pain relief. Insomnia and frequent awakening can be eased with Benadryl (diphenhydramine, as in Simply Sleep or Sominex), also available in various pediatric strengths. The many over-the-counter medications for symptoms such as diarrhea, gas, and painful urination need only be checked for salicylates. In general, children's compounds don't contain aspirin because of the danger of Reye's syndrome. (Pepto-Bismol is a rare exception, but is clearly marked.) Because children use fewer products than adults, finding salicylate-free products and teaching about them is quite simple. Tom's of Maine makes three children's toothpastes—Silly Strawberry, Orange Mango, and Grape—and many enjoy the Citrus, Pineapple, or Cranberry Grace Fibro-Smile or Lemon Lime Personal Basics by

Andrea Rose. Since sunscreens for children should be carefully checked for ingredients that protect from skin cancer, those without the salates are better choices anyway.

Children should be encouraged to interact with friends and stay as active as their illness allows. No matter how often you have to repeat it, it's encouraging to hear that nothing's so seriously wrong that time won't fix it. Parents walk a bit of a tightrope at this point. They must display compassion while remaining resolute that symptoms will be revisited and must be endured. They might need the wisdom of Solomon and the patience of Job to steadfastly hold a sick child to certain standards of achievement and behavior. But in truth, applying common sense and an attentive ear to the child's needs serve as admirable substitutes. Older children quickly learn how to pace themselves and work hard during better periods and rest when they feel worse. Smaller children can't be expected to understand—but then their lives are less stressful, and missed opportunities have fewer negative consequences.

Most children test the system once they're feeling well. At some time or another, expect them to stop their medication. Each of our children has done exactly that; even Malcolm, the original guinea-kid, has done it more than once despite his pride at being the first fibromyalgic treated with guaifenesin. We have to expect that as they grow older, they feel that great surge of invincibility required to propel them into lives of their own. Rest assured, they'll grope their way back to the medicine shelf and that bottle of guaifenesin when they feel bad enough. Luckily, since they're young and haven't fallen far behind, they respond as before and quickly make up lost ground.

In summary, guaifenesin is safe at any age. The return road from fibromyalgia is a shorter journey if begun in the early stages. For the sake of our children we, their parents, must trust ourselves to diagnose the illness perhaps sooner than physicians. We're fortunate enough to have a reliable medication that so swiftly restores our youngsters to normal. Looking at our affected progeny, those of us with fibromyalgia will inevitably reflect on our own lives. We'll always wonder how different our lives might have been had we been given an early diagnosis and effective treatment. For most of us, life would certainly have included considerably less suffering and fewer broken relationships. Instinctively as parents, we surely recognize that if our experiences have given us the strength and insight to help our children, they were not entirely wasted.

> "I suggest you get and read Dr. SA and Claudia's book *What Your Doctor May* Not *Tell You About Pediatric Fibromyalgia.* Because they clear so quickly on Guai if started early, I would rather my child had FMS than many other chronic illnesses. We were thrilled when Dr. St. Amand diagnosed my fourteen-year-old granddaughter with both FMS and HG. Otherwise she would have been labeled bipolar and on meds the rest of her life. Instead she is phasing off her antidepressant and doing so well in many ways. No more hating PE or being unable to go to school after walking home six blocks the day before. She also has the energy to do her homework and the memory to turn things in on time."
>
> —*Sandy, Idaho*

Part III

Strategies for the Road Back

Unlike the chapters included in part II, the following chapters are not specifically about treating fibromyalgia or its syndromes. Rather, they are about practical, everyday matters that affect your life, such as coping with your job, family, home, and other medications or treatments.

We hope that the information and suggestions in the following chapters will help you contend the disease on a daily basis. Undoubtedly, you will learn some things that your doctor has not told you, or that you have not learned through other sources. We hope this section will help you while you're waiting to begin (or are in the early stages of) guaifenesin treatment.

Chapter 14

Medical Band-Aids: Currently Promoted Treatments for Fibromyalgia—What You Don't Know Can Hurt You

"Neither my general practitioner nor my rheumatologist would talk to me about guaifenesin (to treat my fibromyalgia). My rheumatologist told me I would have to learn to live with the pain and illness for the rest of my life. I agree that this may happen, but if there is anything that can help slow it down or reverse it, why not try? No medication can be any worse than some of the medications I have tried."

—*Bonnie Jean, Arizona*

WHY OUR PROTOCOL IS NOT WIDELY PRACTICED

Durham Medical Center

"Ms. W. presents today in follow-up for depression. States she is significantly better. Feels like a different person and thinks she may have fibromyalgia and has been taking guaifenesin twice a day from a book she red [sic] and states that she is doing much better also. Patient is eager to discuss this novel or book by someone in California about the treatments of fibromyalgia which she states have saved her life. A/P 1) Depression: Patient is significantly better and I am happy for her.

2) Myalgias: Also better. Encouraged the patient to continue to take the guaifenesin if it is effective for her."

—*Actual medical records of patient*

There is no mystery to the standard approach to treating fibromyalgia. The party line is echoed throughout medical literature over and over, and little or no dissent is heard. Therapeutic options arise in scholarly journals such as the *Journal of Rheumatology* and work their way down into publications for general practitioners, chiropractors, nurses, and physical therapists. All footnote the same studies, and the same advice is given tailored slightly for each target audience.

It's virtually impossible to get published in rheumatology journals when your ideas differ from the accepted norm or if you are an outsider—not a researcher at a university. The peer review process is part of this obstacle. Before being approved for publication, manuscripts go to two experts in the field for comments and recommendations. These "peers" are either editors of other publications or close associates who correspond with journal editors, who also scrutinize papers for fraudulent conclusions. By nature, all of these specialists are especially leery of new and contrary ideas that spring up from any source other than full-time academia—where they've been conditioned to believe that all new discoveries originate. What peer reviewers and editors say goes; there is no place to appeal their decision, nowhere else to be published that's considered a reliable source. While, for the most part, this is an admirable system, procedurally sound, and designed for patient safety, it also stifles innovations that might arise from practitioner rank and file, or those in the trenches who treat patients full time and don't have access to laboratories.

I've commiserated with more than a few practicing colleagues who've unexpectedly stumbled onto something not offered in textbooks. Although they were trained to be alert and respect their own serendipity and the experiences they've acquired dealing with real live patients, most avenues are closed for propagating their observations. This is unfortunate. I believe it's rare to find a physician who, after a lifetime of practice, couldn't relate at least one better way of doing medicine. As we'll discuss later in this chapter, the FDA trusts physicians to use medications in any way they feel is appropriate once they are on the market. However, if they stumble upon something that works, there's no way to share this information with others. Lacking laboratories and funding, it's not an option for them to explore the chemistry or the reasons that would explain what they've learned.

For medical journals and their editors, there's a single gold standard when it comes to introducing new therapies. This is the so-called double-blind study in which half of the subjects are given the new compound, the other half an inert tablet, or placebo. Neither the physicians nor the enrollees know who is taking the active drug. At the end of a predetermined time, results are tabulated; if the subjects taking the new drug have improved more than those who are not, the study is considered a success, and thus suitable for publication. It's been documented time and time again that placebos, or sugar pills, help patients about 30 percent of the time, so that's the actual number a new discovery has to better.

For practicing physicians attempting to help fibromyalgics, this is a huge obstacle to surmount. First of all, they obviously can't give half the patients who come to see them for treatment a sugar pill. Second, without a drug company financing a large study with lots of patients, positive outcomes are hard to come by. Seeing ten or fifteen patients improving is just not going to cut it. Furthermore, top researchers or big names in the field routinely get hefty sums of money to be consultants to test new medications. A private physician can't possibly compete financially for their time. When the therapy in question isn't a moneymaker for drug companies or institutions, substantial funding is nearly impossible to find. A new use for a drug still under patent or exclusively produced by a single company would probably titillate interest, but barring that, the establishment just isn't interested. It's these limitations that keep many physicians from investigating previously unexplored problems—no matter their magnitude.

It's no secret that medical research in the United States is driven increasingly by a huge respect for the financial bottom line rather than for patients' welfare. Very few of the "new" medications brought to market are actually innovative, or different. Instead, huge sums are put into producing chemical cousins of existing drugs: variations on antidepressants, statins for cholesterol, stomach acid blockers, or blood pressure drugs.

As Dr. Sharon Levine, an associate director of the Kaiser Permanente Medical Group, put it: "If I'm a manufacturer and I can change one molecule and get another twenty years of patent rights, and convince physicians to prescribe and consumers to demand the next form of Prilosec or weekly Prozac instead of daily Prozac just as my patent expires, then why would I be spending money on a lot less certain endeavor which is looking for brand new drugs?" We've encountered these obstacles for many years. Facing this reality in 1999, we wrote the first edition of this book because we knew of no other way to get our observations and our results to patients and their physicians. We didn't want our protocol to die with this physician. Enough patients now have the message and sufficient energy to teach physicians and to help each other when necessary. And, as we'd hoped, a reverse approach is working from the bottom up, from patient to professionals. While this certainly rubs some professionals, especially researchers, the wrong way, others are simply overjoyed to find something to share with patients that actually offers them a chance for improvement. When they see the results we've predicted, they, too, become believers. Each year, physicians from all over the world fly to California to work with us in our office and to learn firsthand what it is we do. There's no doubt that there's hope.

THE ACCEPTED TREATMENT

> "It may well be better not to treat patients with our well-known but hardly effective armamentarium of drugs. . . . Treatments with antidepressants, tricyclics, formal exercise programs—particularly because they do not seem to work—prolong medicalization and dependency, the opposite of what we should wish to accomplish."
>
> —*Frederick Wolfe, MD,* Journal of Rheumatology[1]

So what's the predominantly accepted way to manage fibromyalgia? We already know that at best it's only partially effective, because disability claims, alternative treatments, and self-help groups abound. To make matters worse, the deplorable choices patients are being offered by many doctors are not great improvements over simply suffering in silence. We might say that at least these practitioners admit there's an illness and they're trying to help, but that doesn't much change the outcome of their approach. Too few of my colleagues agree that multidrug prescribing is a dangerous trade-off over the prolonged course taken by this disease.

The current majority plan or party line for treating fibromyalgia is to:

- Maintain a positive attitude about the chances for recovery.
- Assure patients that fibromyalgia is not going to kill or maim them.
- Advocate exercise for resurrecting energy.
- Endeavor to restore normal sleep patterns.

- Relieve as much pain as possible using medications the physician feels comfortable prescribing. (This varies greatly from doctor to doctor.)
- When those fail to restore health, help patients file for disability.

On the surface, we can't imagine anyone quarreling with these noble goals. They sound simple enough and, were they achievable, for some patients they might be the solution. Or would they? Look closely and you'll notice that, despite their appeal to common sense, not one even aims at altering the basic, metabolic malfunction of fibromyalgia. None of them is designed to fix the problem or even allude to what it might be. Except for exercise, none of them will keep patients from getting worse. It's also unlikely that sick individuals can push through the pain of even a minor workout. If they can't, what's left is a life of prescription medications that over time will need to be stronger, and with side effects that add more complaints to an already long list. On top of that, the very last item—"Help a patient to file for disability"—implies that despite optimism of the first part, it's accepted that many will have to face getting more and more incapacitated until they are legally disabled. We must ask ourselves, finally, should disability be a desired goal of those who come to a doctor looking for help and guidance?

PAIN

The official position of the American Medical Association is to use the lowest possible dose necessary of a medication for as short a duration as possible.

By the time patients visit doctors, they have more pain than they can handle by themselves. The brain gives pain priority over other sensations because it is such an important warning signal. Tissue destruction is what triggers the alert, and the body demands an immediate and dramatic response with the goal of preventing further injury.

Reflex withdrawal of fingers from flame illustrates that principle. Yet, as we've seen, there is no damage in fibromyalgia: The pain is chronic, or something that goes on day after day. The result is a brain that has exhausted its resources. Evidence is ample that the body responds in a different way to pain that is consistently present. We just don't get the benefit of the same potent hormones released in the acute scenario.

Even before arriving for an initial consultation, patients will have tried most over-the-counter analgesics such as aspirin, acetaminophen (Tylenol), and nonsteroidal, anti-inflammatory drugs (ibuprofen, naproxen, and a host of others). A physician may have already prescribed mild muscle relaxants such as carisoprodol (Soma) or cyclobenzaprine (Flexeril). The initial relief most patients experience with these medications has already worn off—that is, if they can tolerate the main side effect of fatigue. Before tossing his hands up, a previous doctor may have raised the doses a bit—accepted collective medical wisdom concludes that this is appropriate.

When this approach fails, the harried physician is frustrated and refers the patient to a specialist who is more comfortable writing stronger prescriptions. Hopes are raised: a new doctor! Simply taking the complicated history will fill the twenty to thirty minutes. Then, in a testimonial to the age of computers, the frustrated but hopeful patient produces a file, stuffed with documents listing every doctor who's been seen, each medication that did nothing much, and even the sequential dates when symptoms first appeared. Perhaps included are surgery reports and gruesome details of accidents. Sheets of laboratory results—tests done on every obtainable bodily fluid—are next, sometimes with hair or saliva analyses thrown in for good measure. Added to the stack are results of X-rays, MRIs, ultrasounds, scans, and copious notes inscribed by a variety of medical examiners. Nearly all tests are normal, but here and there slight deviations have been circled. Everything is there.

> "Last night before going to bed I took some sleeping pills (trazodone) and an anti-inflammatory (Voltaren). By the side of the bed I put some Bonine because I was feeling a little dizzy, Ambien because I come wide awake every night between 2:30 and 5:30 and if it's earlier rather than later I knock myself out so I can get a little rest, Tylenol because my spine aches terribly after lying in bed, Pamprin because menstrual cramps can be awful in the middle of the night and a heating pad (because a few nights before I woke up with a severe calf cramp that crippled me for three days afterward). I ask you, is that normal? I've always hated taking pain pills; even after I ruptured a disc I refused to take painkillers and sleeping pills. I got through it with difficulty but I survived. Now I am so worn down that I'll take anything if it will help me get some sleep. Every morning I wake up expecting to be normal again. It's a bad dream."
>
> —*Susannah, Maryland*

What do you suppose the I've-heard-it-all-before doctor is thinking? He knows people are in his waiting room rechecking their watches for the umpteenth time and have finished last year's newsmagazines. Just about now they're plaintively asking the receptionist, "How much longer do you think?" There's probably another expectant soul in an adjoining exam room freezing to death underdressed in a crumpled paper "gown."

The physician must think quickly. "She needs pain relief; she's already tried a bunch of over-the-counter drugs. I've got to do something." Out comes the Rx pad; it's time for the trump card, something more powerful than the patient's ever had before. That might be propoxyphene (Darvocet-N), tramadol (Ultram), or perhaps a new type of nonsteroidal anti-inflammatory such as celecoxib (Celebrex)—whatever isn't on the patient's intimidating, already-done-that-doesn't-work list. The patient leaves clutching the new prescription hopefully.

Unfortunately, the medications most doctors prescribe don't work for long. Pretty soon, the resourceful physician must again pull out the ever-ready prescription pad. It's time to get serious and turn to bigger guns, narcotics. They're all close cousins with different names, some natural and some synthetic, and are marketed alone or in combination with aspirin, acetaminophen, or ibuprofen. Readers may already be closely acquainted with some of them: codeine, Vicodin, Lorcet, Lortab, OxyContin, Percocet, and Norco, for example. At first, the pain is certainly dulled, and patients slowly learn to deal with side effects: a little fatigue, nausea, dizziness, and constipation. Some of the side effects lessen a bit with time, with the exception of constipation.

The first problem with narcotics is that the body gradually builds a tolerance to them. There's only a certain amount of time nature allows for the efficacy of any particular pain reliever. So narcotics aren't really designed for long-term use. But faced with unyielding pain, physician and patient succumb. What choice is there but to raise the dose when the drug no longer gives relief? And here comes the catch. The path toward stronger, longer-acting narcotics is one well trodden. When searching for relief from pain, danger lurks at every step, and patients trip on insignificant obstacles. They take what are marketed as safer pain pills, achieve temporary relief, develop tolerance, and move on looking for more powerful help. Unless fibromyalgia is treated at its root cause, the hourglass runs down. The opportune window is closed if individuals have run the analgesic gamut and are already radiating the happy flush of addiction. We know that look all too well, and it dejects us each time we face it. Even doctors quick to prescribe narcotic drugs admit "nearly all patients on opioids become physically dependent."[2] Some physicians neglect to tell patients their new prescription is an opiate that will surely make them physically drug dependent. Often they are prescribed by brand or chemical names that unsuspecting patients, in their desperation for pain suppression, don't recognize.

Even after a few weeks of using narcotics regularly, certain patients may not be able to muster the willpower to stop. Even if pain levels improve, the brain can't see it that way anymore. It has adapted to its marriage with the narcotic, which occupies receptors in the emotional part of the brain, where it produces pleasurable feelings. The body doesn't have to work to produce its own feel-good chemicals, endorphins, anymore. A pill is doing it the easy way. When the plug is pulled, the brain becomes petulant: *You ration me and I'll give you pain like you've never felt before!* Withdrawal means greater fatigue, insomnia, cognitive wipeout, severe anxiety, and even salivation or itching as parts of the ploy. That's true drug dependence, a physical reaction beyond the control of the conscious mind. The plot is this: When it's time for drugging, the brain reproduces every mental and physical symptom the individual has ever experienced. Fibromyalgics can't discern the difference, since their brains have been expressing identical complaints for years. The reasoning goes: *I feel all the same things, so my fibromyalgia isn't a bit better.* It's nevertheless brain-speak and duplicity. No longer are muscles, sinews, gut, and bladder sending distress signals; the brain now *initiates* them. Even after guaifenesin has sufficiently reversed the illness, the brain keeps duping the individual with its cornucopia of ruses. Once narcotics have been discontinued, it takes some time for the body to begin producing its own natural endorphins again, which makes this period very difficult.

In medicine, we sometimes play with words. *Habituation* and *dependence* versus *addiction* are examples of this. Like everybody else, doctors like clear separations—black and white suits us much better than gray. We have a preference for findings and solutions that can be accurately filed into distinct categories. When fibromyalgia presents its spectrum and hops disconcertingly from one system to another, we're far less comfortable. We're very insecure if we have to calm a conglomeration of symptoms all at once. We know we should relieve pain. That's part of our oath, but *primum no nocere*—above all do no harm—should supersede our need to be heroes trying to curb every discomfort no matter the cost.

Since escalating drug use often ends up badly, we direct you to an old medical maxim: *For chronic diseases, avoid giving addictive drugs if at all possible.* In fibromyalgia, this can only be accomplished by early diagnosis and treatment. Some of you probably want to slam this book down in anger just about now, but don't. Hear us out. We judiciously prescribe pain medications if we must, but only non-narcotic varieties. We stress to our patients: *Bear with us and let's treat the disease instead of only mental and physical anguish.*

Dependency can become a secondary issue for fibromyalgics, because the side effects of narcotics are often easier to tolerate than the never-ending pain. Fibromyalgics can't discern the difference, since their brains have been expressing identical complaints for years. On this emotionally charged topic, it's hard to get both sides to listen to scientific fact and reason. Dependency is not the same as addiction, which by definition means that drug use is causing a problem in certain social ways. Dependency simply means that the body has come to depend on an outside chemical to fulfill a normal function. As we've seen, the body converts narcotic pain medications to morphine, and this morphine occupies pain receptors in the brain, ones that were designed for natural endorphins. When this happens on a daily basis, the brain is fooled and the body cuts normal production levels drastically, in some cases to next to nothing. There's no problem as long as the body continues to get the artificial supply, but when a dose is skipped or delayed, no natural chemicals replace it. The body will reproduce pain, and any modest pain such as a headache or muscle strain that would be a slight annoyance normally is sensed as much worse. Since endorphin receptors are largely in the emotional part of the brain, depression and apathy also occur. This is the reason that many patients have been put on even more potent and long-acting narcotics such as OxyContin or morphine. The rationale is simply that since these compounds don't wear off as quickly as say, Vicodin, the patients are spared the discomfort of rebound pain every four to six hours. The bad news is that when narcotics are discontinued completely, it takes several months for the body's own natural endorphin levels to return to normal. Other hormones related to the hypothalamus (such as estrogen) are also reduced and may be one of the reasons for fatigue and weight gain.

There are no medications in the *Physicians' Desk Reference (PDR)* designated for long-term relief of chronic pain, defined as lasting longer than six months. That's because these medications aren't safe or devoid of serious side effects. In general, chronic pain is more difficult to treat than the acute kind. In normal responses to trauma, the brain masterminds the release of endorphins and other specific hormones to deal with hurting. These naturally occurring painkillers are actually members of the opioid family. They sneak in, attach to pain receptors, and try to block pain perception, but this does not work for long. Nature's idea is to blunt the pain for long enough so the injured body can get to safety. Then pain is a necessary warning in order to persuade the injured to rest and heal while respecting necessary limitations. The brain isn't programmed for dealing with prolonged hurting, because it regards pain as an important messenger.

Long-term releases of endorphins promote desensitization. As we've seen before in other systems of the body, unrelenting messages are eventually ignored as if they are a malfunction. In this case, they wear down endorphin-producing cells, which finally refuse to respond. The brain gradually produces less, and unneeded receptors recede into the depth of cells, where many are destroyed. Steady narcotic use meets that same kind of ultimate stonewalling: Brain cells tire, reject the opiate signals, and keep right on hurting. Mounting complaints make doctors think fibromyalgics are very sensitive to pain and must obviously need heavier dosages. Eventually, most physicians balk at the quantity they now must prescribe for even modest relief and send the poor patient packing.

So what do you do if you swear off narcotics? Cumulative studies are showing that acetaminophen (Tylenol) can lead to kidney or liver damage if taken regularly over several years. That same study found no such problems with some nonsteroidal anti-inflammatory drugs (NSAIDs) such as ibuprofen or naproxen. We remind you there's no inflammation in fibromyalgia, but the drugs can still cut pain somewhat. The entire group may, however, induce bleeding ulcers, liver damage, and symptoms that mimic fibromyalgia or even disrupt deep-sleep patterns. This class had the added dangers of causing gastrointestinal bleeding. The newer anti-inflammatories that are kinder on the stomach appear to be harder on the heart. One of them, rofecoxib (Vioxx), was recently pulled by its manufacturer from the market due to increased risks of heart attacks. Recent references suggest that all NSAIDs, along with acetaminophen, can interfere with energy production in mitochondria. If taken before exercise, they can actually interfere with some of its strengthening benefits.

AN OVERVIEW OF MEDICATIONS COMMONLY USED FOR FIBROMYALGIA

"For 30 years I have taken Ativan at night to deal with interstitial cystitis (which got much better with the guai) and for about a year I got used to taking a Vicodin a day to keep coping with everything. It seemed to give me just the energy I needed. I want you to understand that before treatment no amount of Vicodin, Ultram, Ativan, etc. would work. Dr. St. Amand kept insisting I dump the Ativan for sure. He felt I was getting rebound fa-

> tigue. I finally listened to him five months ago. It is amazing that even one milligram at night would cause such trouble, not to mention Vicodin, just one a day. The first two weeks I was really uptight. I took up knitting and it got me through. Then lo and behold I felt this feeling lift right out. That was five months ago. The fatigue is gone, the anxiety gone, and yet I can still deal with my main stress issue every single day."
>
> —*Tammy, California*

Since the mid-1980s, low-dose antidepressants have been used for fibromyalgia. Side effects include weight gain, dry mouth, constipation, and fatigue. Some studies suggest that one type, the tricyclics, gave relief in only 30 to 40 percent of patients (see the quote by Dr. Goldenberg below)—clearly not much better than the placebo response. Newer, specific serotonin-reuptake and norepinepherine-reuptake inhibitors are being prescribed as though they were no more dangerous than after-dinner mints. A very recent paper suggested they had no advantage over placebo. That's suspect because at least clinically, significant numbers of patients have surely been helped. In those for whom such drugs are effective, sleep patterns are somewhat restored, depression eased, and pain perception diminished up to 50 percent. Notwithstanding that, some people get adversely wired up and suffer serious disruption of stage four sleep. Desperate physicians continue prescribing them despite the unpromising statistics; making combinations of the various types of antidepressants is increasingly popular. Side effects for these newer classes vary greatly but most common are drowsiness, nausea, headache, and dry mouth. For fibromyalgics, particularly disturbing can be hair loss and lowered libido in both males and females.

The above paragraph is discouraging—and it gets worse! Antidepressants have no lasting benefits for fibromyalgia, even though pain and depression are temporarily masked. Their effectiveness lessens after about nine weeks, and unfortunately, the disease marches on. Nothing has been done to alleviate the cause, and symptoms simply burst through the drug suppression at some point. Dosages should not be titrated upward. Studies show that if low potencies don't work, then higher amounts won't prove much more effective.

Drug interactions are another concern with antidepressants. While they do help with a number of symptoms to a certain degree, quite often they are contraindicated with other therapies. The tripan migraine medications (Imitrex, Maxalt, and so on) should not be used within five weeks of some antidepressants. Used with sleeping medications, both prescription and over-the-counter versions may cause oversedation. Other therapies that have an effect on serotonin levels such as 5-HTP are considered dangerous in conjunction with any antidepressant. Tramadol (Ultram) is also considered risky in combination. Narcotics and central nervous system depressants such as muscle relaxants and benzodiazepines (for anxiety) should be used with great caution if you are taking an antidepressant.

> "Although tricyclic medications, notably low doses of amitriptyline and cyclobenzaprine, have been beneficial in controlled therapeutic trials in fibromyalgia, overall effectiveness in patients has not been impressive. Patient self-rating of medicinal therapy has been no better than such non-medicinal treatments as physical and chiropractic therapy. Only 30 to 40 percent of our patients described medications as very effective. In the only long-term longitudinal study reported in FMS we surveyed 39 patients for three consecutive years. Although 83 percent of them continued to take some medications, usually multiple, during the three years, only 20 percent felt well."
>
> —*Don L. Goldenberg, MD,* Journal of Rheumatology[3]

Muscle relaxants, sedatives, and anti-anxiety drugs round out the list of drugs commonly prescribed for fibromyalgia. Patients tolerate them only in limited quantities because of the hangover fatigue they generally induce. That and mental fogginess are two reasons patients give for discontinuing them. Confirming their value by double-blind studies is difficult, because sedative effects are too flagrant compared with placebo. At least they don't interfere with our protocol and are helpful for those who handle them well. As time goes by, more and stronger drugs are casually added to the arsenal. Zanaflex (tizanadine hydrochloride)—a potent drug designed for serious medical conditions that cause muscle spasticity—may be prescribed instead of the older, surely safer Soma (carisoprodol) or Flexeril (cyclobenzaprine). Neurontin (gabapentin), a drug designed for epileptic seizures that do not respond to other medications, is handed out for nerve pain despite the potential for serious side effects. In desperation, physicians and patient are being pushed to try something new because nothing has worked well thus far.

Recently, a trend has begun largely in response to the fatigue, mental slowness, and lethargy caused by narcotic pain medications, especially the more potent ones. It's becoming all too common to see patients of all ages on potent combinations of painkillers offset by a stimulant. Most commonly used are modafinil (Provigil) and amphetamines such as Ritalin, Concerta, and Metadate (methylphenidate), as well as the older dexamphetamine, Dexedrine. Newer compounds include Adderall (amphetamine salts). These are also sometimes prescribed alone when patients complain of deadening fatigue. In fibromyalgia, where energy formation is faulty, these drugs are particularly problematic, especially when used for long periods. Although they'll work initially, the cells eventually become exhausted and fail to respond to even higher doses of stimulants, rather like beating a dead horse. The body's energy stores are dragged farther back into deficit spending, and it takes time to recover when these are finally stopped because of lack of efficacy. Other drugs that are sometimes used to promote daytime alertness are the antidepressants fluoxetine (Prozac) and buproprion (Wellbutrin).

If there were any drugs that always worked for pain and fatigue, we'd all know about them. The vast amounts of drugs and supplements patients take are ample proof that none is very effective. People who come to us are frequently taking amazing combinations; it's common to see patients on ten or more medications. The saddest part is that even with all those compounds, they are still searching for relief. These days, five brain-altering drug mixtures are almost the norm. Each of them is offered in various dosages. Even mathematicians couldn't easily calculate the possibilities of drug interactions in that interplay. For us, it's mind boggling!

New patients arrive with their drug stockpiles and, to get them to join our protocol, we don't try to interfere with their products. Once they're doing better, it's time to discuss the notion of purging the list one drug at a time. We're happiest with newcomers who are taking no such products. When we explain their unappealing side effects weighted against the scant relief, most of them opt to confine intakes to over-the-counter analgesics. Luckily, we also see patients who have tried everything and concluded that strong medications are of no benefit and only result in more symptoms and feeling less like themselves. Common sense dictates that you should avoid chemical Band-Aids when at all possible, especially because there is reversal treatment at hand. Polypharmacy, or multiple medications, are a very real problem when suffering has gone on without relief for a number of years. Eventually, medications alone are reason enough for a patient to be considered disabled. For example, a patient taking heavy narcotics such as methadone, fentanyl, or MS Contin should not operate a car. Many states consider this "driving under the influence." At work, narcotics certainly make people accident prone and a possible danger to themselves or others.

Prescription drugs aren't the only thing commonly used for

fibromyalgia. In response to the lobbying efforts of the multi-billion-dollar "dietary supplement" industry, Congress in 1994 exempted their products from FDA regulation. Since then, products of all description—animal, vegetable, and mineral—have flooded the market, subject only to the scruples of their manufacturers and rashly promising all sorts of miracles. The so-called scientific facts on labels are often indistinguishable from advertising jargon. Dietary supplements may contain the substances listed on the label in the amounts claimed, but they need not, and there is no one to police them and prevent their sale if they don't. The much-touted coral calcium products, for example, which claimed to treat everything from cancer to fibromyalgia and arthritis, were found to contain dangerously high levels of lead when finally subjected to independent laboratory testing.

> "In an analysis of ginseng products, for example, the amount of active ingredient in each pill varied by as much as a factor of 10 among brands that were labeled as containing the same amount. Some brands contained none at all. . . . The only legal requirement in the sale of such products is that they not be promoted as preventing or treating disease. To comply with that stipulation, their labeling has risen to an art-form of doublespeak."
>
> —*Marcia Angell, MD, and Jerome P. Kassirer, MD,*
> The New England Journal of Medicine[4]

It's not within the scope of this book to agonize over herbal medications, their safety, and their efficacy. Since plant concentrates totally block guaifenesin, it's a moot point for us. We've previously questioned the wisdom of taking tablet concentrates from crushed leaves, roots, or other plant parts that contain at least one hundred thousand various compounds. The dangers of individual idiosyncrasies mount with that volume of chemical contents. While herb users are seeking help from just a couple of these chemicals, they are consuming many more by ingesting the entire extract. The nonmedicinal portions exponentially raise the likelihood of hypersensitivity reactions and consequent liver or renal damage—increased with frequent dosing and questionable purity.

While some herbal formulas, taken in concert with a doctor or health practitioner's guidance, can certainly be beneficial, the vast majority of users self-medicate, which can be a recipe for disaster. As these supplements are used more widely, interactions with prescription drugs have been documented as well as side effects—the same as with any medicinal compound, no matter the origin. Despite what advertising would have you believe; *natural* is not a synonym for *safe*. Medications, quite simply, are poisons judiciously administered. We suggest that any compound that has a medicinal effect on the body should be treated with respect.

Hormones such as DHEA, thyroid, progesterone, testosterone, growth hormone, and estrogen will not block guaifenesin, and are used by some doctors. Lamentably, they're given because one of them turned up low on a single test, and sometimes not even the appropriate one. Just as often, they're handed out for boosting a metabolism desperately trying to scrape together energy while dealing with the ravages of fibromyalgia. As an endocrinologist, I strongly suggest that patients do extensive research before considering hormone therapy of any kind. These are powerful and too often mishandled with disrespect for their full effects. Be sure you're abnormal on repeated testing, done at the proper time of day, before embarking on such misadventures. Also bear in mind that many hormone levels are *meant* to decline with age, and boosting them to youthful levels in older patients may cause severe problems. The newest vogue, "bio-identical" sex hormones, is a case in point. Although these have not been shown to have the same risks as synthetic or animal compounds, they also have not been studied to the same extent. The portion of the name *identical* signifies that these must attach to at least most of the same receptors in the body. What is known about them is less than what is unknown, yet the widely held, non-FDA-endorsed "consensus" is that they must be safer.

Research will also turn up other problems with some of the compounds on the market. Some hormones such as growth hormone cannot be taken orally but must be injected. Thus any oral preparation touted as growth hormone couldn't be effective. Abnormalities of other hormone levels (such as cortisol) must be diagnosed by tests administered at appropriate times of the day, as normal levels vary widely depending on the hour.

We repeatedly issue warnings about ingesting excess vitamins and supplements. Very little is known about consuming large quantities, and unbalanced components may interfere with the others. Fat-soluble ones such as K and E might pose minor risks; D shouldn't be abused, however, and A (beta-carotene) seems downright dangerous in the quantities customarily marketed. Minerals won't block guaifenesin. They can interfere with some prescription drugs, though, especially the absorption of thyroid hormone. Calcium is known to partially block the action of some antibiotics, and magnesium the effects of Neurontin. Magnesium is often taken for muscle relaxation but can cause diarrhea. Larger amounts of others such as zinc have been questioned for safety by some Alzheimer's disease researchers. Vitamin C in large doses can increase the risk of weight gain when taken with tricyclic antidepressants.

> "I should tell you that not only have I improved due to guaifenesin, I have also thrown out all the other stuff I was on. Now, I use no sleeping pills, no antidepressants, no steroids, and I used to think I needed all three of them for the rest of my life. I only take a little Tylenol now and then for headaches, and of course, guaifenesin."
>
> —*Jeri Lynn, California*

To recap, we steadfastly advocate a single, simple medication for the treatment of fibromyalgia—guaifenesin. It's been around for a very long time and devoid of side effects, so we unhesitatingly prescribe if for persons of all ages. We're especially pleased when new patients come to us with the desire to stick to just one protocol. This way, there is no confusing what gets them well. In time, they'll realize that guaifenesin is what got them there and not some weird combination. Although it's tempting to reach for every new golden promise or astounding miracle, it's wise to stick with one modality at a time. Wiser still is to research the proposed treatment thoroughly for safety. When it comes to this issue, guaifenesin wins hands-down.

SLEEP

> "Difficulty falling asleep and staying asleep long enough to reach the Stage 4 phase of restorative sleep is the first major hurdle that we face in dealing with the other symptoms of FMS. I absolutely cannot nap no matter how hard I try, and going to sleep at night requires a ritual of sleep aids, a calming atmosphere, total darkness in the room, numerous pillows piled around my body, a light-weight cover. I would like to trade a day with a normal person who goes out like a light, sleeps deeply and wakes refreshed. Oh I wish. . . ."
>
> *—Elizabeth R., Georgia*

The desire for restful sleep eventually leads exhausted fibromyalgics to demand sleeping pills. By that time, an expensive mattress, contoured pillows, blackout curtains, and white-noise tapes haven't made much difference. Pre-bedtime rituals such as warm baths, dimmed lights, soothing music, or meditation that initially helped no longer work. My own experience was that nighttime inactivity further stiffened my already contracted muscles, tendons, and ligaments. Every time I'd lie in one position for a few minutes, my pain mounted progressively. At first it was subliminal—just enough to make me restless. As the night progressed, I hurt enough to awaken from whatever stage of sleep I'd managed to reach. My nights were a bit like the Indianapolis 500, moving to and fro, constantly steering for position. I could make a rare victory lap only if I got a good night's rest. As I recall, I rarely won.

The earliest studies of modern fibromyalgia by Drs. Moldofsky and Smythe concentrated on the poor sleep patterns that more than 70 percent of patients complained about. Most commonly, the complaint is the inability to stay asleep for more than three or four hours. Because articles about sleep disturbance were the first to make it into medical journals, nearly all physicians are willing to prescribe sleeping compounds and are aware that fibromyalgics have problems getting enough rest.

We urge patients to try the over-the-counter sleeping aids—diphenhydramine (brand name Benadryl) and doxylamine (Unisom). These old antihistamines made people so drowsy, they were abandoned as allergy treatments, but they were rediscovered as sleeping aids when they went over the counter. They are non-habit-forming and safe in small amounts, even for children. Benadryl is often allowed by obstetricians during pregnancy. It's marketed in 25 mg capsules, but the dosage can be titrated up to 100 mg a night. Diphenhydramine is the sleep-inducing ingredient in products such as Tylenol PM, Sominex, and Unisom. It helps reach delta, deep-sleep levels. About 10 percent of people get adverse effects such as jitters and excitability and for those, these two antihistamines should be avoided. Others find that these compounds make them excessively tired the next morning. If this is the case, you should purchase them in liquid or tablet forms so that very small doses can be used and titrated on a nightly basis.

Melatonin is a hormone released by the pineal gland. It has

many effects in the body, where it eventually becomes serotonin. As of this writing, it appears safe and helps many people reset their sleep clocks for better rest. Travelers have used it for years to offset jet lag. Levels of the hormone decline with age, which may explain some of the insomnia of the elderly. Its safety has not been established for children or teenagers because they already produce large amounts. We concur that it works best for older individuals who may require a higher dose than younger patients because their own levels are lower to start with. A recent paper recommended taking the hormone nightly for at least two months if you are trying to readjust the brain's time clock, the so-called circadian rhythm.

The sublingual form of melatonin provides quicker action and makes for smaller dosages. It dissolves and absorbs within ten minutes under the tongue. This introduces it directly into the bloodstream and avoids the digestive tract. Fibromyalgics should be aware that the minted variety will block guaifenesin, but orange flavoring is also available. (The tablets, which are swallowed, contain no flavor at all.) We've had some success combining melatonin with diphenhydramine when neither alone worked, and there's also evidence that it enhances the action of amitriptyline (Elavil). High dosages of melatonin may invoke unpleasant dreaming that suggests lowering the intake. Depression has also been listed in various places as a possible side effect.

Another nonprescription compound is 5-HTP, short for 5-hydroxy-tryptophan. Like melatonin, it eventually becomes serotonin in the body. Doses generally begin at 20 mg before bed, but lower doses are sometimes taken by day to help control pain. Doses as high as 100 mg three times a day have been studied, but some patients are sensitive to it so doses should be started very low and moved up slowly. Side effects include dry mouth, daytime fatigue, dizziness, and constipation. Most pharmacies and health food stores carry 5-HTP, which has been used since L-tryptophan was taken off the market when contaminated batches caused some fatalities. This should not be used within five weeks of treatment with an SSRI antidepressant.

If patients still can't sleep or don't tolerate the above compounds and their combinations, we reluctantly turn to prescription medications. These vary greatly in their habit-forming propensities, yet all have the potential to create dependence. If our patients must take them, we suggest taking the tiniest effective amount and diligently avoiding nightly use. Although this results in inferior sleep on alternate nights, it spares the probability of habituation and loss of efficacy. The exact type of sleeping problem should be explored as well. Do you have a problem falling asleep or remaining asleep? Is early-morning awakening the problem? Different medications work on these various problems so that solutions can even be addressed on a night-by-night basis if necessary.

Sedatives may produce side effects such as a central nervous system depression leading to morning hangover. This compounds the problem for fibromyalgics, who already have difficulty functioning at that time of day. Sleeping potions may also cause rebound effects the next afternoon when the fatigue can actually be quite intense. If patients are forced to nap as a result, they may get into a vicious cycle that further intensifies nighttime insomnia. Other side effects are mental confusion, slowed thinking, dizziness, and malaise.

Many other medications, such as muscle relaxants, tranquilizers, anti-anxiety drugs, antidepressants, and narcotics, greatly add to an already overwhelming fatigue. Some of these are used to promote sleep because the side effect of drowsiness helps patients fall asleep and remain so for hours. Fibromyalgics are given many of these compounds in diverse combinations. It's a toss-up whether or not the enhanced sleep they provide is worth the energy-sapping side effects. We urge patients with unrelenting fatigue to review their medications with their physicians or pharmacists. Ever-present fatigue should not always be blamed on the illness—symptoms of fibromyalgia are usually variable from day to day at least to some extent. Over-the-counter anti-inflammatories and analgesics must also be viewed in context, since they can easily contribute to persistent drowsiness by cutting energy production.

Some of the more common drugs used to aid sleep are hypnotics such as estazolam (ProSom), flurazepam (Dalmane), temazepam (Restoril), and triazolam (Halcion). They are the older drugs in this class, and since they are available as cheaper generics, they are preferred by insurance companies over the newer compounds. They have longer duration of action, which may cause more morning fatigue. Ambien (zolpidem) has been shown to have fewer side effects. Zaleplon (Sonata) has the shortest half-life of all and can be used to permit easier morning awakenings. For the last two listed, you may have to petition for insurance coverage, but if rebound fatigue is a problem it is worth the time and effort.

At the very end of 2004, a new sleeping medication, Lunesta (eszopiclone), was approved by the FDA indicated for difficulty falling asleep as well as staying asleep. It is nonnarcotic and not limited to short-term use like other compounds for insomnia. Since is has not been widely used, data are limited, and because it is expensive it's unlikely to be covered by many drug plans.

Commonly Prescribed Medications for Sleep Disturbances in Fibromyalgia

Tricyclic and polycyclic antidepressants (the most studied drugs in fibromyalgia)—Possible weight gain is a side effect, as well as early-morning grogginess, constipation, and dry mouth. Benefits are seen two to four weeks after initiation. If efficacy starts to fade, a monthlong break may be taken every four months. Most common: amitriptyline, doxepin, cyclobenzaprine, nortripyline, and desipramine. Of the polycyclic antidepressants, side effects include drowsiness, nausea, headache, constipation. Trazodone—both a sedative and an antidepressant—is the most commonly used. Small doses should be used in the beginning, and often that's all that is necessary. Other classes of antidepressants such as the SSRIs generally do not help as well with sleep problems.

Benzodiazapines—Side effects include drowsiness, poor coordination, constipation, mental confusion, and short-term memory loss. These have higher addictive potential and must not be discontinued abruptly. They were designed to reduce anxiety and agitation. For this reason, they induce sleep. Most common are clonazepam, lorazepam, and alprazolam.

Muscle relaxants—Used to reduce muscle tightness and spasm and help relaxation. Since fatigue is the major side effect, they are often prescribed indirectly for sleep. Most common are the older cyclobenzaprine and carisoprodol, which have been well studied. A newer addition is the much more potent Zanaflex (tizanidine hydrochloride)—actually marketed to decrease spasticity of muscles in serious conditions. Side effects include mental confusion and hallucinations; they should be used with care. Insurance companies regularly prefer the older drugs for which generics are available.

A new medication, ramelteon, will soon be on the market. It is the first novel drug in thirty-five years of sleep research and will be indicated for insomnia. It targets specific receptors in the brain, MT1 and 2, which are critical in regulating the body's sleep–wake cycle. It is still being studied in long-term trials to determine its potential for abuse and addiction.

"Although we've learned that it is better to take only guaifenesin, for many it is difficult to do so. Many of us started on a number of different medications. I was diagnosed with FMS in 1988 and have been on plenty of medications since then. My symptoms began in 1977. I was taking Elavil for three years and Ambien for two. I tried to stop taking both of these a number of times before guaifenesin but I was in such sad shape I would have to start up again. I very slowly weaned myself off the Elavil. That was not very hard to do. I had no real reaction from stopping. I was concerned with the Ambien because I needed to sleep, so I cut way back, usually only taking ¼ of a tablet at night except when I was feeling well. Then I stopped taking it. The first few nights I used Benadryl, it made me very groggy. Then I tried melatonin and got the same results. I also tried a combination that made me groggy too. So, after a week of messing around I went to bed without anything and I fell asleep just fine. . . ."

—Linda P., Ohio

EXERCISE

"I also have a problem with pain the day after [sexual] intercourse which, just like any other type of exercise, makes me hurt for days and may send me into a flare."

—B. J., Arizona

The recommendation for exercise is one of the few truly useful ones. It's near and dear to the hearts of most researchers and medical practitioners, and is the most commonly prescribed treatment for fibromyalgia. Endless studies tout its benefits as well as the difficulty in persuading patients to begin a program and stick with it. Advice is soundest when gentle stretching and pool workouts are suggested. We heartily endorse these types of gentle versions that don't overstress the already weakened body. They're a great way to start, but more effort will be needed later—as you will learn.

The problem is that well-meaning physicians try to push patients into an immediate athletic program that very few can handle even though it may be labeled "low impact." A huge number of fibromyalgics can't even tolerate walking a few blocks without bracing for the physical price they'll pay the next day. We understand why this is true. It's our contention that aches and pains of fibromyalgia are caused by intracellular metabolic debris actually caused by steadily working cells. As long as those residues remain in affected cells, they stand at attention in a perpetually alert state. In short, fibromyalgia is an overexercised, energy-stealing disease that seriously impedes rest. Any significant workout creates more of this debris, which must recruit other tissues to act as dump sites. This intensifies the condition, and the body doesn't have the capacity to make energy to clear the problem. Further malfunction follows as expressed by more pain, fatigue, and, finally, systemic collapse.

The rationale behind prescribing heavy exercise is understandable. Stress releases brain opioids—endorphins—in response to muscular aching. As they latch onto receptor cells, pain perception is dulled, thus allowing us to push on with the activity. Yet their positive effect is nullified when the pain caused by exercise lasts too long. That's even more predictable if the would-be athlete takes narcotic pain medication before exercise. As we've seen, these drugs depress the brain's ability to produce natural endorphins and grow new, bodywide mitochondria to add energy (ATP). It should also be remembered that upon discontinuing narcotics, it takes the body some three or four months to begin producing natural endorphins again. Chronic use of opioids depresses natural levels to about 5 percent of normal. During this period, if you begin an exercise program, be aware that your tolerance for pain is abnormally low, and you may feel far worse. Muscle aches, which under normal circumstances would be minor, will seem more intense until endorphin levels return to normal.

Disciplines that work well in healthy patients fail substantially in fibromyalgia. Exercise is intended to make you feel better, and that goal should be kept in mind. The rules are simple: Keep muscular workouts light and within tolerable discomfort zones. Treat the underlying disease, wait for improvement, and only then expand muscular efforts to tolerance. That's when you can go for the gold and finally break the self-perpetuating, sedentary-begets-fatigue cycles.

We can't emphasize enough that muscles, tendons, and ligaments must be treated gently until guaifenesin has cleared them. Until that time, care is needed. Exercise cannot heal tendons and ligaments, and as long as they are affected, they may not provide adequate support for joints. Until ligaments are strengthened and tight muscles are relaxed, endurance exercises should not be undertaken. In the beginning, a warm shower or bath may be helpful before stretching. Gentle walking is another way to begin an exercise session. The goal is not to yank hard on contracted structures lest injury occur and derail the program.

Earlier we stressed that totally sedentary people wipe out up to 80 percent of the mitochondria in their muscle cells. Without them, the energy-generating capacity of the body is compromised and cannot be remedied. Reversing fibromyalgia with guaifenesin restores the efficiency of those last few standing, but only endurance exercise can promote mitochondrial rebirths and resurrect dormant ones. Extra mitochondria result in more abundant energy and growing stamina. While it doesn't happen overnight, exercise will begin the process of making both body and brain more functional. The key is to start with realistic goals and expand them as guaifenesin cleans the tissue and makes more activity possible.

> "I spoke to you five years ago. I had begged my pain doctor to let me try guaifenesin but he refused to believe in it and then so did I. I am much, much worse since five years ago. I now use a cane and can't work anymore. I am willing to try again now but my doctors do not recognize that it works. I am very close to a wheelchair and being bankrupt and now I am taking two anti-depressants because this disease has ruined my life. Don't worry; I don't have the guts to kill myself. I just wish the pain would stop. I take 100 mgs of methadone a day and today is a bad day."
>
> —*April, Pennsylvania*

DISABILITY STATUS: A RAGING CONTROVERSY

> "When it comes to disability determination, anyone who has to prove he or she is ill will be rendered more ill in the proving. When a physician participates in the process it becomes worse than counterproductive, it becomes iatrogenic. At issue is the growing numbers . . . for whom self respect in the work-place is so elusive that the gauntlet of disability determination seems an easier path."
>
> —*Nortin Hadler, MD*[5]

In 1987, the American Medical Association acknowledged that fibromyalgia (or fibrositis, as it was then called) is a condition capable of causing disability or, rather, the inability to work at a job with regular demands. Despite this straightforward statement, qualifying for benefits remains a major challenge for patients and, by extension, for us, their physicians. Unique problems exist in fibromyalgia because of the subjective nature of complaints and total lack of diagnostic tests. It's impossible to prove someone is actually sick with a disease from which he or she will not improve or recover. Obviously, and for good reasons, the establishment is a little leery of "the patient says he [or she] hurts too much to work." There remains no way to measure pain—to prove it exists (or doesn't), or where it's located—and the same goes for fatigue. Equally elusive are the symptoms of irritable bowel, bladder, muscle stiffness, and problems with memory and concentration!

As physicians, we have an obligation to care for patients. That much is clear. If patients say they can't work, can we deny it? It's our duty to help, but how do we verify it? The absence of an unequivocally accepted yardstick to measure this illness relegates us to hedging statements: "The patient *states* she is too tired to work, and describes daily headaches"; "the patient *says* sitting at her computer makes her back hurt too much to concentrate." Fibromyalgia is known to cause cognitive problems such as impaired memory and concentration. Under pressure to control costs, insurance companies balk and demand proof of disability that meets *their* criteria. The fact is, patients, doctors, lawyers, third-party insurers, and governments are locked in a complicated struggle with no easy solutions. Currently, disability law is structured so that if you can perform your job, even though it hurts to do it, you're not eligible for benefits. The younger you are, the harder it will be for you to convince a judge that you can't do any kind of work. While it's easy for fibromyalgics to take this situation personally, it should be mentioned that only a terminal illness allows for immediate granting of benefits. Missing an eye or a limb or a hand doesn't guarantee you'll win your case—despite these obvious limitations. Everyone else is in for a struggle, especially one with an illness as invisible as fibromyalgia. It can be a long process with less-than-satisfactory results and no guarantee of final vindication. Reports of depression beginning when benefits are granted are also common. With the fight behind you, the ramifications of what being legally disabled means can be very difficult to accept. Finding a meaningful life in the aftermath is a challenge that must be faced and appreciated.

Physicians' letters are no longer adequate to qualify for insurance benefits or Social Security disability. They're only first steps in a long and costly process. Initial denials are routine, even with a lawyer's expertise. Second appeals are often summarily dismissed as well. At this point, persistent fibromyalgics who haven't already done so end up hiring attorneys for their third appeal or the trip to federal court that follows if it fails. There is no question that this is a dismal and demeaning situation for the severely incapacitated individual who must face a long and expensive fight. To top it off, many must fight the embarrassment and stigma they feel on the inside as well. On the other side, extensive paperwork and phone interviews steal time from busy physicians who are far more adept at treating the sick. Report upon report is demanded, for which charges must be made because of the time involved in writing them. Resentment can grow on both sides easily: Physicians buried under piles of paper can't always answer questions honestly the way the patient demands. Records are copied multiple times, and new questionnaires arrive daily by mail. These piles of papers are a real burden to a medical office when multiplied by many patients. Applicants can expect the ordeal of being examined by physicians working for insurance companies and the state. More reports are generated, requiring yet another round of letters repudiating other findings.

> "FMS cases have reached near epidemic proportions in the courts, in U.S. Social Security disability claims, workers' compensation, and accident litigation. As many as 25 percent of U.S. patients with FMS have received some sort of disability or injury compensation."
>
> —*Frederick Wolfe, MD*[6]

On the other side of the situation, insurance companies and governmental agencies are justifiably terrified. Many fibromyalgics are young, and granting permanent disability will prove horribly expensive. The sheer number of them is frightening, too, especially as the baby boomers push into their fifties and sixties. The workforce would be decimated if agencies didn't fight every applicant. One and a half million people filed for disability in 2004, and it's obvious that there has to be some kind of gatekeeping. But what kind? One long-term disability insurance carrier notoriously maintains that fibromyalgia is due to a mental impairment, since nothing ever shows up on accepted tests. Records are combed for words such as *depressed, anxious,* and even *sad.* This permits enforcement of the fine-print clause limiting coverage for psychiatric illnesses. Dirty? You bet! There's a not-too-funny cartoon circulating of a physician reading Miranda rights to a patient sitting on an examination table: "Anything you say may be used against you in a court of law."

But no company is in business to go broke. Most take the not unreasonable position that everybody with a job is tired, has aches and pains, and yet continues to function. Taxpayers and their legal representatives in the legislature are frightened, too. Some states have gone so far as to introduce legislation banning fibromyalgia as a compensable condition, at least under workers' compensation programs.

We doctors also pay taxes and are aghast about the impact of fibromyalgia on the economy. Yet our concern is tempered by our oath to care for our patients, and what we should be asking ourselves: What is best for each individual? Is long-term disability really in a patient's best interest? We instinctively know that remaining active and functional in some capacity is an integral part of self-esteem. Pride in accomplishment is essential, and so is the sense of usefulness. A job well done, no matter how small, feels good. Long-term disability, like some of the current solutions for fibromyalgia, begins or is party to a downward spiral. Too often, patients enter this slide by expending energy and resources trying to prove disability. Even if the legal battle is won, it takes a lot of time, and afterward they must find ways to restore meaning and challenge to everyday life. They can't undertake restorative physical activity in public for fear of being videotaped by an insurance private eye. No matter how much they might improve in the future, they must behave sickly enough to merit regular medical attention. The cards are stacked against them, and too often if improvement is managed, rehabilitation is out of the question. It's too difficult to find a way back into the workforce even if it becomes possible. Having been disabled, they are uninsurable, and a poor risk for a potential employer to hire and train.

Several things are clear. We badly need assessment criteria that would accurately measure levels of disability in FMS. It's commonly accepted among specialists that working with the current evaluation forms is futile because they rely on measurements of motion and strength. Yet it is repetition of tasks that causes the exhaustion and pain—something standard forms do not address at all.

> "I am not a senior citizen. But regardless, I would like to comment about the high cost of prescription drugs. I am not on a 'fixed' income. Rather, I am on a 'broken' income. I am disabled due to FMS, chronic fatigue, and mercury poisoning. I have not worked since 09-01-01. I was a self-employed attorney with a comfortable (not rich) income. Now I am a disabled attorney with no income. I filed for SS disability, but was denied. My insurance plan pays eighty percent of nothing. (That's my attempt at humor!) I have no coverage for migraine headaches, as they are a pre-existing condition. I have suffered with migraines for 33 years. I cannot afford 'Amerge' tablets which cost $22 per pill. So, I tough it out."
>
> —*Kim, Ohio*

> "Right now, I can work a full time desk job, but if my brain fog gets worse, or my pain gets worse, I don't think I want to be at work. I have a highly stressful job. I work as a Mkt/Adv. Manager for 18 automotive dealerships and I am under constant deadlines and pressure to get it done. Mistakes aren't tolerated, and I'm afraid of being fired if I start making too many. This Automotive field of work is full of work-a-holics. I used to be the same way, but I just can't do it anymore."
>
> *—Debbie, Arizona*

Most of all, as healers we know that we need to keep each person as productive as possible. The best way to accomplish this is by early diagnosis and effective treatment. It's hard for us to side with a middle-aged person who just wants to stay home and uses fibromyalgia as an excuse to escape from the workforce. Somebody's got to pay for the contemplated lifetime of relative leisure. Yet it is also an inescapable conclusion that we, the public, will have to rework the disability system if it's to survive. There are people who are truly ill who have fought long and hard to remain working at jobs they enjoy and cherish until the day that it just can no longer be done. Their reward for this is to have to fight even harder for help. The answer may lie in more flexible workplace policies mandated by law. More jobs should be tailored for the partially handicapped that successfully bolster productivity and maintain self-esteem. We must do this for the government, and for patients it would be a real win–win situation.

Despite compassion, physicians should feel that every patient requesting permanent disability represents a major defeat for medicine. If at all possible, we should fix them before they ever finger an application form. Fibromyalgia reversal is swift in younger people and can be completed long before such thoughts are considered. Victories will only come with early diagnosis and treatment directed at the cause and not symptom patchwork. Too often, one of the reasons disability is necessary is because of the side effects of multiple medications that cannot be discontinued easily or effectively replaced. We know some of the preceding paragraphs will hurt readers who are on disability or in the process of trying to get it. But our bottom line is simple. Look back and remember a time when you could have healed. Had you known of a reversal protocol, would you not have jumped at the chance?

We hope this chapter has answered some questions, but, more importantly, that it has also underscored our basic tenet. First and foremost, we've got to diagnose patients before they are incapacitated, and then fight for treatments that get patients well. Each and every patient should be offered the chance to have the most productive, successful, and complete life possible. Nothing less should be acceptable to us both as medical professionals and as human beings.

> "Having a reversal protocol has changed everything. I now see it as a wake-up call and one I have used to empower myself and to heal myself. I feel strong and confident. Without [this] it would be a dreary time of self-blame if not outright depression."
>
> —*M. K., Hawaii*

Late-Breaking News

Probably, by the time this book is printed and in the years to follow, there will be some serious and other frivolous additions to this list. We will try to keep up with them on our Web site: www.fibromyalgiatreatment.com. Though they belong in the Band-Aid group, here are recently released medications that are being touted for fibromyalgia:

Lyrica (pregabalin)—The manufacturer, Pfizer, says that there is a "strong possibility" it may ask for fibromyalgia designation for this drug, which is a chemical cousin of Neurontin, designed for epileptic convulsions, pain, and anxiety. It's used primarily for nerve pain. It may be the first medication actually indicated for fibromyalgia.

Cymbalta (duloxetine)—A dual-action antidepressant (SSNRI) from Eli Lilly similar to Effexor (venlafaxine) and Remeron (mirtazapine) that was approved in August 2004 for depression. Some studies on pain showed a slight efficacy, but only in female patients. It has not been compared with other antidepressants that act on serotonin and norepinephrine—just with placebos—and other studies showed it is as effective as other antidepressants. It may have a shorter half-life, allowing it to be discontinued more abruptly than older drugs. Side effects include nausea, dry mouth, constipation, headache, insomnia, and sweating. In men, especially, it lowered blood pressure.

Thalomid (thalidomide)—Trials are slated to begin for severe chronic pain. Obviously, this medication (from Celgene Corporation) will be strictly controlled. In cancer studies, it appeared to reduce pain. Originally marketed as a sleeping pill, it would obviously help sleep. It will never be available for women capable of bearing children because of the severe birth defects it is known to cause. This is an emotional issue that must be addressed before trials begin for anything other than for cancer that has failed to respond to other therapies. (This is the only currently allowed application.)

Milnacipran—A dual-action antidepressant like Cymbalta. Cypress Bioscience hopes to have this on the market by 2006. It belongs to a class called NSRIs or norepinephrine- and serotonin-reuptake inhibitors. It is similar to the currently available venlafaxine (Effexor). It may work better than other classes of antidepressants on pain, but this remains to be seen in head-to-head trials not yet concluded. It has currently only been tested against a placebo.

Are new drugs rushed to market without adequate testing? Do current methods of studying safety and efficacy of new compounds leave something to be desired? These questions remained to be answered, although books such as these raise serious questions.

Recent withdrawals of Rezulin (diabetes), Lotronex (irritable bowel), Redux and fen-phen (diet), Baycol (cholesterol), and Vioxx (NSAID) certainly underscore concern. There's really a dual issue: Is a new medication more effective than existing ones, and is it safer? In general, our feeling is that the longer the track record of a drug, the safer it is. No study showed Vioxx more effective than ibuprofen for pain, and yet heavy advertising sold it!

To bring things into perspective, Russell Portenoy, MD, chair of the Department of Pain Medicine and Palliative Care at Beth Israel, says: "When I started in pain management, apart from narcotics and anti-inflammatory drugs there were only two medications commonly used—Tegretol and Elavil. Now I have more than 50 medications to pick from. I have no way of knowing which a patient will respond to."

Chapter 15

Coping with Fibromyalgia: What Will Help While Guaifenesin Heals Your Body?

> "I have been on guai since July 1997—I probably have another two to three years to clear. The past 14 months have not been hell at all. They have been the best 14 months in a long time for me. I know I am healing. I have more energy. I have more stamina. I can do more things, socially, physically, and mentally. So for me, if this is hell—bring it on!"
>
> —*Linda P., Ohio*

IN A VERY real sense, the first day you take guaifenesin is the birthday of your new life. You've read testimonials throughout this book. They're all good and true. Yet you must wonder: Authors would hardly include bad ones, would they? It would be more helpful if you knew someone who's run through the protocol and is responding well to guaifenesin. If you aren't that lucky, you'll just have to trust us and the online support group. Wonderful possibilities lie ahead, and for the first time in what seems forever we hope that we have given you hope. If so many others get well, why can't you? The flip side to this is the worry, *But what if it doesn't work for* me*?*

By now you're also aware there's more to this treatment than just swallowing a pill. We haven't hidden the fact that fibromyalgia reversal is demanding, takes time, and requires both perseverance and dedication. You may encounter people who think this protocol is too restrictive or too complicated. Guaifenesin is, after all, not for the faint of heart; we've said that before, haven't we? If it's any consolation, we'll tell you straight out: Since you've bought this book and read this far, don't fret over your resolve—you've got the guts to persevere!

What's left now is to think about what you can do for yourself while waiting for guaifenesin to do its job. We think it important enough to repeat: If you're taking the correct dose and you aren't blocking, guaifenesin will work. You don't need to take any other medications. Everything else, as far as we're concerned, is optional or only temporarily useful. But there are certainly things you can do mentally and physically to pave the way toward your new life.

> "Nothing could stop me from trying guaifenesin. I was diagnosed in 1988—have tried everything—they all helped to some degree, but not like this. I've had symptoms since at least 1976. I leaped at the chance for this. I have been through so much with this disease over the years—I wanted a chance to get well. The fear of a little more pain was not going to stop me. Besides what guarantee do you have now? My FMS seemed to be getting only worse over the years and here is a chance to change that."
>
> —*Jerri, South Dakota*

REDUCE STRESS

Poor stress! It's blamed for everything untoward that happens to us. For years, it was even thought responsible for inducing fibromyalgia. There's no doubt that chronic pain makes you battle your body even to get up and dress in the morning. That's real stress! Add to this the other things you can't get done; things you regularly forget to do; the neglect you impose on your family and relationships. These are all enough to keep you on edge and at fever pitch. Undoubtedly, mental strain intensifies symptoms of FMS or, for that matter, any chronic illness. That's no surprise, is it? Being sick is stressful. You may have already considered many of the coping strategies we'll suggest, but we think it still helps to see them collected in writing.

As a priority beginning, get other health worries out of the way. Make sure your doctor has checked carefully for coexisting conditions. Treat anything that overlaps and confounds fibromyalgia. If you're hypoglycemic, don't duck the issue. Start the corrective diet without hesitation. In just a few days, you'll have more energy, shed some depression, think better, and find your irritable bowel considerably placated. Within two months, all of the carbohydrate-related problems will be gone. Thyroid function should be checked and only treated if it's abnormal. Anemia can make you feel tired and weak, and can greatly block especially the muscular clearing of fibromyalgia. It's usually an easy situation to reverse. Your worries about having more serious conditions as the root cause of your many symptoms can only be put aside by a reassuring professional. So discuss your underlying fears with your doctor.

Remember that the Internet contains both accurate information and scams and is not a diagnostic tool to replace an astute physician. That's why we stressed in the first chapter the importance of working with someone you respect and trust.

Review your medications and remember that some of them are certainly compromising your recovery due to side effects. Some depression is normal in chronic illness. Do you really need to take an antidepressant? Such medications are often handed out with very little reasoning the minute a doctor suspects fibromyalgia. Maybe you can you cut the dosage? Study the effects of the mood-altering drugs and tranquilizers that have stripped your personality of its highs and lows. We acknowledge you must make some compromises just to continue functioning, but it's also logical to reflect on how much a drug is actually helping. For this process, you will need the wisdom only your doctor can offer. Ask how should you go about sequentially reassessing your medications for both value and side effects. You might wonder what this has to do with stress, but it's pertinent for several reasons. Deep down you're probably worrying about the effects and long-term risks of multiple compounds. Most people really don't like taking drugs. For most people, paying high pharmacy bills each month doesn't make life any easier. Finally, until you reduce drugs to minimal needs, you can't estimate how this polypharmacy is affecting your mental outlook.

Besides your prescription drugs, look at the over-the-counter stuff and the supplements you've added over the years. These are even more expensive because your insurance doesn't cover them. Wonder a bit about their side effects and safety, especially since they aren't tested for interactions with prescription drugs. This is a new beginning: A good time to repack the baggage you'll carry into the future. If something hasn't been very helpful, ask your doctor's opinion about discontinuing it. We understand the fear of stopping anything on the chance it might make you feel worse. Dwell on this thought a bit. If you stop something and you learn it was actually useful, you can always add it back. Your target is to make your regimen as simple as possible. Removing the worry about what medications are doing to your system should certainly lessen your stress.

> "Please don't worry about what may or what will be, and take each day/moment one by one. The anxiety you cause yourself will not serve you in a positive way, as you may be surprised how your cycling goes. Taking guaifenesin could quite possibly lift the symptom you are most worried about and how you re-

experience it may not be on the same level you already experience it. It was that way for me as I could much easier handle cycling depression versus depression caused by my past problem."

—Kim, Pennsylvania

STRESS AT HOME

"One day I asked my husband what was the hardest part about being married to someone as sick as I was. I expected him to say working all day, then coming home to do the cooking, cleaning and wait on me. But he didn't, he said it was the loneliness!! I had no idea. At that time I wasn't able to give anything to him, I was a blob. He took care of me and loved me unconditionally. Maybe not perfectly, [but] to the best of his ability. See, I am the luckiest girl in the world!"

—Susie, California

Next, carefully examine where life is the sweetest—your home. Ask those who share that comfortable retreat to understand what you're about to undertake. If they're interested in reading about your illness and the protocol, you can share parts of this book or materials from our Web site: www.fibromyalgiatreatment.com. The site also contains a "Letter to Normals." Read and adapt it for your own use if you're interested in putting your feelings on paper and sharing them that way.

Everyone in the household should be given a chance to understand what's happening with your health. Keep explanations simple with the children. Remind them you're going to get better. It may seem a bit scary at first for juvenile minds. The fear of losing a parent is always present. Let them know there'll be things you just can't do right now; it isn't your fault or theirs. If you express yourself simply, even very young children can understand and face the circumstances by making up activities you can mutually share. Keep in mind that time spent with kids is not only instructive but will also be kept in the nostalgia file for review in their adulthood. Our time is truly a precious thing that we have to give. Long after cherished toys are broken and forgotten, children remember the day Mom taught them how to bake cookies. Board games can substitute for outdoor playing. If your children are old enough, let them read to you out loud. Watch movies with them, or work on simple projects. On better days, as energy permits, short walks together can be marvelously bonding and refreshing.

Let family members know what help you need. Be specific and explain why you need it. If they understand that you are seriously beginning a demanding protocol for getting well, it will be hard for them to refuse you. There are three secrets for getting help. First, learn how to ask and be specific about what you want. Don't expect clairvoyance from your significant other when it's time to mop a dirty floor. Children won't automatically volunteer to haul trash all the way to the curb just because you wish they would. Second, if someone is trying to do something helpful, don't supervise the task. Not only does this expend energy you don't have, it's annoying to those around you as well. If it's not exactly the way you would've done it . . . oh well. There are more ways than one to accomplish things, and perfection in household tasks is not essential. And third, of course, say thank you. Express your appreciation even to a child who made you a cup of tea or drew you a picture. Be grateful to a spouse or friend who cooked dinner and even cleaned up afterward. Let each know you view their efforts as wonderful. "Do you know what that means to me?" goes a long way as a reward and makes them participants in your recovery.

Simplify is a golden cane for support. *Lower your standards* would make a good motto when you face house and garden chores. This last phrase might contain words of wisdom for the new millennium—even healthy people have too much to do these days. Everyone, not just fibromyalgics, feels stressed out and pressured from all sides. Changes you cultivate during guaifenesin treatment may turn into much healthier habits useful for the rest of your life.

Consider simple meals and eating them off paper plates. Save some energy by cooking bigger batches of familiar recipes when you feel up to it. Freeze the extra portions for energy-deprived days that are sure to come. Find easy recipes—women's magazines and cookbooks have plenty of them; some are printed on package labels. Especially in the winter, Crock-Pots can be used for one-dish dinners requiring less cleanup and no supervision. Low-carbohydrate recipes are available on the Net and also in cookbooks if you are hypoglycemic or on the weight loss diet.

Stop worrying about what's accumulating behind the refrigerator or under the stove. Remind yourself over and over that there's a time for everything, and this is yours for healing. A spotless house should be low on the list of priorities in life, but health at the very top. You've already lost your well-being, so we don't need to remind you what you're looking for. When you regain that, you'll have plenty of energy to play catch-up with all of those dusty corners.

Perhaps you can afford to pay someone to help with housework. We're not insensitive to the fact that some budgets won't allow it. Just having someone come in every two weeks or once a month to do the heavy stuff is lifesaving. Another possibility is to let your kids earn extra money by doing housework. You know it won't be to your satisfaction, but it'll be a learning experience for them. They'll undoubtedly do it in fits and starts, but so what? It's at least a little break when you're about to collapse.

> "Even my spouse could see the incredible difference. He now felt guilt-free to serve me with divorce papers. How kind of him. He was going to anyway, he says, but he had been feeling painfully guilty about it. Look how guai even helped *his* pain!"
>
> —*Iris, California*

If your relationship didn't survive the chronic pain and other symptoms of fibromyalgia, there's probably nothing you can do about that right now. Some couples get lucky and mend the rift. Try not to chastise yourself or the escaped partner—that's another stressful mind exercise, and it wastes what little energy you have. Fibromyalgia is a great stressor, but so are many other situations in life. If your relationship wasn't strong enough to survive this illness, it might well have faltered anyway. It's not so bad to have learned that now. Dedicate yourself to getting well. When that happens, you'll have time enough to build a new relationship if that's something that you want to do.

> "Have faith, not only in guai, but also in yourself. You would not be trying it if you lacked the one vital trait necessary to heal. That is a determination to see it through. At the end of this road you will find your life again. Is this not worth anything you have to endure? It is similar to the process of birth. At the end of the agony of labor you are gifted with a new life. The pain is forgotten in the joy. The reward is the most precious thing you can possess—your health. If you have your health, you have everything you need. Nothing else compares, as good health enables you to do whatever you desire in life."
>
> —*Kathy Shuller, Florida (pain-free, and on my way out the door)*

STRESS IN THE WORKPLACE

> "Emotionally I'm still very depressed by having so little education, work experience, and future financial security at my age. And I am simply lonely from so many years of isolation. I don't know how to make or keep friends. Dr. St. Amand assured me that my mind would heal along with my body and that I simply couldn't imagine the positive changes I would experience in my emotions. I hope this is true. I will simply have to rely on the same hope that caused me to start the guai in the first place."
>
> —*Iris, California*

Job stress from overwork and anxiety is sure to magnify your symptoms and make fibromyalgia worse. It's important not to let work situations weigh you down. We don't recommend quitting, but perhaps a sympathetic boss will let you cut your hours temporarily. Or possibly you could do some paperwork from home. Computers have made it much easier for employees to telecommute or simply bring home work where it can be completed in a more comfortable chair and more peaceful surroundings. When you're working at home, you can take breaks when you need them, move around and stretch.

The problem with this simple advice is that by the time many fibromyalgics are diagnosed or begin treatment, they may already be having problems at work. Some have taken too many sick days; others have fallen behind and performed badly on days when fibrofog and other symptoms were at full fury. If it's feasible, schedule a meeting with your supervisor to discuss fibromyalgia and the treatment you're about to start. Keep it simple and honest but stress that you're going to improve. You can finally promise that in good faith; all you ask is tolerance for the weeks that lie ahead.

If you've been told that your job is in jeopardy if you call in sick just one more time, you might need to take some specific actions when you start guaifenesin. Your possibilities will be different depending on the size of your company and your benefits package. It's not a bad idea to consider the option of taking time off at the beginning of treatment if you feel you won't be given any help. The Family and Medical Leave Act (FMLA) became law in 1993 and may apply to you if you work for a company that employs more than fifty people. It was enacted to permit up to twelve weeks of unpaid leave for you to reverse a serious health condition. It does require continuing treatment by a licensed health care provider. You'll need to provide documentation from your doctor. The law also mandates you be restored to the same or an equivalent position with the same pay and benefits. You can get better information from your state's Board of Equalization (by whatever name) or your employer's Human Resource Department, where you can learn about your personal options in detail.

On the other hand, it's still important not to be too frightened or overreact in advance, especially if your options are limited when it comes to time off. Despite what you may have heard or read, the vast majority of patients continue working during the initial days on our protocol. Only a few require a period of absence, and typically that means just a month or two off. We're not all endowed with the same strength, but certainly most of our patients cope with jobs successfully throughout reversal. That's one of the reasons why we've advised you to start on a small amount of guaifenesin and titrate up slowly to find your proper dosage. Taking more medication than you actually need will make you cycle harder. It's far better for you to take the correct amount and sooner attain good days. When these start appearing, it will make it possible for you to catch up with some of your work.

In the United States, employers are becoming much more sensitive to those with disabilities. There are now many resources available, and often a simple note from your physician will help you make changes. More comfortable chairs, wrist supports for computer work, footstools, and cushions are all things your employer might provide. New laws require them to make reasonable accommodations, and a little research on your part can promote cooperation. The best approach is to do some research on your own and present options that you believe will help you to be more productive. Try to be realistic about what your employer can afford and keep demands at a minimum.

Relationships with co-workers might benefit if you simply tell them that you're beginning a difficult new treatment for your fibromyalgia. Share your hopes and fears and explain that you intend to do your best and continue working as hard as you can. Most people will respond to such a direct approach and will be more inclined to help. Try getting them to understand that a medical problem is the basis of your struggles and that you're doing your best to get it under control. Reassure them that you won't be ill forever.

> "Normal are the hours when I forget I am a sick person. Normal is when I keep up with a fit person my age and don't pay for it big time. Normal is when I cry for a normal reason. Normal is when I laugh without being macabre or cynical. Normal is when I don't burn when I think about doctors. Normal is when I *want* to do something besides watch TV. Normal is not being in pain all the time. I have these normals now and you will too."
>
> —*Janet, Canada*

THINGS YOU CAN DO FOR YOURSELF

> "Before the protocol I was not able to sleep because I would have deep wrenching spasms in my legs right in the middle of

my deepest sleep. The pain was almost intolerable. I would jump out of bed screaming. Often with my foot contorted with a spasm that would not release no matter what. I no longer have spasms of that magnitude at all. Once in a great while I will have a charley hourse at night but if I get up it immediately goes away. And that is rare."

—Laura, Arizona

Get Enough Sleep

We all clean out the metabolic debris created by simply existing during our sleep. That's the time when cells do their housekeeping. Fibromyalgic muscles compile overabundant metabolic leftovers because they're kept constantly contracted and prevent the restorative rest needed for a good nighttime cleansing. To a lesser extent, it's the same for the rest of the body, particularly the brain. It follows that a prominent complaint in fibromyalgia is insomnia and the dominant exhaustion that this imposes. No matter how tough you are, fitful sleeping makes it impossible for next-day function. Rest is crucial, so get as much as you can—but realize that it won't entirely solve the problem of fatigue.

When you've had a bad night, occupy the next day with less demanding tasks. Although this is not always possible, choose the simplest ones from your must-do list. On those bad days, send your kids on the errands they can do. Now is the time for simple meals such as grilled cheese sandwiches, soup, or takeout. If you've frozen a casserole or portions of a larger meal, this is the time to thaw them out. Conserve what strength you have for the most basic and urgent tasks. Remember that mental and emotional workouts are also tiring.

A good general rule is to grab what rest the disease allows whenever you can. Snatch naps when you have to if at all possible. Keep them brief and find a way to awaken yourself before you lapse into a prolonged coma. You've got to remain tired enough to sleep that night. When you start yawning in the evening, forget the next TV show and go to bed earlier than usual. Sometimes it requires a Herculean effort to propel yourself from your chair into the bedroom, but do it. Dozing in your chair or on the couch is not as restorative as sleeping in a quiet room. Your husband isn't enjoying your company, especially if you're snoring. He won't mind if you beat a calculated retreat. Your workplace may have a back room or a private area where you can rest at lunchtime or during breaks. A small, inexpensive futon can be stashed on a shelf along with a small pillow. Even half an hour can make a difference if it's spent stretched out with your eyes closed.

Schedule sufficient bed hours; it's counterproductive to aim for seven hours when you know you need nine. Set your alarm half an hour earlier than usual if you really must finish some task from the night before. You'll complete it much more rapidly when you're rested. It may also help to set the alarm earlier, take the morning dose of pain medication, and then press the snooze button while waiting for it to take effect. In this way, you'll feel better when you finally have to get up and start moving.

If you're a light sleeper, relaxation tapes, quiet fans, and white-noise machines can make it easier to stay asleep. Make sure your bedroom is dark and your mattress comfortable. When purchasing a new one, ask for a trial period and a money-back guarantee—there's no one kind of mattress that helps everyone with FM. On painful nights, little adhesive heat pads for muscle pain may be used or apply a simple old-fashioned hot-water bottle. You do not want to use electric heating pads because of the danger of burning yourself. Don't overlook simple aids such as earplugs or sleep masks if your room has features that keep you from fully relaxing. Exercise in the afternoon will also help, as will gentle stretching after a shower or a bath before bed.

Without medical reversal of fibromyalgia, everything gets even worse, including insomnia, and nocturnal tissue cleansing remains incomplete. During guaifenesin reversal, you'll still have to temporarily make do with whatever downtime you can muster. Making rest a priority and finding workable solutions to avoid unwanted wake cycles are essential for restoring your ability to cope on a daily basis. (See chapter 14 for guidance on getting better sleep.)

> "I am sleeping through the night right now without the aid of medication and I am dreaming again, oh what a wonderful thing! It's amazing what a good night's sleep does for a person! Speaking of sleep, last year I couldn't sleep on my sides because my hips hurt so bad. Now I only sleep on my sides. I can make it through a day without needing a nap or needing to lie down. Last year if I didn't lie down at least once in the afternoon I couldn't make it to dinner. Restless legs plagued me for years. It was one of the first things to go so now my husband sleeps better too."
>
> —*Gina, New York*

Take Warm Baths

> "I recently spent a week at my mother-in-law's apartment in New York City. Because the shower had variable temperatures in the space of a few minutes I couldn't deal with it, so I took a bath. I was immediately sold on the idea because it made me stop and relax and also made my muscles feel much better. I vowed to make the time for at least one bath a week, and I do. Bubbles in the bath help me relax more because I can't see my body and it's like being in a cloud."
>
> —*Valerie, Nevada*

Hot or warm baths will soothe sore muscles or joints and ease the aching pains of the FMS day. They're quite relaxing and may help you fall asleep. Epsom salts, powdered milk, cornstarch, or mineral or emu oil should be added to the water. They do nothing medicinally, but they do protect your skin from getting all puckered up as you soak. Turn off and dim as many lights as possible to set a pleasant atmosphere in the bathroom or bedroom.

Heavy fragrances should be avoided in bath products. Even if you can tolerate the smell, the added chemical can irritate the skin and even make it difficult to relax. Some patients report that a mildly scented candle is a wonderful addition to this quiet time, and there are many available on the market. If you have noisy children or a spouse who likes a loud TV, play a relaxation tape or quiet classical music to make your bath more soothing.

Warm showers work best in the morning. That's when you must loosen muscles that stiffened during the night, yet not so relaxed that you want to go back to bed. Baths do their best work at night, showers in the morning. Newer body lotions designed to be used in the shower can soften and moisturize your skin for the entire day. They also help calm the itchy skin so common in fibromyalgia. If you have long hair, wear your shower cap: It will keep you from having to wash and style it each day. This alone can save a bunch of energy. Some of you find taking a shower simply too exhausting; try gentle stretching for about ten minutes instead.

Understand Your Depression

"It's crushing when people we love treat us this way but I think you are absolutely right to avoid being around these negative folks, family or not. Remember that old saying that living well is the best revenge? Well, in our case, getting well is the best revenge. We can hope that one day your mother and your sister realize how much pain they have caused you but until that time you still need to get well. And you have to do that one day at a time. How sad that your mother thinks that as a sick person you are supposed to be miserable all time. And how pathetic."

—*Cris, Michigan*

A certain amount of depression and frustration is normal with chronic illness. Most patients instinctively understand and don't want to take medication for milder forms. Antidepressants certainly have a place in serious depression, but as we've seen, they have effects on the body that are less than desirable if there are other choices.

Try a few tricks to coax your brain out of depression while you're waiting for guaifenesin benefits. Easier said than done, but you can better learn to fend off some of its facets. It's perfectly normal to chafe against your limitations, mourn losses, and feel sad at being deprived of stamina to do what you've previously enjoyed. You can nevertheless find activities to replace some lost capacity and, in less demanding ways, still spend time with those you love. Overcoming such obstacles will let you cope far better.

Depression in fibromyalgia may stem from feeling defeated in trying to meet some unrealistic standards, self-imposed at home or work. Recognizing limitations is a good place to start and might also lessen stress by letting you erase self-inflicted rules. Concentrating energy on doing what you do best helps immensely. Find relief from the tasks you dislike such as housework and save your efforts for what fulfills you. You're not alone: Many women say that looking around their unkempt homes puts them into an immediate funk. If the deplorable state of your house is a major cause of your anguish, put changing this at the top of your priority list. Lower your standards and remember that most people with children and busy lives don't live in magazine-picture-perfect rooms either. Perhaps your budget can afford occasional outside domestic help for such chores. If being in an imperfect home is that depressing to you, paying for a little help should take precedence over less important things.

Worth thinking about is using your talents to supplement your income while doing something you enjoy. For example, if you're adept at sewing, you might earn extra money to help pay for a cleaning helper. Embroidering school and club uniforms or costumes might be right up your alley. Holiday tablecloths or place mats might be sold at craft fairs or accepted for sale by small boutique stores. You could even make presents of your wares. Besides just earning compliments for your skills, some recipients and their friends might well offer to pay you for similar productions.

Exercise is a fantastic way of fighting depression and feeling blah. Simply getting out for a walk can really make a difference. Walking to or sitting outside in a park, weather permitting, is a great change of pace. Joining an exercise group at the YMCA or recreation department will also get you out of the house and give your mind and body breaks. An operation called Curves is very popular with fibromyalgics because the workout can be tailored on a daily basis. It's also inexpensive and easy for women of all sizes, shapes, and ages. Especially if you have a bad back, water aerobics is another option that will pull you out of the emotional dumps. Do you remember that exercise produces those important chemicals, our feel-good endorphins?

Shun doing what can be avoided, especially if you're not too good at it. Reassuringly, most of our patients shake off a lot of depression between reversal cycles. Remember that there are culprit chemical abnormalities causing the symptoms of fibromyalgia. So keep in mind that down days will reappear during your pain and fatigue cycles. After you've felt good for a while, the onset of a new round of symptoms can be really difficult. There's nothing more fundamentally awful than not being able to trust your own body. During such periods, recall and concentrate on those better moments. Convince yourself as best you can that they're sure to return and will last even longer.

Join a Support Group or Start Your Own

> "Be careful. There are some groups claiming to be support groups that are actually venting grounds. That is, the people in the group do little more than moan and groan about what a lousy hand life has dealt them. A little venting is good for the soul and the health of everyone. But if the entire discussion is centered on moaning and groaning, it will drag you down into the depths of negativity. Avoid negative groups."
>
> —*Devin J. Starlanyl,* The Fibromyalgia Advocate[1]

Communicating with other fibromyalgics is very comforting. Connecting with others is inspirational and offers steadfast encouragement. You can end your isolation and quite likely help others in the process. Our Web site, www.fibromyalgiatreatment.com, keeps a list of groups designed to support the guaifenesin protocol. Local newspapers publish calendars with weekly schedules of other groups dedicated to helping various medical conditions. If you have trouble locating one in your area, call The Arthritis Foundation for a listing it might have. Health care professionals who deal with the illness may usually know of such groups. Your hospital may already be providing space for meetings and can put you in touch. If you live in a sparsely populated area, remember that any chronic pain or arthritis groups might serve you well.

If you live in a large city, you may find more than one fibromyalgia support group. Visit each and select the one that provides you positive feelings. Ideally, a group serves two functions. First, it should afford members a venue for expressing feelings and releasing frustrations. Unfortunately, this is where too many of them stop. Meetings are full of sad stories strongly accentuated with moans and groans, week after week. Tales of pains, failed therapies, and poor spousal and family support are part of each person's litany. It sounds like a competition for who's the worst off! These are negative organizations. Forget them! You're already low enough emotionally. The second important benefit you want from a support group is dedication to improving the quality of lives. The group should be a forum for suggestions that help you in coping with daily functions. Members can share resources and information about fibromyalgia, good care providers, and ways to make day-to-day life easier. Some even organize car pools, shared child care, or potluck meals. They do just what the name implies—unrelenting support for members. When one individual isn't feeling well, others will come to the rescue. Helping with household chores, doing a little shopping for you while doing their own—just a few practical things that an understanding friend can provide. Loneliness is terrible but brightens when you call a buddy and speak to an empathetic ear.

> "I call people by the wrong name. I called my new daughter-in-law by her sister's name and then a few weeks later I called her by my own sister-in-law's name. It's embarrassing. I must come across as a total idiot to a lot of people in those situations when I can't recall the simplest things, fumble, drop, and spill things, and ricochet off walls and doorways.
>
> "But I've learned that when I'm in a group of people who share my experiences that all falls away. It is so wonderful to know that everyone there understands exactly what I'm talking

about and why I can't remember my own name or what day it is and there is so much warmth and acceptance that I can soak it up and coast on it for a long time afterwards."

—Anne Louise, Minnesota

If no acceptable support group exists in your area, consider starting one of your own. We must stress *acceptable.* Many of our patients have gone to more than a few and left disenchanted. Discussions too often center on a new pain pill, sleeping potion, antidepressant, "my doctor said," and the hot new herbal concoction of the day. You're far better off with a guaifenesin support group devoted to a single protocol designed to heal you, not simply applying patches to your symptoms. It's not an enormous task starting an organization, so don't be frightened at this thought. As with everything else, simplicity is the notion of the day. You can start by getting together regularly with a fibromyalgic friend or two. You'll be amazed how quickly that sprouts into a sizable group—Jane will know Suzie, who knows her mother and a neighbor with fibromyalgia . . . Once under way, work on constructive things: Discuss the protocol and where to find good salicylate-free products; collect simple recipes and helpful tips for improving the quality of your lives. Groups from all over the world are now linking up, and soon there'll be an international organization. You and your friends can help yourselves and millions of others. It will take many missionary leaders to spearhead and support the awesome task ahead. As soon as you start your group, a simple post to the online support group or a member of the administration team will get you a listing so that others may find you and pitch in.

Of primary interest to readers is The Fibromyalgia Treatment Center headed by Claudia Marek, coauthor of this book. It's a tax-deductible, charitable foundation with fundamental purposes: to seek out competent researchers, and to help fund studies of the altered chemistry and genetics of fibromyalgia. The center is under way with such a project at this time. A more immediate goal is to get the success of our protocol into medical literature. We've included it several times in these pages but, once more, here's the Web site: fibromyalgiatreatment.com. Claudia and her administrative team are dyed-in-the-wool guaifenesin protocol supporters and totally knowledgeable about the disease and its treatment. They handle copious e-mail inquiries daily. The center is also dedicated to spreading the word among patients and interested practitioners about seminars and symposiums that are scheduled all over the world. You can keep track of them on the same Web site. Mapping instruction, formal and informal gatherings, and meetings are exceptionally inspiring and must be experienced to be believed. It's wonderful to meet fellow fibromyalgics in your own area, but better still to kick off your own support group.

> "I had to quit telling my mom things that I knew she wouldn't be supportive about. But it took me 40 years! We always think that 'surely' our families will support us and say the right things. Instinctively we know the truth. It's hard to accept. I rarely talk to anyone about my FMS but my support group."
>
> —*Kathy, Oregon*

Get Some Exercise

> "I understand how hard it can be to exercise when you hurt badly but you must understand that even the slightest exercises such as gentle stretching will help you to be not so stiff. The more you can do without overdoing it, the better for your body. Everyone needs to learn what they can handle and celebrate the small victories as the small victories lead to big ones in time. You may gain weight having this chronic illness and some factors such as medications can cause you to gain. That

> may be out of your control, but you can still choose to eat right and exercise to the best of your ability. If you can control small things you will not feel so depressed but feel instead you are making steps in the right direction. Celebrate all your victories no matter how small or insignificant they might seem."
>
> —*Kim, Pennsylvania*

In this high-tech age, we often forget how simple things can be. Exercise doesn't require fancy-colored tight-fitting designer togs, shiny equipment, hundred-dollar shoes, or a racing bike. You don't need to join a gym or even buy weights that match your leotards and sweatbands. The sight of well-toned athletes working out with huge resistance equipment is intimidating and looks too hard to try. The reality is that very few people look that good. Most of us don't have those perfect bodies, fashionable outfits, or fetchingly placed perspiration. Many more people stay healthy by taking long, peaceful walks, especially with a calming partner. There's no doubt even modest exercising will make you feel better. We've discussed this fairly extensively in the previous chapter. Besides improving pain thresholds, releasing endorphins, and rebuilding mitochondria, exercise has a positive effect in ameliorating depression.

You can begin exercising early in the treatment, but go easy and start out moderately. Ambitious jump starts are predictors of certain defeat. You can begin by walking around the block or gently stretching on your living room floor with a videotape, DVD, or book to guide you. Some are designed particularly for fibromyalgics; we've designated a few in the Resources section of this book. You'll appreciate hints that help you recognize and abide by your own limits of tolerance.

Exercise should never be done when your muscles are cold or tired. Do some mild stretching, or take a warm-up walk or even a warm shower before you begin. In her book *The Fibromyalgia Advocate*, Devin Starlanyl offers an excellent rule of thumb for evaluating an exercise program: "If mild soreness disappears after the first day, you can repeat it on the second day. If it persists to the second day, postpone any exercise until the third day. If soreness persists on the third day, your exercise routine must be changed. This rule of thumb is true for any treatment, such as massage or electrical stimulation."[2]

> "I started slow, walking around the block. One day I walked five blocks to buy a lottery ticket (hope blooms eternal) and five blocks back. It almost did me in, but I survived. Now I can walk to the grocery store and if I am too fatigued I take the bus part-way to save a few blocks. It's like Claudia once said—you will be in pain whether you are home or not. You will be worn out at home or you can get out and be just as tired. Sometimes it is like I am moving in a fog but at least I am moving. A few times I've called my friend in San Diego on my cell phone and the walk doesn't seem as long because we are talking the whole time."
>
> —*Janice, Minnesota*

For those who prefer structured programs, The Arthritis Foundation will direct you to those that meet your needs. Ask for descriptive brochures. The recommended aquatic program is often the easiest and most sustainable. It's designed for those with limited mobility and empowered by enlisting the soothing buoyancy of warm water. There are beginner group workouts that offer exercise in class-like settings. They're not hard to find. One secret is to join a class designed for senior citizens; the pace is usually slower. Yoga, tai chi, and other disciplines all have advocates. The value of any exercise is determined by the number of people who stick with that particular modality. We encourage patients to keep searching until they find a regimen they can both enjoy and tolerate. The consensus is that carefully graduated workouts that avoid overdoing things progressively promote energy and a wonderful sense of well-being.

> "After about three months on the guai I decided to try exercising on my stationary bike again. . . . I have found that when I am really hurting, if I ride the bike for at least 15 minutes the pain begins to ease up. It is really hard to convince myself to get started when it hurts to even walk, let alone really exercise. But the benefits are worth it. Evenings are my worst times and I find that if I ride my bike for about 30 minutes just before bedtime, I get rid of a lot of my pain and become very relaxed. This promotes a good sleep that often leads to a better day afterward."
>
> —*Marilyn J., North Carolina*

Try Massage and Body Work

> "I have had pain all my life but was told it was growing pains. I have chronic back pain at times so severe I can't function. The muscle spasms are so bad it feels like I have ropes in my back. This was much worse during pregnancy. I discovered then that if I roll on a tennis ball in the areas where it felt just like knots it would make the pain radiate somewhere else or it hurt right where it was, but either way it always felt better. What I have read tells me I am actually rubbing on trigger points."
>
> —*Liz, Kentucky*

Body work is done by licensed practitioners who use teaching, touch, and repetitive stroking for healing. Practically no one discounts the soothing power of human hands. Only a few hypersensitive people cannot tolerate being touched. If you're one of these, you know it and can skip this section until you feel it becomes applicable to you. For most people, trained therapists who understand fibromyalgia and use gentle massage can magically ease muscular pains and pacify jangled nerves. As long as you both bear in mind that the benefits are transient, you'll do fine.

Carefully avoid deep-tissue work and stay away from Rolfing—these techniques will increase pain. The wrong kind of massage can bring immediate pain that may last for days. Other times, you won't realize until much later how badly you've been hurt. Bear in mind that the lumps and bumps of fibromyalgia can't be jackhammered out by using bare-knuckled attacks. That can cause tissue damage and greatly disturb already distressed structures. Make sure that any practitioner you visit understands fibromyalgia. Read printed material about the proposed treatment before you submit to it and be sure it's appropriate for your condition. Some patients get relief from acupuncture, and many medical researchers support its partial benefits. As it is with chiropractic approaches, other investigators have found little lasting benefit. Ask your doctor and support group for recommendations if you don't know where to start. When using chiropractic services or acupuncture, make it absolutely clear that you cannot use any herbal products as medications or on the skin. Even though you think you've explained this thoroughly, be vigilant to make sure that you were understood and your practitioners comply.

Highly endorsed by fibromyalgics is the Feldenkrais Method. In a series of lessons, patients are taught how to integrate their body movements so they can function with less effort and pain. Instructions are individually structured as a series of altogether smooth and gentle activities. Similar disciplines such as the Alexander Technique and Bowen Therapy also have staunch supporters, but our experience with these is minimal. After any kind of treatment, except massage, plan on resting. Your body has just had a significant workout. If your muscles are already getting tight, take a warm shower to relax them.

Unfortunately, the above therapeutic approaches are expensive. Not every patient has insurance coverage, and even sound, hands-on treatment is often rejected as unnecessary. Prepaid medical carriers usually regard massage as a luxury except following an accident, and not for extended periods. However frustrating this is, it will help to accept that these modalities will, at best, provide only brief comfort, and that none of these disciplines is required for healing.

> "There are colleges of massage therapy that charge much smaller fees than do the professionals. I had my second visit at my local school and I am still sold on the idea. I even took my sisters-in-law and the four of us got in on a two-for-one special: $10 a person! They are now sold on the idea too. One important note: although there may be one main address for the school, there are often additional locations of that school in different cities in your state. Take Utah for example—there is one school but it has three different locations throughout the state. Contact the schools in your state for more information on additional locations."
>
> —*Sharon H., Utah*

Do Something You Love Every Day

> "I used to put 'baking cookies with my son' on my list almost every week because we would talk while we were cooking, and he loved that. I would tell him about when I was a little girl and how I used to watch my mother bake, and it made me happy to remember good things. If I did nothing else at all that day, at least I did that. I made a vow not to flog myself for what I could not do—not to sit and watch other mothers running after their kids and beat myself up anymore. Instead I focused on the tasks I had made for myself . . . and counted myself lucky when I could do them."
>
> —*Cathy, California*

Most detrimental of all to your emotional health is to stop doing things important to you. That's the quickest way to lose hope and face permanent entrapment in a sinkhole of a life without pleasure. You must somehow keep in touch with yourself and the person you were before fibromyalgia took over your entire being. That's hard to do when you feel so rotten—very hard. As the disease progresses, many people retract into some inner sanctuary that conserves strength for essential activities that can't be shoved aside. Such a move is logical but ultimately counterproductive. Far better to streamline unavoidable chores by trimming wasted effort while still retaining everything that lends charm to a life. Energy conservation is necessary, but only a modest beginning.

> "I found that there were activities I had stopped doing long ago, such as playing the piano and sewing, that really make me feel good. . . . If I am sad or stressed, perhaps experiencing early warning signs of an approaching flare, I make sure to spend some time involved in such an activity. It makes me feel better and my life feels enriched."
>
> —*Mary Ellen Copeland, coauthor,* Fibromyalgia and Chronic Myofascial Pain Syndrome[3]

Start by deciding what you really enjoy doing and makes you feel good. You have to provide some time for your partner and children, but of similar importance, what do you particularly love to do? What makes you feel better? Is it just anticipating a particular activity? Possibly it's gardening, painting, reading, or solving crossword puzzles. Do you like strolling in the evening or just sitting quietly in the morning sun sipping a cup of tea? Choose something so wonderful that it usually makes you lose track of time.

Make a list of all the things that were important to you when you still felt well enough to do them. If you love watching your son play soccer, jot it down. Logging onto a newsgroup that serves the needs of others may be to your liking; that's a major joy to include. Going to the library, art museums, concerts in the park . . . which of these pastimes do you miss? Many music schools and colleges provide plays and entertainment at reasonable prices in a less rigid setting. Maybe you haven't considered these lately.

Finish the list and get a calendar with unusually big spaces. For each day, make a simple entry. Write in what you plan to do for yourself. It might be working in the garden for whatever time you can safely expend, or going in the afternoon to watch your daughter practice softball. It could be a morning trip to a farmer's market or renting a movie you've been meaning to see. If it's an outdoor activity, you could run out of steam; have a standby book you've always wanted to read.

It's true that life isn't just made up of fun time. So you'll have to add a chore or two to the daily schedule. At least they also give satisfaction of a mandatory job completed. That could be changing bedsheets, cleaning out the car, or organizing the refrigerator. Marketing and errands could be necessities for another day. Con yourself into thinking that vacuuming is part of your exercise program.

Every day, try with all your might to satisfy your plan. If you can muster such discipline, you'll start getting in touch with the wonderful person you were and still are. Even if no one else praises your effort, pat yourself on the back for the strides you've made. Life will be enriched and more meaningful to you. You'll subdue some of your recent demons and gain respect for your steadfast resolve. You're now a doer, not just a viewer. Mounting confidence will smooth your interactions with friends, family, and even doctors. Your new focus is on the road ahead, and you're now unstoppable on your drive to health.

Conclusion

One Author's Last Word

IF YOU'VE READ this far, from beginning to end, despite your fibrofog, pain, and fatigue, I'm impressed. As I was helping to write these pages, I wondered how to end this book. I also pondered how long some of you would bear with us. We've offered you reversing cycles of fatigue, disturbing cognitive symptoms, and added pain; possibly taken away your favorite herbs, cosmetics, and, for some of you, chocolate, potatoes, pasta, bread, and favorite desserts. Yet here you are, preparing to close down with us.

Presented with a well-detailed medical history, more physicians are sooner suspecting fibromyalgia and becoming adept at confirming the diagnosis. This is good, hopeful news and a change since we first started working with and writing about the illness. With diligence and persistence, you should be able to find caring doctors to work with you. While it's still true that many physicians are not aware of our protocol, that, too, is changing. Some have heard of our premises, but remain unconvinced. They might willingly allow you to be their guinea pig and wait for you to report success or failure. In this case, you hold the futures of others in your perceptions. We're counting on you to make them positive. Your doctor or physical therapist might be sufficiently curious to examine your body for the contracted tissues we find in such predictable patterns. Maybe you can teach one of them the value of the famous left thigh, always present in adults and first to clear within one month.

It's unlikely that you'll find a doctor who will accept the shortcut method we've described for diagnosing hypoglycemia. If the opportunity presents, remind the physician that you're suffering the same acute adrenaline symptoms diabetics get with insulin overdoses. If you have full-blown hypoglycemia, the treatment is black and white. We've listed what you can eat and drink and what you must assiduously avoid. It's all very straightforward and has worked for my patients for more than forty years. Sure, it takes perfect discipline for at least two months. Muster the remnants of your willpower and accept no excuses: You can do it. Approach the diet with a positive attitude. There is no other way to rid yourself of many of your symptoms.

Another 30 percent of you are carbohydrate intolerant though not actually hypoglycemic. You'll have to recognize that fact on your own, curtail your cravings, and try either the liberal or the strict diet for a few weeks. You should feel a swell of energy and considerable relief from irritable bowel syndrome if you change the way you eat. In the future, you won't need professional reminding that excess carbohydrates don't set well.

A few of you are wondering: *How can I possibly do all of this?* Unfortunately, you're not alone. We've grown accustomed to hearing from those who just can't do it. Almost all of the hypoglycemics are successful because rewards are so swift in coming. Fighting fibromyalgia is tougher and benefits more slowly reaped. Yet the majority of you will adopt the protocol. We hope you can muster enough reserves to pay the highway toll for the road back to destination health.

Very few professionals will give you the requisite warnings about salicylates; that's something you'll have to learn for yourself. Identifying and avoiding them will be your responsibility, so prepare to do some homework. That's the hardest part for women, but it must be done. The initial search demands time and patience. Once completed, even currently safe products may change and demand meticulous label reviews when buying replacements.

We're well aware of some who've failed on the protocol. When we can get to them, we almost invariably find the reasons are blocking or insufficient dosage. This is why Claudia and her team created and maintain a Web site. Seek online help if you must, because one failure is far too many. After product check is behind you, treatment is simple enough: Just take guaifenesin, find your dosage, and give it time to work. Getting guaifenesin is as simple as walking into a pharmacy. The intensity of the reversal cycles will vary for each of you. When it seems most difficult, it may help to remember a few facts:

- You weren't well before you started, and were probably getting sicker.
- You'll likely feel worse initially, but since guaifenesin has no significant side effects, intense cycling pain means the drug is working.
- It took time to develop fibromyalgia. It will take less to get rid of it, but it will surely take time.
- Your first good hours will tell you that your body is capable of recovery. Bunch a few good days together and you'll become a strong advocate of our protocol.
- We define happiness as freedom from pain—mental and physical. There are such days ahead for you.

Each of us who has conquered the disease owes something to those still sick. As wonderful as it is to feel well, we remain sad for those who are still miserable. As long as we receive e-mails and letters detailing lifelong struggles with pain, fatigue, and relationships, our victory is not complete and our job is not yet done. We hope this book will provide the initiating core for a chain letter. As you get well, you progressively incur a debt, and you should plan to repay it. You can best do that by helping others who are still searching for the path you've already walked. Please, won't you help?

—R. Paul St. Amand, MD

Appendix

Technical Appendix

THIS TECHNICAL SUPPLEMENT is intended for medical personnel who are already familiar with the disease. We offer the following in support for our theory concerning the physiologic and biochemical basis for fibromyalgia. We also extend the description of the illness and our success in reversing it. Please refer to the text for comprehensive details of the following summary.

Patients focus on dominantly affected tissue as their chief complaint. Variations are as follows. *Musculoskeletal* (pain in any muscle, tendon, ligament, joint, and leg cramps); *brain* malfunction (fatigue, irritability, depression, apathy, nervousness, anxiety, insomnia, suicidal ideation, impaired memory and concentration); *irritable bowel* (nausea, gas, bloating, cramps, deep aching, constipation or, alternativly, diarrhea); *genitourinary* (dysuria, pungent urine, recurrent bacterial or interstitial cystitis, vulvodynia); *dermatologic* (rashes such as hives, eczema, pruritic vesicles, acne, rosacea, seborrheic and neurodermatitis, scattered maculopapular red or colorless lesions, brittle nails, defective hair, paresthesias, itching); *head, eye, ear, nose, and throat* (varieties of headaches, dizziness, vertigo, imbalance, dry eyes, blepharitis, conjunctivitis, gritty discharge, blurred vision, nasal congestion, postnasal drip, bad or metallic tastes, painful tongue, scalded mouth, tinnitus or low-pitched sounds); *miscellaneous* (patches of numbness and tingling especially digits, weight gain, low-grade fevers, water retention, restless leg syndrome, hypersensitivity to light, sounds, and odors).

Differing pain thresholds and clinical presentations have been used to create artificial groupings that share identically distorted physical findings. We consider the above symptoms as well as chronic fatigue, myofascial pain, and chronic candidiasis as variants within a spectrum that merge imperceptibly with fibromyalgia. The term *energopenia* would be more inclusive. We examine in greater detail than the limited search recommended by the American Academy of Rheumatology seeking "eleven-out-of-eighteen-tender-points" at predetermined sites. We regularly palpate multiple swollen areas and depict them on a body caricature to provide visual evidence of lesion size, shape, and location. Most affected areas are tender, but expressions of pain do not influence such body mapping. Our method is totally objective and not influenced by purely subjective tenderness. It avoids the pitfall of individual pain thresholds. We remap patients each visit to substantiate progress. Certain tissues are preferentially affected—for instance, the earliest lesions usually appear in the sternomastoid and trapezial areas. Furthermore, 100 percent of adults display spastic involvement of the left thigh (vastus lateralis and rectus femoris) to provide accurate diagnostic validation. With effective dosage and patient compliance, the same lesions reliably clear within the first month, predicting success.

Contracted muscles, tendons, and ligaments are working tissues. Biochemical aberrations obviously exist to force fibromyalgic cells into unrelenting overdrive. Any theory seeking to explain such physical findings must encompass the plethora of symptoms arising from nonpalpable tissues. We propose the following.

Forty-five years ago we began treating a then unnamed illness with the uricosuric agents probenecid and sulfinpyrazone. Thirteen years ago we realized the therapeutic value of guaifenesin, a minimally uricosuric and totally safe drug. Observations with this medication now include more than six thousand patients. Reversal of the illness begins at the following cumulative dosages: 300 mg twice daily is effective for 20 percent of patients; 600 mg bid, for 80 percent; 1800 mg per day for 90 percent; only 10 percent require 2,400 mg or more. Devoid of decongestants and cough suppressants, guaifenesin has no significant side effects. There is debate whether it increases the urinary metabolite of serotonin, 5 HIAA (5-hydroxyindoleacetic acid) or simply induces a false positive determination.[1]

Lesions reverse in retrograde cycling. Purging reproduces most of the previous symptoms, similar to clearing gouty joints of uric acid deposits. It proves far worse for fibromyalgics due to the extent of tissue involvement. Individual responsiveness and duration of the illness determine the time needed for recovery. The slowest responders reverse a minimum of one year's accumulated lesions for every two months of treatment. Low-dosage patients (300 mg bid) greatly accelerate the process. Improvement is initially felt for only a few hours, later for days, and eventually weeks.

Uricosuric agents as well as guaifenesin are totally blocked by aspirin and all sources of salicylate. The chemical readily absorbs through intact skin, and significant amounts ultimately concentrate in the proximal renal tubules. All plants make salicylates, using them for repairs and for repelling soil microorganisms and pests. Thus, topicals with plant derivatives such as aloe, ginseng, castor, or camphor oils (lipsticks, chapped-lip preparations, and deodorants) contain such blockers. The mint family (muscle pain balms, mouthwashes, and candies) deliver the compound into the system within seconds. Toothpastes almost all contain unlisted mint and/or salicylates.

Herbal medicinals readily overwhelm hepatic conjugating capacities, which normally suffice to render vegetable salicylates harmless. Plant juices adhere to skin, so gloves and closed shoes must be worn when gardening or walking on grass. The text fully exposes these blocking sources, as does our updated Web site: www.fibromyalgiatreatment.com.

Susceptibility to fibromyalgia is multigenetic, allowing various combinations of dominant and recessive genes. We have treated four patients aged two and others with late onset in their seventies. There is equal frequency in prepubertal boys and girls, but a strong female preponderance (85 percent) exists in adulthood. Obviously, either parent may transmit defective genes. Our theory casts strong suspicion on altered phosphate metabolism (see below). This important anion would likely be under the control of several genes scattered on different chromosomes. Puberty usually affords prolonged or permanent relief in men due to the massive need for phosphate during testosterone-induced growth and to sustain tissue structures of adulthood. Most women enjoy some respite at that time but sooner succumb to the illness.

Forty percent of patients recall the misnomered "growing pains" before age ten. They usually clear during the accelerated growth of puberty. Other symptoms begin spontaneously anytime after full development. Some patients date the onset following stress, infection, surgery, or trauma, but memories can often be nudged into recalling earlier symptoms. The cycling nature of fibromyalgia initially intersperses good and bad days. Gradually and progressively, incapacitating times prevail without significant respite. Older family members recall similar past symptoms that have now progressed to joint pains, suggesting that unresolved fibromyalgia deteriorates into osteoarthritis. Such individuals display the same mapping lesions as their affected offspring and relatives.

Fibromyalgia is unrelated to uric acid or gout, but we theorize it is also a retention disease. As stated above, we implicate inorganic phosphate (P_i), something that invokes no inflammatory response. In sufficient concentration, that anion would induce systemwide metabolic misadventures. Some clinical evidence supports our premise. Signs and symptoms of the disease cleared equally well using four older medications and more recently, guaifenesin. None of this benefit was related to effects on uric acid. Limited urine studies have shown increased twenty-four hour excretion of phosphate after instigating treatment with either guaifenesin or probenecid. Each effective drug has induced some lysis of dental calculus and progressively improved peeling or chipping fingernails. Both structures are mineralized by calcium phosphate. Adding calcium or magnesium to meals binds P_i, thereby increasing bowel excretion and allowing slight reductions in guaifenesin dosages. Beneficial effects of calcium make it an unlikely cause of the illness, though we think it abets the crime.

Biochemical research supports a primary defect in phosphate metabolism. Exercise-induced fatigue is erroneously attributed to lactic acid and falling pH. Lactate is, however, recycled for energy within muscles, and lowered pH sensitizes fibers to calcium, combining to increase endurance. Exercise produces copious H^+ that is promptly buffered into an enervating metabolite as shown in one study. Mitochondrial pH stabilized at 6.2 with no further decrease as subjects continued heavy bike exercises. Ultimately, exhaustive fatigue paralleled a *ninefold increase in diprotonated phosphate* ($H_2PO_4^-$).[2] Obviously, inorganic phosphate co-transports with H^+ and successfully buffers further assaults on pH, thus preventing apoptosis. Unrelenting spasms in sinews of fibromyalgia likely produce similar by-products. Additionally, it is well known that excess P_i blocks ATP formation as follows:

$$\Delta G = \frac{ATP}{ADP + P_i} \quad (\Delta G = \text{energy change}) \; (P_i = \text{inorganic phosphate})$$

Many papers address energy deprivation in fibromyalgia, but we refer to only a few. Bengtsson and Henriksson biopsied swollen and tender areas in trapezii and found a 20 percent reduction in ATP as well as phosphocreatine, the high-energy phosphate reservoir. The situation was actually worse because normal tissue was included in specimens.[3] Adjacent, unaffected muscle tissue was barely altered. This was confirmed by Lindman.[4] Strobel found increased P_i, as well as decreased phosphocreatine and pH, in contracted spinal erector muscles of fibromyalgia using ^{31}P magnetic resonance spectroscopy.[5] Other studies support this, including one on patients at rest.[6] Low-erythrocyte ATP has also been documented. Such cellular fatigue easily explains all the symptoms of fibromyalgia. Tired cells must hibernate and thereby shirk their biochemical duties.

The name *fibromyalgia* only infers pain in muscles and fibers and does not address the basic plight suffered by patients and cells. *Energy deprivation syndrome* has been suggested; we previously offered *dysenergism syndrome*. We readily yield, however, to a savant Greek colleague who coined the word *energopenia*. The currently accepted name hardly encompasses the following. Intermittent, nondiagnostic, and unreliable laboratory aberrations have been uncovered: *decreased* growth hormone, IGF-1, serotonin, free ionic Ca^{2+}, calcitonin, free urinary cortisol (weak cortisol response to ACTH), certain amino acids, neuropeptide Y; defective T cell activation, poor TSH response to TRH; *increased* serum prolactin, damaged mast cells releasing contents such as histamine, heparin, cytokines, and inserting IgG into the epidermis; elevated homocysteine and substance P in cerebrospinal fluid; plasma angiotensin converting enzymes. Obviously, the metabolic error is very fundamental if it affects so many systems. Other high-energy phosphate suppliers (ITP[3], GTP[3]) probably share the failure to provide adequate energy for the accelerated metabolism of fibromyalgia.

These abundant reports testify to widespread deficits and excesses of hormones, enzymes, and cytokines. Scant attention is given, however, to the fundamental reason: Energy-deprived organs malfunction. Cycling fibromyalgics at times almost meet energy demands, on occasion barely, and often not at all. Tiny surpluses within energy banks occasionally permit bursts of effort but rapidly deteriorate into renewed deficit spending. Wanton energy expenditures demanded by accidents, emotional stress, infections, or surgery sometimes provide the final insult initiating the first attack of fibromyalgia.

Ingested phosphate (P_i) is 80 to 90 percent absorbed. Retention or excretion is tightly controlled by the proximal renal tubule according to systemic needs. Our postulated renal defect is possibly shared by cell membranes in other tissues (enzyme, receptor, or pump) that ultimately permit excess intracellular phosphate accumulations. Cells readily absorb P_i from extracellular fluids and rapidly apportion it between the cytosol, endoplasmic reticulum, and outer mitochondrial chamber, where it rises as phosphoric acid in ratio with $P_i^=$. Such H^+ excess in the outer chamber destroys the inner membrane proton gradient and blunts H^+ egress from the matrix. ATP is normally generated when that proton returns through the inner wall back into the matrix via ATP synthase. If this action is blocked, the Krebs cycle remains operational but perforce activates uncoupling proteins 2 and/or 3, producing heat instead of energy. Such function alteration invokes fibromyalgia in a cascade determined by tissue susceptibility.

An increased serum pyruvate and normal or low lactate have been reported in some fibromyalgics, suggesting an intact aerobic metabolism.[7] Sufficient pyruvate, acetyl CoA, and citrate obviously exist for completing the Krebs sequence within the mitochondrial matrix. Attesting to the P_i/H^+ blockade of ATP formation is the spontaneous flushing and sweating in fibromyalgia that indicate production of heat rather than energy. Low cellular ATP and phosphocreatine (PCr) accompanied by rises in adenosine mono- and diphosphate (AMP and ADP) are powerful distress signals that beg for energy augmentation. Despite accelerated food intake, the dearth and malfunction of remaining mitochondria cannot fully respond. Insulin nevertheless reacts to increase renal reabsorption of phosphate and drive it into affected cells. Biochemical distress of fibromyalgia is thus accelerated.

Cellular entry of the negatively charged P_i^{2-} requires buffering with positive charges, mainly provided by $calcium^{2+}$. Water is drawn in by sodium, chloride, and other elements to cause swelling and adds to the pain produced by overworked tissues. ATP-driven pumps normally extrude calcium from cells or to storage within mitochondria and endoplasmic reticula. This is how cells end any stimulated activity peculiar to their function. Nanomolar calcium sparks (oscillations) are sufficient for minuscule and limited responses to extra- or intracellular signals. Greater impulses induce more forceful and graded efforts up to rigor mortis, the ultimate ATP surge from dying cells. ATP-depleted tissues of fibromyalgia cannot fully man the pumps (ATPase) that extrude calcium. The goading effects continue and readily outstrip dwindling energy supplies. Basic physiology and biochemistry dictate: The palpably spastic structures of fibromyalgia are steadily working tissues that can only be sustained by abnormal calcium levels within their cytosol or sarcoplasm.

Many body secretions attempt to eject offending ions. Tears may burn and permit formation of morning "sand." Outbursts from salivary glands produce bad or metallic tastes and lingual irritation, finally precipitating as dental calculus (calcium phosphate). Urinary sediments are amorphous crystals composed of calcium phosphate, oxalate, or carbonate that accumulate at the trigone. They abrade the distal bladder or urethral mucosa upon urination to cause dysuria. Excreted acids of fibromyalgia bathe denuded surfaces, precipitating symptoms of interstitial cystitis or facilitating bacterial invasion. Vaginal involvement leads to dyspareunia, vulvitis, vestibulitis, and overgrowths of microorganisms or *Candida.*

Other mucosal surfaces in the eye, lids, or mouth share hyperacidity and energy deprivation. The mucosal counterpart, the integument, suffers similar irritation that introduces paresthesias, defective nail formation, and inferior hair texture and growth. Dermal attacks by mast cells are matched in bronchial, vaginal, and bladder walls.[8] Histamine provokes rashes and pruritus; heparin surges account for easy bruising witnessed in 75 percent of fibromyalgic women.

Persistently working tissues of fibromyalgia continuously burn fuel and induce sugar craving. Yielding to this urge is a futile attempt to restore lost energy. Carbohydrate intake generates little extra because of delinquent ATP formation. Consequent insulin surges only add to pathology. About 40 percent of fibromyalgic women and 20 percent of men become hypoglycemic, as manifested by adrenaline surges. Symptoms include frontal headaches, tremors, sweats, heart palpitations (pounding or tachycardia), and bursts of anxiety or panic attacks. If insulin-dependent diabetics listed these complaints, physicians would have no difficulty in determining hypoglycemia. We suggest the cluster is sufficiently diagnostic in any patient without further testing. *Acute* symptoms appear a few hours postprandially, often nocturnally, and last twenty to thirty minutes. We describe the *chronic* carbohydrate-induced symptoms in the text. CNS and IBS complaints of fibromyalgia strikingly overlap, but epinephrine bursts readily distinguish the two entities. Patients improve by treating either condition separately, but both must be controlled for full restoration of energy.

Glucopenia is more descriptive than *hypoglycemia* since it refers to tissue, particularly brain, levels of glucose. During five-hour glucose tolerance tests, plasma glucose may not drop below the accepted 50 mg standard for diagnosis. Genter and Ipp sampled blood every ten minutes to study counter-regulatory hormones in twenty young, healthy subjects during glucose tolerance testing. Nine of them suffered epinephrine releases despite normal glucose levels.[9] Patients have varying thresholds that individually mandate corrective neuroendocrine responses. Diagnosis is somewhat impeded when repeated bouts of hypoglycemia dull the brain from evoking appropriate counterattacks. Progressively lower glucose levels are required to initiate customary responses.[10] The low-carbohydrate diet described in the text restores normal signaling within two weeks.

Many fibromyalgics gain weight arguably due to diminished activity imposed by the disease. Additionally, there are documented decreases in muscle mitochondria in sedentary individuals, as much as 80 percent compared with well-honed athletes. Not only is there a dearth, but the remaining ones are sick and barely produce sufficient ATP for survival. Hoping to make energy, patients yield to carbohydrate craving, suppress glucagon, and increase insulin secretion—an ideal combination for weight gain. Insulin recruits malonyl CoA to hasten the conversion of glucose to fatty acid and also prompts storage of any immediately unused fuel as fat.

Beyond burning calories, the customarily prescribed exercises restore mitochondria. As soon as patients are able, we urge walking to rebuild the bulkier muscles of the lower torso. Such aerobic efforts restore type I muscle (red meat), the main dysfunctional fibers of fibromyalgia that are normally most heavily endowed with mitochondria. Anaerobic workouts such as resistance training enhance type II fibers (white meat) that are less in need of restoration. Not only healing mitochondria but also newly generated ones better burn unused calories, augment energy availability, and facilitate weight reduction.

In summary, this paper is long in theory but based on many facts, some we have not discussed due to space limitations. Guaifenesin is highly effective but, like uricosuric agents, is totally blocked when salicylates enter the body orally or topically and concentrate in proximal renal tubules.[11] Even tiny amounts in cosmetics, toothpastes, and botanicals slow or negate the drug's benefits, as they did all of our previous agents. We have thousands of serial maps to prove this contention. Susceptibility to blockade seems genetically determined and highly variable. Many fibromyalgics are carbohydrate intolerant and must temporarily diet. Though too painful without treatment, patients are eventually able to exercise sufficiently to resurrect mitochondria. Adherence to our protocol must be meticulous or there will be no improvement. Physicians who deviate from this design expose their patients to an undeserved failure.

We have described the only effective treatment for fibromyalgia and hope to wean physicians from prescribing dismal "threatment" with the habituating or frankly addicting medications currently promoted. Our protocol uses a nontoxic, over-the-counter drug that works to mitigate the metabolic error. Recent research has too often focused on deficient cell products rather than basic malfunctions shared by all affected cells. It is my mission to disseminate information gleaned from my forty-nine years of experience.

R. Paul St. Amand, MD
Assistant Clinical Professor of Medicine
Endocrinology—Harbor/UCLA
Los Angeles, California, 2005

Notes

Chapter 1

1. Frederick Wolfe, "The Fibromyalgia Problem," *Journal of Rheumatology* 24, no. 7 (1997): 1247–9.

2. W. R. Gowers, "A Lecture on Lumbago: Its Lessons and Analogues," *British Medical Journal* 1 (1904): 117–21.

3. F. Wolfe, H. A. Smythe, and M. B. Yunus, "Criteria for the Classification of Fibromyalgia," *American College of Rheumatology* 33 (1990): 160–72.

4. The Copenhagen Declaration, "Consensus Document on Fibromyalgia," *The Lancet* 240 (September 12, 1992). Incorporated into the ICD on January 1, 1993.

5. F. Wolfe, J. Anderson, and D. Harkness, "The Work and Disability Status of Persons with Fibromyalgia," *Journal of Rheumatology* 24 (1997): 1171–8.

Chapter 2

1. A. Bengtsson and K. G. Henriksson, "The Muscle in Fibromyalgia: A Review of Swedish Studies," *Journal of Rheumatology* 16, supplement 19 (1989): 144–9.

Chapter 3

1. Medical Economics, *Physicians' Desk Reference* (Montvale, NJ: Medical Economics, 1999). Entry for Humbid, 1698.

2. C. M. Ramsdell, A. E. Postlewaite, and W. Kelley, "Uricosuric Effect of Glyceryl Guaiacolate," *Journal of Rheumatology* 1, no. 1 (1974): 114–6.

3. Julia Lawless, *The Encyclopedia of Essential Oils* (Lanham, MD: Barnes & Noble, 1992), 106.

4. Medical Economics, *Physicians' Desk Reference for Herbal Medicines* (Montvale, NJ: Medical Economics, 1998).

5. Medical Economics, *Physicians' Desk Reference* (Montvale, NJ: Medical Economics, 1999). Entry for Humibid, 1698.

Chapter 4

1. P. Morra, W. R. Bartle, and S. E. Walker, "Serum Concentrations of Salicylic Acid Following Topically Applied Salicylate Derivatives," *Annals of Pharmacotherapy* 9 (September 1996): 935–40.

2. *Science Journal,* November 18, 1984.

3. A. R. Swain, S. P. Dutton, and A. S. Truswell, "Salicylates in Foods," *Journal of the American Dietetic Association* 85 (August 1998): 950–9.

Chapter 5

1. P. Genter and E. Ipp, "Plasma Glucose Thresholds for Counterregulation After an Oral Glucose Load," *Metabolism* 43, no. 1 (January 1994): 98–103.

2. Janette Brand Miller, "International Tables of Glycemic Index," *American Journal of Clinical Nutrition* 62 (1995): 871–90.

3. Robert C. Atkins, *Dr. Atkins' New Diet Revolution* (New York: M. Evans and Co., Inc., 1992); Richard K. Bernstein, *Dr. Bernstein's Diabetes Solution* (New York: Little Brown and Co., 1997).

Chapter 7

1. Harvey Moldofsky, "Nonrestorative Sleep and Symptoms After a Febrile Illness in Patients with Fibrositis and Chronic Fatigue Syndromes," *Journal of Rheumatology* 16, supplement 19 (1989): 150–3.

Chapter 10

1. J. J. Yount and J. J. Willems, "New Direction in Medical Management of Vulvar Vestibulitis," *Vulvar Pain Newsletter* (fall 1994): 5–7.

Chapter 11

1. S. Enestrom, A. Bengtsson, and T. Frodin, "Dermal IgG Deposits and Increase of Mast Cells in Patients with Fibromyalgia: Relevant Findings or Epiphenomena?" *Scandinavian Journal of Rheumatology* 26, no. 4 (1997): 308–13.

Chapter 13

1. Origin unknown. The guaiacum entry is from an old book sent to us from a patient in Washington State.

Chapter 14

1. Frederick Wolfe, "The Fibromyalgia Problem," *Journal of Rheumatology* 24, no. 7 (1997): 1247–9.

2. Robert Bennett, "Q & A with Robert Bennett, M.D.," *Fibromyalgia Network Newsletter* (October 1998): 13.

3. Don L. Goldenberg, "A Review of the Role of Tricyclic Medications in the Treatment of Fibromyalgia Syndrome," *Journal of Rheumatology* 16, supplement 19 (1989): 137–40.

4. Marcia Angell and Jerome P. Kassirer, "Alternative Medicine: The Risks of Untested and Unregulated Remedies," *New England Journal of Medicine* 339, no. 12 (September 17, 1998): 839–41.

5. Nortin M. Hadler, "Fibromyalgia: La Maladie Est Morte. Vive la Malade!" *Journal of Rheumatology* 24, no. 7 (1997): 1250–1.

6. Frederick Wolfe, "Disability and the Distress in Fibromyalgia," *Journal of Musculoskeletal Pain* 1 (1993): 65–87.

Chapter 15

1. Devin J. Starlanyl, MD, *The Fibromyalgia Advocate* (Oakland, CA: New Harbinger, 1998), 227.

2. Ibid., 169.

3. Devin J. Starlanyl, MD, and Mary Ellen Copeland, *Fibromyalgia and Chronic Myofascial Pain Syndrome: A Survival Manual* (Oakland, CA: New Harbinger, 1996), 161.

Technical Appendix

1. Medeva Pharmaceuticals, Inc. PDR, 1999. "Humibid," 1698, Drug/Laboratories test interactions.

2. Wilson JR, McCully KK, Mancini BB, Chance B. Relationship of Muscular Fatigue to pH and Diprotonated Pi in Humans: A 31–P–NMR Study. J App Phys 1988: 64–2333–9.

3. Bengtsson A, Henriksson KG. The Muscle in Fibromyalgia: A Review of Swedish Studies. J Rheum 16 supp 19 (Nov 1989):144–9.

4. Lindman R, Hagberg M, Angqvist K-A, Soderlund K, Hultman E, Thornell L-E. Changes in Muscle Morphology in Chronic Trapezius Myalgia. Scan J Work Env Health 17 (1991):347–55.

5. Strobel ES, Krapf M, Suckfull M, Bruckle W, Fleckenstein W, Muller W. Tissue Oxygen Measurement and 31P Magnetic Resonance Spectroscopy in Patients with Muscle Tension and Fibromyalgia. Rheum Int 16 (1997):175–80.

6. Park JH, Phothimat P, Oates CT, Hernanz-Schulman M, Olsen NJ. Use of P-31 Magnetic Resonance Spectroscopy to Detect

Metabolic Abnormalities in Muscles of Patients with Fibromyalgia. Arth Rheum 41(3) (Mar 1998):406–13.

7. Eisinger J, Plantamura A, Ayavou T. Glycolysis Abnormalities in Fibromyalgia. J Am Coll Nut 13(2) (1994):144–8.

8. Enestrom S, Bengtsson A, Frodin T. "Dermal IgG Deposits and Increase of Mast Cells in Patients with Fibromyalgia." Scan J Rheum 26 (4) (1997):308–13.

9. Genter P, and Ipp E. Plasma Glucose Thresholds for Counter-regulation After an Oral Glucose Load. Met 43 (Jan 1994):98–103.

10. Hvidberg A, et al. Impact of Recent Antecedent Hypoglycemia on Hypoglycemic Cognitive Dysfunction in Nondiabetic Humans. Diabetes 45 (8) (1996).

11. Delaney TP, et al. A Central Role of Salicylic Acid in Plant Disease Resistance. Science 266. (Nov 18, 1994). Winter R. A Consumer's Dictionary of Cosmetic Ingredients. New York: Crown Trade Paperbacks, 1994. Taylor JR, Halprin KM. Percutaneous Absorption of Salicylic Acid. Arch Derm 3(6) (June 1975):740–3. Brubacher JR, Hoffman RS. Salicylism from Topical Salicylates: Review of the Literature. Tox 34(4) (1996):431–6. Yip AS, Chow WH, Tai YT, Cheung KL. Adverse Effect of Topical Methylsalicylate Ointment on Warfarin Anticoagulation: An Unrecognized Potential Hazard. Postgrad Med J 66(775) (May 1990):367–9.

Resources

CHAPTERS 1 AND 2

ASSOCIATIONS

The Arthritis Foundation
National Office
PO Box 7669
Atlanta, GA 30357
800-283-7800
www.arthritis.org

The National Fibromyalgia Association
2200 North Glassell Street, Suite A
Orange, CA 92865
714-921-0150
www.fmaware.org

BOOKS

Cunningham, Chet. *The Fibromyalgia Relief Handbook.* Encinitas, CA: United Research Publishers, 2003.

Marek, Claudia Craig. *The First Year: Fibromyalgia. An Essential Guide for the Newly Diagnosed.* New York: Marlowe Books, 2003.

Russell, I. Jon. *The Fibromyalgia Syndrome: A Clinical Case Definition for Practitioners.* Oakland, CA: New Harbinger, 2004.

Starlanyl, Devin J. and Mary Ellen Copeland. *Fibromyalgia and*

Chronic Myofascial Pain Syndrome, 2nd edition. Oakland, CA: New Harbinger, 2001.

Staud, Roland, MD, and Christine Adamec. *Fibromyalgia for Dummies.* New York: Wiley Publishing, 2002.

Williamson, Miryam Ehrlich. *Fibromyalgia: A Comprehensive Approach.* New York: Walker & Co., 1998.

Videotapes

Depper, Joel, MD. *A Rheumatologist's Approach to Fibromyalgia.* Arizona Symposium, 2004. Available from the Fibromyalgia Recovery Group (Brenda Frandsen, president), 2814 East Mallory Street, Mesa, AZ 85215-1714; 480-832-5733; www.fibromyalgiarecovery.com; brenda@fibromyalgiarecovery.com.

Starlanyl, Devin J. *Chronic Myofascial Pain Syndrome: A Guide to the Trigger Points.* Oakland, CA: New Harbinger, 1977.

Wymore, Marian, MD, and Claudia Marek. *Working with Your Doctor.* Arizona Symposium, 2004. Available from the Fibromyalgia Recovery Group (Brenda Frandsen, president), 2814 East Mallory Street, Mesa, AZ 85215-1714; 480-832-5733; www.fibromyalgiarecovery.com; brenda@fibromyalgiarecovery.com. Both Dr. Wymore and Ms. Marek have fibromyalgia and work with fibromyalgic patients.

Web Sites

www.immunesupport.com. Newsletter and information.
www.sover.net/~devstar. The site of Devin Starlanyl.
www.nfa.org. National Fibromyalgia Association's online newsletter.

CHAPTER 3

Books

St. Amand, R. Paul, and Claudia Craig Marek. *What Your Doctor May* Not *Tell You About Fibromyalgia Fatigue.* New York: Warner Books, 2002.

Newsletters

The Fibromyalgia Treatment Forum

Claudia Marek, editor
PO Box 64339
Los Angeles, CA 90064
www.fibromyalgiatreatment.com
The newsletter costs $32 for six issues a year.

Support Groups

Guai Group: www.fibromyalgiatreatment.com

An online support group. List owner: Clauda Marek; administrative team: Jan Houp, Anne Louise, Char Melson, Gretchen Parker, Cris Roll; Webmaster: Char Melson.

Videotapes/DVDs

Depper, Joel, MD. *The Use of Guaifenesin in a Rheumatologic Practice.* Arizona Symposium, 2004. Available from the Fibromyalgia Recovery Group (Brenda Frandsen, president), 2814 East Mallory Street, Mesa, AZ 85215-1714; 480-832-5733; www.fibromyalgiarecovery.com; brenda@fibromyalgiarecovery.com.

St. Amand, R. Paul, MD. *The Chemistry and Treatment of Fibromyalgia.* Arizona Symposium, 2004. Available from the Fibromyalgia Recovery Group (Brenda Frandsen, president), 2814 East Mallory Street, Mesa, AZ 85215-1714; 480-832-5733; www.fibromyalgiarecovery.com; brenda@fibromyalgiarecovery.com.

St. Amand, R. Paul, MD, and Claudia Craig Marek. *The Guaifenesin Protocol for Fibromyalgia: Diagnosis, Treatment, and a Demonstration of the Mapping Technique.* Available as a Video/DVD from The Fibromyalgia Treatment Center, PO Box 64339, Los Angeles, CA 90064; www.fibromyalgiatreatment.com. The cost of $25 includes priority shipping and handling.

CHAPTER 4

AUDIOTAPES/DVDS

Marek, Claudia. *Salicylates: Key to Recovery.* Arizona Symposium, 2004. Available from the Fibromyalgia Recovery Group (Brenda Frandsen, president), 2814 East Mallory Street, Mesa, AZ 85215-1714; 480-832-5733; www.fibromyalgiarecovery.com; brenda@fibromyalgiarecovery.com. Claudia Marek explains the importance of salicylates, and how to avoid them.

BOOKS

Begoun, Paula. *Don't Go to the Cosmetics Counter Without Me,* 5th edition. Seattle: Beginning Press, 2003.

Winter, Ruth, MS. *A Consumer's Dictionary of Cosmetic Ingredients,* 4th edition. New York: Crown, 1994.

PRODUCTS

Grace Fibro-Smile Products

Flora Stay, DDS, and Andrew Stay, founders
321 Aviator Street, Suite 113
Camarillo, CA 93010
888-883-4276 or 805-383-3776
www.fibrosmile.com

Grace Fibro-Smile operates via distributors and is designed to help those with FMS. For information, contact Lou@myfibrosmile.com. Products include dental products, skin and hair care, makeup, lip balm, breath mints, and guaifenesin.

Illuminaré Cosmetics

Ruthie Molloy, founder
4970 Windplay Drive, 71st Floor
El Dorado Hills, CA 95762-9659
866-999-2033 or 916-939-2033
www.illuminarecosmetics.com

ruthie@illuminarecosmetics.com
Beautiful mineral makeup.

Marina del Rey Pharmacy
Jim Zelenay, pharmacist and owner
4558 South Admiralty Way
Marina del Rey, CA 90292
310-823-5311
www.fibroconnection.com
Products including vitamins, supplements, guaifenesin, skin care, makeup, salicylate-free progesterone cream, sunscreens, toothpastes, and more are available and shipped worldwide from this pharmacy.

Martinez FMS Products
Gloria Martinez, owner
Cosmetics, personal products, guaifenesin, and treatment information for Spanish speakers.

Mary Kay Inc.
PO Box 799045
Dallas, TX 75379-9045
800-627-9529
www.marykay.com
Operates via distributors. Mary Kay keeps a list of salicylate-free products that's updated annually and anytime new products are introduced.

Paula's Choice
Paula Begoun, founder
1030 Southwest 34th Street, Suite A
Renton, WA 98055-4813
800-831-4088 or 425-988-6068
www.paulaschoice.com
Use *only* products tagged SALICYLATE FREE.

Paula's Choice, Australia
within Australia: 800-819-566
outside Australia: 613-8742-2303
www.paulaschoice.com.au

Paula's Choice, Singapore
+65 9068 3333
paulas@starhub.net.sg

Personal Basics by Andrea Rose
Andrea Rose, owner
888-712-ROSE
www.andrearose.com
All the basics, from skin care to cosmetics to toothpaste.

Pro Health, Inc.
2040 Alameda Padre Serra, Suite 101
Santa Barbara, CA 93103
800-366-6056
international: 001-805-564-3064
www.immunesupport.com
Guaifenesin, and some salicylate-free vitamins, supplements, and other products. (Not all products are salicylate-free.)

Sunblocks.com
Sunscreen International
Steve and Lisha Finley, owners
PO Box 384813
Waikoloa, HI 96738
808-883-8400
www.sunblocks.com
Salicylate-free sunscreen.

Tom's of Maine
PO Box 710
Kennebunkport, ME 04343
800-367-8667
www.tomsofmaine.com
Acceptable toothpastes are the nonmint varieties: strawberry, orange, grape, apricot, unflavored, and the fennel without myrrh oils. Do not use the orange with menthol.

Women's International Pharmacy
12012 North 111th Avenue
Youngtown, AZ 85363

623-214-7700 or 800-279-5708
2 Marsh Court
Madison, WI 53718
608-221-7800
info@womensinternational.com
Will make salicylate-free compounded topical products.

> Be aware that except for the companies listed in this section, all products should be rechecked each time they are purchased to make sure there have been no ingredient changes.

Web Sites

To find material data safety sheets for household products:

- www.ilpi.com/msds

All cosmetics companies have Web sites, and some list ingredients. Most also include 800 numbers on the packaging. Try the following sites:

- www.avon.com
- www.physiciansformula.com
- www.suave.com

Web sites that list ingredients for multiple products include:

- www.beauty.com
- www.drugstore.com
- www.ulta.com
- www.walgreens.com

The following sites also list ingredients and carry product lines normally sold by dermatologists:

- www.dermstore.com
- www.mydermdoctor.com

To check your own products and find lists of acceptable products, information is available at:

- www.fibromyalgiatreatment.com

- in Australia and New Zealand: www.voxau.com
- in the United Kingdom: www.froguk.com

Claudia's Salicylate Search Resource

Salicylates may be known as:

- Salicylate
- Salicylic acid
- Octisalate
- Homosalate
- Any chemical with *sal* in the name
- Menthol
- Any chemical with *men* in the name
- Mint flavor
- Oils with a plant name (exceptions: soy, wheat, corn, oats, rice)
- Gels with a plant name (exceptions: soy, wheat, corn, oats, rice)
- Extracts with a plant name (exceptions: soy, wheat, corn, oats, rice)
- Pycnogenol
- Camphor
- Bisabol (barks)
- Meradimate

If none of the words on this list is present, the product is fine. However, if you see:

- [something] oil,
- [something] gel, or
- [something] extract

and you don't know whether the accompanying word or phrase is a plant name, look it up on dictionary.com (www.dictionary.com). If it is a plant name, you can't use it.

If the word or phrase is Latin and is not listed on Dictionary.com, search the Internet using Google (www.google.com). For example, you might search "Pinus sylvestris oil" or "Melissa officinalis gel" or "Nepeta cataria extract." Be sure to enclose the entire phrase in quotation marks. The first entry will usually identify the substance. Then you can recheck it against the above list.

For medications, look up the chemical name of the medication on drugstore.com (www.drugstore.com) or any of the drug information sites. If the name has *sal* in it, you cannot use it. If the chemical name does not contain the phrase *sal*, then you can use it.

In vitamins, look for bioflavonoids, flavonoids, rutin, quercetin, hesperidin, and any herb. These are forbidden.

CHAPTER 5

ASSOCIATIONS

The Hypoglycemia Support Foundation
PO Box 451778
Sunrise, FL 33345
www.hypoglycemia.org

AUDIOTAPES/DVDS

Meshorer, Gwen. *Low Carbohydrate Diet Ideas.* Arizona Symposium, 2004. Available from the Fibromyalgia Recovery Group (Brenda Frandsen, president), 2814 East Mallory Street, Mesa, AZ 85215-1714; 480-832-5733; www.fibromyalgiarecovery.com; brenda@fibromyalgiarecovery.com. The editor of *The Fibromyalgia Treatment Forum* newsletter presents ideas for creating low-carb meals for hypoglycemics.

St. Amand, R. Paul, MD. *Diet Considerations in Fibromyalgia.* Arizona Symposium, 2004. Available from the Fibromyalgia Recovery Group (Brenda Frandsen, president), 2814 East Mallory

Street, Mesa, AZ 85215-1714; 480-832-5733; www.fibromyalgiarecovery.com; brenda@fibromyalgiarecovery.com. Dr. St. Amand explains the interplay between fibromyalgia and hypoglycemia and why a low-carb diet makes the majority of fibromyalgics feel better.

Books: General

St. Amand, R. Paul, and Claudia Craig Marek. *What Your Doctor May* Not *Tell You About Fibromyalgia Fatigue.* New York: Warner Books, 2003.

Starlanyl, Devin J. and Mary Ellen Copeland. *Fibromyalgia and Chronic Myofascial Pain Syndrome,* 2nd edition. Oakland, CA: New Harbinger, 2001.

Williamson, Miryam Ehrlich. *Blood Sugar Blues: Overcoming the Hidden Dangers of Insulin Resistance.* New York: Walker & Co., 2001.

All books by Robert Atkins, MD, contain information about insulin, blood sugar, and carbohydrates. Recipes and resources are available online at www.atkins.com. Make sure that all the recipes you use are acceptable for the hypoglycemia diet. For weight loss, they do not need to be reviewed.

You can get a catalog of Atkins products from:

Atkins Nutritionals Inc.
2002 Orville Drive North, Suite A
Ronkonkoma, NY 11779
800-2-ATKINS
www.atkins.com

Books: Low-Carb Recipes

Not all low-carbohydrates are the same. Be sure to check all recipes to make sure they're compatible with our diet.

Carpender, Dana. *The Low-Carb Barbecue Book: Over 200 Recipes for the Grill and Picnic Table.* Gloucester, MA: Fair Winds Press, 2004.

———. *15-Minute Low-Carb Recipes: Instant Recipes for Dinners, Desserts, and More.* Gloucester, MA: Fair Winds Press, 2003.

———. *500 Low-Carb Recipes: 500 Recipes from Snacks to Dessert That the Whole Family Will Love.* Gloucester, MA: Fair Winds Press, 2002.

———. *500 More Low-Carb Recipes: 500 All New Recipes from Around the World.* Gloucester, MA: Fair Winds Press, 2004.

———. *200 Low-Carb Slow Cooker Recipes: Healthy Dinners That Are Ready When You Are!* Gloucester, MA: Fair Winds Press, 2005.

Grad, Marcia. *A Taste for Life: Recipes for a High-Protein Diet* (introduction by R. Paul St. Amand, MD). New York: Charles Scribner's Sons, 1975. (Out of print.)

Long, Sharron. *Extreme Low Carb Cuisine: 250 Recipes with Virtually No Carbs.* Avon, MA: Adams Media, 2003.

McCullough, Fran. *The Low-Carb Cookbook.* New York: Hyperion, 1997.

———. *Living Low Carb.* New York: Little, Brown & Co., 2000.

Books: Diabetes

Bernstein, Richard K. *Dr. Bernstein's Diabetes Solution.* New York: Little, Brown & Co., 1997.

Web Sites

www.diabetes-normalsugars.com.

www.86sugar.com.

www.fibromyalgiatreatment.com. Resources.

www.guaigroup.org. Answers to frequently asked questions and an archive of recipes for both strict and liberal diets, including a full holiday meal.

www.immuneweb.org/lowcarb. For vegetarians.

www.lowcarb.com.

www.mendosa.com. This site, by Rick Mendosa, offers the glycemic index online.

CHAPTER 6

Books

St. Amand, R. Paul, and Claudia Craig Marek. *What Your Doctor May* Not *Tell You About Fibromyalgia Fatigue.* New York: Warner Books, 2003.

DVDs, CDs, and Videotapes

St. Amand, R. Paul, MD. *The Chemistry and Treatment of Fibromyalgia.* Arizona Symposium, 2004. Available from the Fibromyalgia Recovery Group (Brenda Frandsen, president), 2814 East Mallory Street, Mesa, AZ 85215-1714; 480-832-5733; www.fibromyalgiarecovery.com; brenda@fibromyalgiarecovery.com.

St. Amand, R. Paul, MD, and Claudia Craig Marek. *The Guaifenesin Protocol for Fibromyalgia: Diagnosis, Treatment, and a Demonstration of the Mapping Technique.* Available as a CD-ROM DVD from The Fibromyalgia Treatment Center, PO Box 64339, Los Angeles, CA 90064; www.fibromyalgiatreatment.com. The cost of $25 includes priority shipping and handling. A list of mappers and practitioners is also available online at www.fibromyalgiatreatment.com.

International Resources

In Canada: Books, multimedia products, and some salicylate-free products are available at:

www.fibronorth.com
Julie Levy, owner
613-756-3262 or 877-435-7736

In the United Kingdom: Books, multimedia products, and salicylate-free products are available from:

UK FMS Guai Group
Fiona Russell, leader
http://ukfmsguai.tripod.com
E-mail directly at trigleann@aol.com
An online support group.

In Australia, New Zealand, and Asia: Books, multimedia products, guaifenesin, and salicylate-free products are available from:

Positive Living
Jacqui Leeden, owner
PO Box 28-552
Remuera, Auckland, New Zealand 1005
649-578-1958
www.voxau.com
jacqui@voxau.com

Guaifenesin Products

Mucinex (long-acting guaifenesin, 600 mg) available in all stores. Discount pharmacies have the best prices. You can also get excellent prices from:

- Marina del Rey Pharmacy; 800-435-2330; www.fibroconnection.com. Sells all types of guaifenesin, including long-acting perscription dye-free guaifenesin.
- Pro Health; www.immunesupport.com. Pro Health makes a short-acting product called Guaifenesin FA that Dr. St. Amand has tested on patients.

Grace Fibro-Smile Solo Guai 400 mg tablets. No saccharin, no maltodextrin, dye, or vanillin. Formulated by R Paul St. Amand, MD.

- www.fibrosmile.com
- 888-883-4276

Support Groups

www.fibromyalgiatreatment.com. This Web site offers an international online support group and also maintains a list of guaifenesin protocol in-person support groups.

CHAPTER 7

Audiotapes/DVDs

Brandt, Deb, PA, and Claudia Craig Marek. *Coping with Chronic Fatigue.* Arizona Symposium, 2004. Available from the Fibromyalgia Recovery Group (Brenda Frandsen, president), 2814 East Mallory Street, Mesa, AZ 85215-1714; 480-832-5733; www.fibromyalgiarecovery.com; brenda@fibromyalgiarecovery.com. A physician's assistant and this book's coauthor discuss help for chronic fatigue symptons.

Stroup, Angela, RN, MA, Certified Hypnotherapist; 757-714-7375; www.mentorforlife.com. Tapes for relaxation, pain management, and sleep. Custom tapes for individual needs are also available.

Books

Bourne, Edmund, and Corna Garano. *Coping with Anxieties: 10 Simple Ways to Relieve Anxiety, Fear and Worry.* Oakland, CA: New Harbinger, 2003.

Copeland, Mary Ellen, and Wayne London. *The Depression Workbook.* Oakland, CA: New Harbinger, 1992.

CHAPTER 8

Associations

American Pain Society
4700 West Lake Avenue
Glenview, IL 60025
847-375-4715
www.ampainsoc.org
info@ampainsoc.org

Chronic Pain Support Group
http://go.to/ChronicPainSupport.org

National Headache Foundation
820 North Orleans, Suite 217
Chicago, IL 60610
800-643-5552
www.headaches.com

Pain.com
www.pain.com
Many resources and instructional material about pain.

Restless Leg Syndrome
819 2nd Street Southwest
Rochester, MN 55902-2985
507-287-6465
www.rls.org

Books

Catalano, Ellen Mohr, and Klameron Hardin. *The Chronic Pain Control Work Book: A Step by Step Guide for Coping with and Overcoming Pain.* Oakland, CA: New Harbinger, 1996.

Cunningham, Chet. *The Sciatica Relief Handbook.* Encinitas, CA: United Research Publishers, 2003.

Travell, Janet, MD. *Travell and Simons' Trigger Point Flip Charts.* Philadelphia: Lippincott Williams & Wilkins, 1996.

CHAPTER 9

Support Groups

IBS Self Help Group
PO Box 94074
Toronto, Ontario
M4N 3R1 Canada

IBS Support Group and Information
1440 Whalley Avenue, #145
New Haven, CT 06515
www.ibsgroup.org

CHAPTER 10

Audiotapes/DVDs

Willems, John, MD. *Effective Non-Surgical Treatments for Vulvar Pain.* Arizona Symposium, 2004. Available from the Fibromyalgia Recovery Group (Brenda Frandsen, president), 2814 East Mallory Street, Mesa, AZ 85215-1714; 480-832-5733; www.fibromyalgiarecovery.com; brenda@fibromyalgiarecovery.com. Dr. Willems is the head of ob-gyn at Scripps Clinic.

Books

Glazer, Howard, and Gae Rodke. *The Vulvodynia Survival Guide.* Oakland, CA: New Harbinger, 2002.

Laumann, Beverly. *A Taste of the Good Life: A Cookbook for an Interstitial Cystitis Diet.* Freeman Family Trust Publications, 1998.

Stolzfus, Meg, and Joanne J. Young, editors. *The Low Oxalate Cookbook.* The Vulvar Pain Foudnation, 1997. Available from www.vulvarpainfoundation.org; the price of $30 includes postage and handling.

Products

Marina del Rey Pharmacy
310-823-5311
fibroconnection.com.
Emu oil, Prelief, and many other products.
www.prelief.com
Information about the drug Prelief.

Wild Rose Emu Ranch
Joe and Clover Quinn, owners
406-363-1710
wildrose@bitterroot.net

Support Groups and Organizations

The IC Network
Jill Osborne, founder
5636 Del Monte Court
Santa Rosa, CA 95409
707-538-9442
www.ichelp.com

Interstitial Cystitis Association
110 North Washington Street, #340
Rockville, MD 20850
800-HELP-ICA
www.ichelp.com

National Vulvodynia Association
Phyllis Mate, executive director
PO Box 4491
Silver Spring, MD 20914-4491
301-299-0775
www.nva.org

The Vulvar Pain Foundation
PO Drawer 177
Graham, NC 27253
336-226-0704
www.vulvarpainfoundation.org

Treatment

John J. Willems, MD
Scripps Clinic and Research Foundation
10666 North Torrey Pines Road
La Jolla, CA 92037
619-554-8690

CHAPTER 11

Books

Caution: Not all therapies are compatible with guaifenesin use.

Begoun, Paula. *Don't Go to the Cosmetics Counter Without Me,* 5th edition. Seattle: Beginning Press, 2003.

Jacknin, Jeanette, MD. *Smart Medicine for Your Skin: A Comprehensive Guide to Understanding Conventional and Alternative Therapies to Heal Common Skin Problems.* New York: Avery, 2001.

Winter, Ruth, MS. *A Consumer's Dictionary of Cosmetic Ingredients,* 4th edition. New York: Crown, 1994.

CHAPTER 12

Associations

The TMJ Association
PO Box 26770
Milwaukee, WI 53226-0770
414-259-3223
www.tmj.org

Audiotapes/DVDs

Stay, Flora, DDS. *Mouth Problems and Solutions.* Arizona Symposium, 2004. Available from the Fibromyalgia Recovery Group (Brenda Frandsen, president), 2814 East Mallory Street, Mesa, AZ 85215-1714; 480-832-5733; www.fibromyalgiarecovery.com; brenda@fibromyalgiarecovery.com. Advice about oral health specific to those with FMS.

Books

Heller, Sharon. *Too Loud, Too Bright, Too Fast, Too Tight: What to Do if You Are Sensory Defensive in an Overstimulating World.* New York: Perennial Currents, 2003.

Stay, Flora, DDS. *The Fibromyalgia Dental Handbook.* New York: Marlowe Books, 2004.

WEB SITES

www.drstay.com. Flora Stay, DDS, author of two books and countless articles about dentistry, answers questions and offers newsletter and salicylate-free products to help fibromyalgics.

CHAPTER 13

AUDIOTAPES/DVDS

St. Amand, R. Paul, MD. *Pediatric Fibromyalgia.* Arizona Symposium, 2004. Available from the Fibromyalgia Recovery Group (Brenda Frandsen, president), 2814 East Mallory Street, Mesa, AZ 85215-1714; 480-832-5733; www.fibromyalgiarecovery.com; brenda@fibromyalgiarecovery.com. Dr. St. Amand explains the hereditary nature of FMS, the symptoms children experience, and treatment with guaifenesin.

BOOKS

Bell, David, MD, Mary Z. Robinson, Jean Pollard, Tom Robinson, and Bonnie Floyd. *A Parent's Guide to CFIDS: How to Be an Advocate for Your Child with Chronic Fatigue Immune Dysfunction.* Binghamton, NY: Haworth Press, 1999.

Marek, Claudia, and Lou Marek. *Why Can't Sharon Come Out and Play? A Picture Book About a Little Girl with Fibromyalgia.* Available from The Fibromyalgia Treatment Center (www.fibromyalgiatreatment.com) or the Marina del Rey Pharmacy (www.fibroconnection.com).

St. Amand, R. Paul, MD, and Claudia Craig Marek. *What Your Doctor May* Not *Tell You About Pediatric Fibromyalgia.* New York: Warner Books, 2002.

Starlanyl, Devin J., MD, and Mary Ellen Copeland. *Fibromyalgia and Chronic Myofascial Pain Syndrome,* 2nd edition. Oakland, CA: New Harbinger, 2001.

Williamson, Miryam Ehrlich. *Fibromyalgia: A Comprehensive Approach.* New York: Walker & Co., 1998.

Web Sites

www.pediatricnetwork.org. For parents, youths, children, and professionals with fibromyalgia and chronic fatigue, the Pediatric Network offers extensive archives, self-help information, and more.

CHAPTER 14

Associations and Publications

U.S. Department of Justice Americans with Disabilities Act (ADA) Home Page
www.usdoj.gov/crt/ada/adahom1.htm

U.S. Equal Employment Opportunity Commission Clearinghouse
8280 Greensboro Drive, Suite 300
McLean, VA 22102
800-669-3362 (voice)
Publications.

U.S. Equal Employment Opportunity Commission Publication and Information Center
PO Box 12549
Cincinnati, OH 45212-0549
800-669-3362
www.eeoc.gov

Audiotapes/DVDs

Davis, Scott E., PC. *Disability Claims: What Patients and Doctors Need to Know.* Arizona Symposium, 2004. Available from the Fibromyalgia Recovery Group (Brenda Frandsen, president), 2814 East Mallory Street, Mesa, AZ 85215-1714; 480-832-5733; www.fibromyalgiarecovery.com; brenda@fibromyalgiarecovery.com. Scott Davis is a lawyer who specializes in representing those who are disabled from fibromyalgia or chronic fatigue.

Marek, Claudia, et al. *Support Group Ideas and Management.* Arizona Symposium, 2004. Available from the Fibromyalgia Recovery Group (Brenda Frandsen, president), 2814 East Mallory Street,

Mesa, AZ 85215-1714; 480-832-5733; www.fibromyalgiarecovery.com; brenda@fibromyalgiarecovery.com. This book's coauthor and guaifenesin support group leaders from around the world present a workshop about support groups.

Williamson, Miryam. *Sleep Solutions.* Arizona Symposium, 2004. Available from the Fibromyalgia Recovery Group (Brenda Frandsen, president), 2814 East Mallory Street, Mesa, AZ 85215-1714; 480-832-5733; www.fibromyalgiarecovery.com; brenda@fibromyalgiarecovery.com. Miryam Williamson is the author of two books about fibromyalgia.

Wymore, Marian, MD. *Integrative Medical Approaches for Fibromyalgia Symptom Management.* Arizona Symposium, 2004. Available from the Fibromyalgia Recovery Group (Brenda Frandsen, president), 2814 East Mallory Street, Mesa, AZ 85215-1714; 480-832-5733; www.fibromyalgiarecovery.com; brenda@fibromyalgiarecovery.com. Includes acupuncture, chiropractic care, heat, cold, ultrasound, visualization techniques, and more.

Books

Angell, Marcia, MD. *The Truth About Drug Companies.* New York: Random House, 2004.

Jacobs, Greg, and Herbert Benson. *Say Good Night to Insomnia: The Six-Week, Drug-Free Program Developed at Harvard Medical School.* New York: Owl Books, 1999.

Winter, Ruth. *The Anti-Aging Hormones.* New York: Crown Publishing, 1997.

Support Groups

www.fibromyalgiatreatment.com. This Web site offers a setup packet for guaifenesin-oriented support groups, as well as a list of guaifenesin support groups worldwide, both in person and on the Internet.

Web Sites

www.brainbody.com. Ruth Winter, MS, offers information about medications and therapies.

www.consumerslab.com. The Consumer's Lab does independent testing of the potency and purity of medicinal supplements.

www.quackwatch.com. Evaluation of some alternative therapies.

www.rxlist.com. Basic prescription drug information.

CHAPTER 15

Associations

Alexander Technique
PO Box 517
Urbana, IL 61801
217-367-6956
www.alexandertechnique.com

American Academy of Physical Medicine and Rehabilitation
1 IBM Plaza, #2500
Chicago, IL 60611-3065
312-464-9700
www.aapmr.org

American Massage Therapy Association
500 Davis Street, #900
Evanston, IL 60201-4695
877-905-2700
www.amtamassage.org
info@amtamassage.org

American Physical Therapy Association
1111 North Fairfax Street
Alexandria, VA 22314-1488
800-999-2782
www.apta.org

Curves International
100 Ritchie Road

Waco, TX 76712
800-848-1096
www.curvesinternational.com
Work-at-your-own-pace aerobic and resistance training.

Feldenkrais Educational Foundation of North America (FEFNA)
3611 Southwest Hood Avenue, Suite 100
Portland, OR 97239
866-333-6248
www.feldenkrais.com

Pilates: Balanced Body, Inc.
8220 Ferguson Avenue
Sacramento, CA 95828
800-745-2837
in the UK: 0800 015 5620
www.pilates.com
info@pilates.com

AUDIOTAPES/DVDS

Hancock, Ken, moderator. *Relationship Strategies with a Chronic Illness.* Arizona Symposium, 2004. Available from the Fibromyalgia Recovery Group (Brenda Frandsen, president), 2814 East Mallory Street, Mesa, AZ 85215-1714; 480-832-5733; www.fibromyalgia recovery.com; brenda@fibromyalgiarecovery.com. Ken Hancock and the administration team of the Guai Support Group.

Killian, Jeri Lynn. *Getting Your Life Organized.* Arizona Symposium, 2004. Available from the Fibromyalgia Recovery Group (Brenda Frandsen, president), 2814 East Mallory Street, Mesa, AZ 85215-1714; 480-832-5733; www.fibromyalgiarecovery.com; brenda@ fibromyalgiarecovery.com. Tips from a high-powered bank executive with fibromyalgia.

Marek, Claudia, et al. *Support Group Ideas and Management.* Arizona Symposium, 2004. Available from the Fibromyalgia Recovery Group (Brenda Frandsen, president), 2814 East Mallory Street, Mesa, AZ 85215-1714; 480-832-5733; www.fibromyalgiarecov ery.com; brenda@fibromyalgiarecovery.com. This book's coauthor and guaifenesin support group leaders from around the world present a workshop about support groups.

Parker, Gretchen Evans. *Living and Working with Fibromyalgia.* Arizona Symposium, 2004. Available from the Fibromyalgia Recovery Group (Brenda Frandsen, president), 2814 East Mallory Street, Mesa, AZ 85215-1714; 480-832-5733; www.fibromyalgiarecovery.com; brenda@fibromyalgiarecovery.com. Presented by an occupational therapist with fibromyalgia.

Pierce, Renee, BSDM, DNH. *Stress Management.* Arizona Symposium, 2004. Available from the Fibromyalgia Recovery Group (Brenda Frandsen, president), 2814 East Mallory Street, Mesa, AZ 85215-1714; 480-832-5733; www.fibromyalgiarecovery.com; brenda@fibromyalgiarecovery.com.

St. Amand, R. Paul, MD, and Jim Anderson. *It's a Guy Thing: Men with Fibromyalgia.* Arizona Symposium, 2004. Available from the Fibromyalgia Recovery Group (Brenda Frandsen, president), 2814 East Mallory Street, Mesa, AZ 85215-1714; 480-832-5733; www.fibromyalgiarecovery.com; brenda@fibromyalgiarecovery.com.

Books

Bigelow, Stacie. *Fibromyalgia: Simple Relief Through Movement.* Hoboken, NJ: John Wiley & Sons, 2000.

Davies, Clair, Amber Davies, and David G. Simons, MD. *The Trigger Point Therapy Work Book: Your Self Treatment Guide for Pain Relief,* 2nd edition. Oakland, CA: New Harbinger, 2004.

Marek, Claudia Craig. *The First Year: Fibromyalgia. An Essential Guide for the Newly Diagnosed.* New York: Marlowe Books, 2003.

Marek, Claudia, and Lou Marek. *Why Is Mommy Staying in Bed Again Today? A Picture Book Explaining Fibromyalgia to a Younger Child.* Available from The Fibromyalgia Treatment Center (www.fibromyalgiatreatment.com) or the Marina del Rey Pharmacy (www.fibroconnection.com).

Miller, Fred. *Yoga for Common Aches and Pains.* New York: Perigee Books, 2004.

Pellegrino, Mark, MD. *Inside Fibromyalgia.* Columbus, OH: Anadem Publishing, 2001. Information on physical conditioning and some basic exercises, including stretching routines.

Piburn, Gregg. *Beyond Chaos: One Man's Journey Alongside His Chronically Ill Wife.* Atlanta: The Arthritis Foundation, 1999.

Sher, Barbara. *Teamworks: Building Support Groups That Guarantee Success.* New York: Warner Books, 1989.

Silver, Julie K., MD. *Chronic Pain and the Family.* Cambridge, MA: Harvard University Press, 2004.

Starlanyl, Devin J. *The Fibromyalgia Advocate.* Oakland, CA: New Harbinger, 1998.

Starlanyl, Devin J., and Mary Ellen Copeland. *Fibromyalgia and Chronic Myofascial Pain Syndrome,* 2nd edition. Oakland, CA: New Harbinger, 2001.

Williamson, Miryam Ehrlich. *213 Ideas for Improving the Quality of Life with Fibromyalgia.* New York: Walker & Co., 1998.

SUPPORT GROUPS

www.fibromyalgiatreatment.com. This Web site offers a setup packet for guaifenesin-oriented support groups, as well as a list of guaifenesin support groups worldwide, both in person and on the Internet.

VIDEOTAPES/DVDS

Clark, Sharon. *Exercise Videos for Fibromyalgics.* Available from the National Fibromyalgia Research Organization, PO Box 500, Salem, OR 97302; www.nfra.net.

Jaconelli, Liz. *Fitness Training for Fibromyalgics.* Arizona Symposium, 2004. Available from the Fibromyalgia Recovery Group (Brenda Frandsen, president), 2814 East Mallory Street, Mesa, AZ 85215-1714; 480-832-5733; www.fibromyalgiarecovery.com; brenda@fibromyalgiarecovery.com.

MacRae, Catherine. *Gentle Fitness.* Available from Fibromyalgia Recovery, 5083 Grossman Drive, Rhinelander, WI 54501; 800-566-7780; www.fibromyalgiarecovery.com or www.gentlefitness.com. This award-winning video comes with a helpful twenty-page book. It blends yoga, tai chi, and Feldenkrais movement awareness.

Mahaney, Gail, LMT. *Massage Therapy Techniques for Fibromyalgics.* Arizona Symposium, 2004. Available from the Fibromyalgia Recovery Group (Brenda Frandsen, president), 2814 East Mallory Street, Mesa, AZ 85215-1714; 480-832-5733; www.fibromyalgiarecovery.com; brenda@fibromyalgiarecovery.com.

Starlanyl, Devin J. *Chronic Myofascial Pain Syndrome: A Guide to the Trigger Points.* Oakland, CA: New Harbinger, 1977.

Web Sites

www.anxietybookstore.com; 214-672-0564.

www.menwithfibro.com. Information and support for men.

www.relaxation-tapes-music.com; 800-542-7782.

Index

NOTE: Page numbers in italics refer to illustrations

Abdominal pain, *106,* 114–15, *115,* 205, *206,* 207–9
Acetaminophen, 286, 297, 303, 312
Acne, 74–75, 80–81, *115,* 242, 249
Acupuncture, 196, 353
Addictions, 300–302
Adenosine triphosphate (ATP), 31–39, 129, 131, 365–68
  gauifensin and, 59–60
  muscle loss and, 189–90
Adrenaline (epinephrine), 105, 107, 109, 111
Alcohol, 117
Alexander Technique, 353, 398
Allergies, 262, 267
Aloe, 84, 96
Alpha hydroxy, 89–90, 250
American College of Rheumatology, 7, 26
American Medical Association, 296, 320
Analgesics, 286, 297, 312
Anesthetics, 224, 234
Angell, Marcia, 308
Angiodema, 245
Antacids, 210, 212–13
Anti-anxiety medications, 210, 305–6
Antibiotics, 213, 221
Anticholinergics, 215, 237, 246
Antidepressants, 304–6, 327, 344
  for interstitial cystitis, 225
  for irritable bowel syndrome, 214–15
  for skin problems, 246–47
  for sleep disturbances, 315–16
  for vulvar pain, 237
Antifungals, 204, 252
Antihistamines, 225, 236, 246–47, 262, 312
Anti-inflammatories. *See* NSAIDs
Anturane (sulfinpyrazone), 48, 49–50
Anxieties, 24, 114, *115,* 175, 178, 210, 305–6
Apathy, 175, 178
Arthritis, 74, 148, 192–97
Arthritis Foundation, 146–47, 346, 351, 377
Aspirin, 74–75, 76, 80, 81, 297
Asthma, 70, 75
Ativan (lorazepam), 237, 303–4
Atkins, Robert, 142–43, 386
Attention deficit disorder (ADD), 75, 274, 282
Auditory problems, 257, 260–61

Begoun, Paula, 92–94, 380
Benadryl, 225, 236, 286, 312

Benemid (probenecid), 40–41, 46, 48, 49
Ben Gay, 75–76, 80
Bengtsson, A., 32, 366
Benzodiazapines, 316
Bernstein, Richard, 142–43
Beverages, 70, 122, 223
Biochemical basis
  for fibromyalgia, 30–38, 361–71
  for hypoglycemia, 102–5, 107, *108*
Bioflavonoids, 83, 96
Bladder infections, *115,* 218–26, *220, 235*
Bloating, *115,* 201, 203, 205
Blood sugar. *See* Glucose
Blood tests, 147–49, 199, 297–98
Blurred vision, *115,* 257, 258–59
Body fat (triglyceride), 104, 132–33
Body map, 155, 159
Body mapping. *See* Mapping
Body work. *See* Acupuncture; Massage
Bones, 24–25, 187–97, 361, 390–91. *See also* Arthritis
Books, recommended, 377–403
Bowen Therapy, 353
Brain symptoms, 24, 173–86, 361, 390
Breakfast (breakfast foods), 138–39
Brittle nails, 48–49, *115,* 241, 250–53

Caffeine, 117, 141, 223
Calcium, 33–36, 48–49, 218–19, 236, 310
Candida, 68–69, 203–4
Carbohydrates, 102–5, 107, *108,* 116–28
Carbohydrate cravings, 131–37, 151–52, 208
  low-carb diet for, 137–44
Carbohydrate intolerance, 99–110, 113–14, 150–53
Causes of fibromyalgia, 11, 28–39, 361–71
Cells (cell biology), 30–39, 365–70
  guaifenesin reversal and, 52–62, 75–76, 359
Cerebral symptoms, 24, 173–86, 361
Children
  explaining FMS to, 333–34
  with FMS. *See* Pediatric fibromyalgia
Chronic fatigue syndrome (fibrofatigue), 6, 29, 175–79
Clinical trials, 15, 293–94
Codeine, 210, 299
Cognitive problems, 24, 173–86, 361. *See also* Fibrofog
Colas, 70, 122, 223
Cold sores, 264–65
Colognes, 263, 343
Colonoscopies, 199, 200
Colposcopies, 228
Complex carbohydrates, 103, 116–28, 212
Concentration, impaired, *115,* 175, 178–79
Constipation, *115,* 201, 203–4, 207–8, 213–14
Consumer's Dictionary of Cosmetic Ingredients, A (Winter), 85, 380
Contact lenses, 258
Copeland, Mary Ellen, 173–74
Corns, 74–75, 80–81
Cortisone, 245
Cosmetics, 50, 86, 90–94, 380–85
Cough medications, 50–51, 66, 264
Cramps, *115,* 188, 196, 208
Curves International, 345, 398–99
Cymbalta, 327
Cystitis, 219, 221–26. *See also* Interstitial cystitis
Cystoscopies, 221–23

Dairy products, 120, 124, 135
Dandruff, 74–75, 80–81
Definition of fibromyalgia, 6–8, 29–30
Dental care products, 80, 84, 87–88, 93
Depression, 175, 178, 276, 321–22, 343–46, 390
Dermatitis, 242, 247–48
Dermatologic symptoms, 25, 240–55, 361, 394
Desserts, 121–22, 124
Detoxification, 68
DHEA (dehydroepiandrosterone), 254, 309
Diabetes, 142–43, 387–88
Diagnosis
  of bladder infections, 221–23
  of fibromyalgia, 9, 146–50, 297–98
  of hypoglycemia, 110–15
  of irritable bowel syndrome, 199–200, 203–4
  of pediatric fibromyalgia, 279–80

Diarrhea, 201, 203–4, 210, 214
Diet(s), 116–28, 151–53. *See also* Hypoglycemia diet; Low-carb diet
  for carbohydrate intolerance, 116–28, 150–53
  for fibroglycemia, 131–37
  food substitutions, 135
  forbidden foods list, 118–19, 153
  for interstitial cystitis, 223–24
  for irritable bowel syndrome, 209–10, 212–15
Diflucan (fluconazole), 204, 233
Dinner, eating tips for, 139–40
Disability status, 10–11, 320–26
Dishwashing (dish) soaps, 96
Dizziness, *106, 115,* 256
Doctors, selection of, 146–50
Dolorimeters, 26–27
Don't Go to the Cosmetics Counter Without Me (Begoun), 92–94, 380
Double-blind studies, 15, 293–94
Drowsiness, 177
Drug companies, role of, 293–95
Dry eyes, *115,* 258, 259–60
Dry skin, 242, 250, 261, 263
DVDs, recommended, 377–403
Dysenergism syndrome, use of term, 30, 366
Dysuria, 218, 221

Ear symptoms, 25–26, 257, 260–61, 361–62
Eating out, 138, 141
Eczema, *115,* 242, 247
Elavil, 225, 237, 313
Employment stress, 337–39
Endocrine system, 109, 147–48
Endorphins, 179, 300, 301–3, 318
Endoscopies, 199, 200
Energopenia, use of term, 30, 33, 362, 366
Energy (energy production), 31–39, 365–70
Estrace, 233–34
Estrogen, 233–34, 309–10
Exercise, 10, 317–20, 349–52
  for depression, 345
  for insomnia, 179
  for interstitial cystitis, 226
  for musculoskeletal pain and stiffness, 196–97
  for vulvar pain, 238
Exercise groups, 345, 351
Exhaustion, 175, 178–79
Eye symptoms, 25–26, *115,* 257–60, 361–62

Faintness, *106,* 107, *115,* 257
Family and Medical Leave Act of 1993, 338
Family members, explaining FMS to, 333–34
Fatigue, *115,* 175–79, 306–7, 314–15, 390
Feldenkrais Method, 353, 399
Fevers, 268
Fibrofatigue, 6, 29, 175–79
Fibroflux (mood swings), *115,* 184–86
Fibrofog, 22–23, 180–84, 390
Fibro-frustration, 181
Fibroglycemia, 129–34, *130*
  diet for, 131–44
Fibrogut. *See* Irritable bowel syndrome
Fibromyalgia Advocate, The (Starlanyl), 40, 346, 350–51
Fibromyalgia and Chronic Myofascial Pain Syndrome (Starlanyl and Copeland), 173–74
Fibromyalgia Dental Handbook, The (Stay), 93, 265
Fibromyalgia syndrome (FMS), overview of, 19–39
Fibromyalgia Treatment Center, 348–49, 379
Fibrositis, origin of term, 7
Fingernails, 48–49, 241, 250–53
Fisher, Michelle, 98
Flexeril (cyclobenzaprine), 297, 306
Food. *See* Diet
Food and Drug Administration (FDA), 86, 91, 293
Food sensitivities, 203, 257, 263–66
Food substitutions, 135
Foot cramps, *115,* 188, 196
Forgetfulness. *See* Fibrofog
Froriep, Robert, 6–7
Fruits, 117, 120, 123, 126, 135, 223–24

Gardening, 96–97, 160
Gas, *115,* 201, 203, 205, 207–8
Gastroesophageal reflux (GER), 203, 215
Gastrointestinal symptoms, 25, 198–216
Gender differences, 6, 38–39, 44–46, 148, 281
Genes and genetics, 38–39, 134–35, 364
  in pediatric fibromyalgia, 270–73, 286
Genitourinary symptoms, 25, 217–39, 361, 392–93
Genter, P., 112–13
Gingivitis, 264
Glucose (blood sugar), 103–5, 107, *108,* 125–26
Glucose tolerance tests, 110–15, 147
Glycemic index (GI), 125–27
Goldenberg, Don L., 305
Gout (gouty syndrome), 13, 41–48, 50, 364–65
Gowers, William, 7
Growing pains, 39, *115,* 188, 280–81, 284, 364
Guaifenesin, 13–17, 50–71
  beginning to take, 160–69
  blockage of by salicylates, 67–68, 72–73, 75–78
  definition of, 51
  disguising taste of, 285
  dosage, 50–51, 63–64, 66, 162–65, *166,* 285
  drug interactions, 67–68, 72–73, 158
  for fatigue and insomnia, 179
  for fibroglycemia, 136–37
  frequently asked questions about, 65–70
  how and why it works, 52–65
  for interstitial cystitis, 224, 226
  kidney receptors and, 14, 52–62, 69–70, 75–76
  over-the-counter purchase of, 66–67
  for pediatric fibromyalgia, 273, 276–77, 284–88
  pregnant women use of, 69
  remapping while on, 167, *168,* 169
  resources, 379, 388–90
  reversal cycles, 53–65, *61–62,* 164–65, 359
  side effects, 65–66
  storage of, 67
  for vaginal problems, 238, 239

Hadler, Nortin, 320
Hair loss, 253–55
Hair symptoms, 241, 253–55
Headaches, 25–26, 74, 107, *115,* 181, 256, 263
Head symptoms, 25–26, 256–69, 361–62
Hearing problems, 257, 260–61
Heat pads, 196, 341
Hemorrhoids, 207–8, 213–14
Henriksson, K. G., 32, 366
Herbal supplements, 50, 79, 82–85, 158, 307–11, 364
Hippocrates, 73, 109–10
Histamines, 242–43, 246–47, 248, 249–50, 262, 369
Hives, 25, *115,* 240–50
Hoffman, Felix, 74
Home, stress at, 333–36
Hormone replacement therapies, 233–34, 309–10
5-HTP, 313–14
Hypoglycemia, 98–128. *See also* Fibroglycemia
  biological overview of, 102–5, 107, *108,* 370
  carbohydrate intolerance and, 99–110, 113–14, 150–53
  definition of, 99, 104–5
  diagnosis of, 110–15
  fibromyalgia correlation with, 14, *115,* 129–37, *130*
  resources, 385–88
  symptoms of, *106,* 107, 114–15, *115,* 150–51
  treatment of, 100–101, 116–28
Hypoglycemia diet, 116–28
  forbidden foods list, 118–19, 153
  liberal, 123–25, 152–53
  low-carb, 137–44, 151–53, 267–68, 386–87
  strict, 119–23, 151–53

Immunoglobulin G, 37, 243
Insomnia, 175, 177–79, 236, 286, 340–42
  medications for, 311–17

Insulin, 103–5, 107, *108,* 134–35
Insurance companies, 7, 10–11, 321–24, 353–54
Interstitial cystitis (IC), *115,* 219, 221–26, 228–29
Ipp, E., 112–13
Irritability, *115,* 175, 178
Irritable bowel syndrome (IBS) (fibrogut), 25, 198–216, 361
  diagnosis of, 199–200, 203–4
  diet for, 209–10, 212–15
  fibromyalgia as cause of, 204–5, *206,* 207–8, 369–70
  resources, 391–92
  symptoms of, 203–4, 208–9
  treatment of, 209–10, 212–15
Itching, 25, *115,* 240–50

Jet lag, 313
Job stress, 337–39
Joint pain. *See* Muscle and joint pain
Journal of Rheumatology, 50, 292, 295

Kassirer, Jerome P., 308
Kevorkian, Jack, 10
Kidneys, 31–38, 365–70
  guaifenesin and, 14, 52–62, *57,* 69–70, 75–76
  salicylates and, 14, 75–76
Krebs cycle, *34,* 367–68

Laundry detergents, 96
Leg cramps, *115,* 188, 196
Levine, Sharon, 294
Liberal diet, 123–25, 152–53
Ligaments, 24–25, 187–97, 209, 228, 319
Light sensitivities, *115,* 257, 258
Lip balms, 264–66
Lists (list-making), 182–84, 355–56
Low-carb diet, 137–44, 151–53, 267–68, 386–87
Lumps and bumps. *See* Mapping; Tender points
Lunch (lunch foods), 139
Lyrica (pregabalin), 326–27

Magnesium, 210, 213, 310
Makeup. *See* Cosmetics
Mapping, 27–28, 129, 149–50, 153–57, 362
  remapping on guaifenesin, 167, *168,* 169
Massage (body work), 196, 352–54, 398
Mast cells, 242–43, 249–50
Medical history, 149, 297–98
Medical journals, 15, 292–94
Medications, 11–12, 295–317. *See also* Guaifenesin; *and specific medications*
  for fibromyalgia, overview of, 303–11
  for interstitial cystitis, 224–25
  for irritable bowel syndrome, 209–10, 212–15
  late-breaking, 326–28
  for pain, 195–96, 296–303
  reviewing your, 148–49, 331–32
  salicylates in, 81, 86, 158
  for skin symptoms, 245–47
  for sleep disturbances, 311–17
  for vulvar pain, 233–34, 236–38
Melatonin, 312–13
Memory, impaired, *115,* 175, 178–79. *See also* Fibrofog
Menopause, 234, 249
Menthol (mint), 84, 87–88, 158, 160, 363–64
Metallic tastes, 257, 263–66
Milk substitutes, 135
Milnacipran, 327–28
Mitochondria, 17–18, 31–38, 267, 319–20, 365
Moldofsky, Harvey, 312
Mood swings, *115,* 184–86
Morphine, 210, 302
Mouth sores, 264–65
Mouthwashes, 80, 84, 87–88
Mucinex, 51, 66, 239, 389
Murphy, Janis, 10
Muscle and joint pain, 24–25, 114–15, *115,* 186–97, 361, 390–91
  medications for, 195–96, 296–303
Muscle relaxants, 210, 215, 297, 305–6, 316
Muscles, 24–25, 187–97
Musculoskeletal symptoms, 24–25, 187–97, 361, 390–91

Nail fungus, 252
Naps (napping), 340–41
Narcotics, 299–303, 307, 318–19
Nasal congestion, *115,* 257, 262–63
National Vulvodynia Association, 229–30
Natural salicylates, 82–91, 158, 160
Nausea, 65, 201, 203, 205, 263
Nearsightedness, 258–59
Nervousness, *115,* 175, 178
Neurodermatitis, *115,* 247
Neurotonin (gabapentin), 237, 306
Noise sensitivities, 257, 260–61
Nose symptoms, 25–26, 257, 262–63, 361–62
NSAIDs (nonsteroidal anti-inflammatory drugs), 195–96, 297, 298–99, 303, 315
Numbness and tingling, *115,* 188, 196
Nuts, 121, 124

Obesity, 132–33, 143–44, 208
Odor sensitivities, 25–26, *115,* 257, 262–63
Osteoarthritis, 192–97
Osteoporosis, 69
Oxalates, 229
OxyContin, 210, 299, 302

Painful spots. *See* Tender points
Pain relief, 74, 80, 195–96, 286, 296–303
Palpitations, *106,* 107, *115,* 150, 267
Panic attacks, *106,* 107, *115*
Parasites, 68–69
Paxil, 215, 225
Pediatric fibromyalgia, 270–88, 364
  diagnosis of, 279–80
  genetics of, 270–73
  guaifenesin for, 273, 276–77, 284–88
  resources, 395–96
  school problems, 273–75, 285–86
  symptoms of, 279–80, 281–82, 284–85, 286
Peer review, 292–93
Pelvic exams, 228
Pepcid, 213, 246
Pepto-Bismol, 80, 81, 286
Perfumes, 263, 343
Phosphates, 31–38, 365–67
  bladder problems and, 218–19
  children and, 281
  gauifensin and, 52–62, *57*
  insulin and, 134
  muscles and bones and, 193–95
Physical examinations, 9, 149–50. *See also* Mapping
Physicians, selection of, 146–50
Physicians' Desk Reference (PDR), 11, 50, 51, 302
Placebos, 293–94
Plantar fasciitis, 192
Portenoy, Russell, 328
Postnasal drip, 262–63
Potter, Malcolm, 49–50, 51–52
Powder guaifenesin, 161–62
Pregnancy, 69
Prelief, 213, 224, 226, 234, 236
Premarin, 233–34
Prescriptions. *See* Medications
Pro Health, 66, 382, 389
Provigil (modafinil), 274, 306
Prozac (fluoxetine), 307
Psoriasis, 242, 248

Quadriceps muscle (left thigh), mapping, 155–56, 190–91, 362

Ramelteon, 316–17
Rashes, 25, *115,* 240–50
Renal filtering, 56–62, 75–76
Resources, 377–403
Restaurants, 138, 141
Restless legs, *115,* 188, 196
Retinoids, 250
Rheumatoid arthritis, 148
Ringing ears, *115,* 257, 260–61
Rogaine (minoxidil), 254
Rosacea, 242, 248–49, 262–63
Rose, Andrea, 93, 382

Salicylates, 72–97, 363–64
  avoidance of, 14–15, 78–90, 157–58, 160
  blockage of guaifenesin by, 67–68, 72–73, 75–78

in cosmetics, 50, 86, 90–94
dietary, 88–90
frequently asked questions about, 96–97
history of, 72–75
natural, 82–90
resources, 380–85
synthetic, 80–81
uses of, 74–75, 80–81
Salivary glands, 263–64, 368–69
Salt craving, *115,* 241
Saturated fats, 142–43
Schedules (scheduling), 182–84
School problems, 273–75, 285–86
Seborrhea, 242, 247–48
Sedatives, 305–6, 314
Sensitive skin, 25, 240–50
Serotonin, 313
Serotonin-reuptake inhibitors, 215, 304–5, 316
Sexual intercourse, 221, 222, 226, 230–31, 238
Shampoos, 80–81, 84, 254
Showers, 342–43
Shuller, Kathy, 336
Simple carbohydrates, 103, 116–28
Skin symptoms, 25, 240–50
Sleep and sleep problems, 175, 177–79, 236, 286, 311–17, 339–42
Sleeping aids, 179, 236, 311–17, 341
Smoking, 97, 223
Smythe, Hugh, 7, 19, 312
Social Security disability, 10–11, 322–24
Solomons, Clive, 229, 237–38
Soma (carisoprodol), 297, 306
Somers, Suzanne, 143
Sore throats, 265–66
South Beach Diet, 143
Spices, 88–89, 122, 140
Starches, 116–28
Starlanyl, Devin J., 40, 173–74, 346, 350–51
Statistics, 5–6, 100, 133, 175, 201, 218, 241, 256–57
Stay, Flora, 93, 265
Stolle, Mary Ellen, 95
Stress (stress reduction), 185, 330–39
Stretching, 196–97, 226, 238, 318, 350–51
Strict diet, 119–23, 151–53
Sugars (sugar cravings), 110, 116–28, 212, 241
Sugar substitutes, 135
Sunscreens, 75, 80, 287
Supplements. *See* Herbal supplements
Support groups, 346–49
for guaifenesin protocol, 95
for help locating a doctor, 146–47
resources, 379, 390
starting your own, 348
for vulvodynia, 229–30
Sweating, 241, 266–67, 268
Sydenham, Thomas, 42, 43
Symptoms
of cystitis, 219
of fibromyalgia, 8–10, 24–28, 114–15, *115*
of gout, 42, 43, 44
of hypoglycemia, *106,* 107, 114–15, *115,* 150–51
of irritable bowel syndrome, 203–4, 208–9
of the musculoskeletal system, 188
of pediatric fibromyalgia, 279–80, 281–82, 284–85, 286
of vaginal pain, 231, 233
Synthetic salicylates, 80–81

Tampax, 238
Tartar, 40–41, 48, 264
Taste sensitivities, *115,* 257, 263–66
Tears (tearing), 258, 259
Teeth sensitivities, 264–66
Temperature regulation problems, 268
Tender points, 7–8, 26–28, 52, 362
Tendons, 24–25, 187–97, 319
Testosterone, 254, 309
Thalomid, 327
Throat symptoms, 25–26, 257, 263–66, 361–62
Tingling, *115,* 188, 196
Tinnitus, 259–61
Titrate, 213
Tobacco, 97, 223
Toilet paper, 238
Toothpastes, 80, 84, 87–88, 91, 93, 265, 286–87, 363

Topical products, 75–76, 81, 83–84, 87, 96, 158, 160, 245
Treatment protocol, 12–18, 145–70. *See also* Guaifenesin
  addressing carbohydrate intolerance/hypoglycemia factor, 150–53
  diagnosis, 146–50
  eliminating salicylates, 157–58, 160
  for pediatric fibromyalgia, 284–88
Tricyclics, 214–15, 225, 237, 246, 304–5, 315–16
TSH (thyroid-stimulating hormone) test, 147–48
Tylenol, 286, 297, 303, 312

Ultram (tramadol), 298–99, 305
Ultrasound, 199, 200
Uric acid (urate), 41–48, 55, 364–65
Urinalysis, 218, 221, 222
Urinary tract irritation, *115,* 219, *220,* 221–22

Vaginal problems, 218, 226–39
Vegetables, 120–21, 123, 223
Vertigo, 256
Vestibulitis, 226–39
Vicodin, 302, 303–4
Videotapes, recommended, 377–403
Vioxx (rofecoxib), 303, 328
Vision problems, *115,* 257, 258–59
Vitamins, 223, 233, 238, 241, 248, 310
Vulvar Pain Foundation, 229, 231, 238
Vulvar pain syndrome, 218, 226–39, *235*
Vulvitis, 226–39
Vulvodynia, *115,* 218, 226–39

Warm baths, 342–43
Warm-ups, 350–51
Warts, 74–75, 80–81
Water intake, 67, 226, 265
Water retention, 268–69
Web sites, 377–403
Weight gain, 267–68, 370
Weight-loss diets, 86, 119–23, 151–53
Weight maintenance, liberal diet for, 123–25, 152–53
What Your Doctor May Not *Tell You About Fibromyalgia Fatigue* (St. Amand and Marek), 133, 141–42, 188
What Your Doctor May Not *Tell You About Pediatric Fibromyalgia Fatigue* (St. Amand and Marek), 38, 281
Willems, John, 229, 233–34
Willow bark, 73–74, 82–83
Winter, Ruth, 85, 380
Witch hazel, 214
Wolfe, Frederick, 7, 295
Women's health issues, 6, 44–47, 148, 181, 202, 218–19, 221, 226–39, 260
Workplace, stress in the, 337–39
World Health Organization (WHO), 7–8

Yeast infections, 221, 231, 233
Yunus, Muhammed, 7

About the Authors

R. Paul St. Amand, M.D. is a graduate of Tufts University School of Medicine. He has been on the teaching staff of Los Angeles Harbor/UCLA, Department of Endocrinology for fifty years, and is an assistant clinical professor at the UCLA School of Medicine. Presently he is working with City of Hope in Duarte, California, hoping to uncover the genetic abnormality that leads to fibromyalgia. Dr. St. Amand was an early pioneer in fibromyalgia treatment using uricosuric drugs and discovered guaifenesin's effectiveness in 1994. His work is cited wherever the substance is mentioned. He is in private practice in Marina del Rey, California and has treated thousands of patients from all over the world. He has also authored two other books on fibromyalgia: *What Your Doctor May* Not *Tell You About Pediatric Fibromyalgia* and *What Your Doctor May* Not *Tell You About Fibromyalgia Fatigue*, both published by Warner Books.

Claudia Craig Marek is a medical assistant tutored, trained, and taught on the job by Dr. St. Amand. She has co-written medical papers with Dr. St. Amand and maintains a busy schedule traveling and lecturing to support groups around the world. She has worked with fibromyalgia patients for over fifteen years and leads a large internet support group at www.fibromyalgiatreatment.com. In addition to the three books she has coauthored with Dr. St. Amand, Ms. Marek is the author of *The First Year: Fibromyalgia* which was published in 2003 by Avalon Books, and two children's books about the illness which she coauthored with her artist husband, Lou Marek. In 2005 she was honored as a Leader Against Pain by the National Fibromyalgia Association.